KU-209-448

▲

PSYCHOLOGICAL BASES OF SPORT INJURIES

▼

Second Edition

David Pargman, Ph.D.
FLORIDA STATE UNIVERSITY

Editor

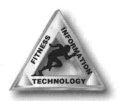

Fitness Information Technology, Inc. • P.O. Box 4425 • Morgantown, WV 26504-4425 • USA

Copyright © 1999, by Fitness Information Technology, Inc.

ALL RIGHTS RESERVED

Reproduction or use of any portion of this publication by any mechanical, electronic, or other means is prohibited without the written permission of the publisher.

Library of Congress Card Catalog Number: 99-71257

ISBN: 1-885693-18-4

Cover design: Pegasus
Copy Editor: Sandra R. Woods
Developmental Editor: Geoffrey C. Fuller
Production Editor: Craig Hines
Printed by: BookCrafters
Printed in the United States of America
10 9 8 7 6 5 4 3 2 1

Fitness Information Technology, Inc.
P.O. Box 4425, University Avenue
Morgantown, WV 25504 USA
(800) 477-4348
(304) 599-3482 (phone/fax)
Email: fit@fitinfotech.com
Web Site: www.fitinfotech.com

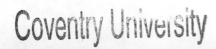
Coventry University

To the memory of my father, Sidney J. Pargman

About the Editor

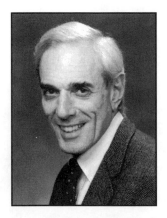

David Pargman is in his 27th year at Florida State University, where he is Professor and Coordinator of Educational Research. Previously, he taught in the Department of Health and Physical Education at Boston University and the City College of New York. Dr. Pargman received a master's degree from Teachers College, Columbia University, and a Ph.D. from New York University.

Dr. Pargman is author and co-author of three other books that deal respectively with stress and performance, fitness and wellness, and sport psychology. He is currently co-writing a textbook entitled *Exercise Physiology*. He has been major professor to 35 Ph.D. graduates, is a member of the American Psychological Association, International Association of Applied Psychology, the North American Society for the Psychology of Sport and Physical Activity, and a Fellow of the Association for the Advancement of Applied Sport Psychology and the American College of Sports Medicine. He is also a Certified Sport Psychology Consultant, the Association for the Advancement of Applied Sport Psychology.

Dr. Pargman has competed in hundreds of road races, was a member of his college track and cross-country team, and continues to train, run, and compete as a distance runner. Consequently, he is often injured and in the throes of mental and physical rehabilitative experiences.

Contents

SECTION 1: INJURY AND SPORT—THE PROBLEM: CONCEPTUAL AND PRACTICAL APPROACHES

Chapter 1
Sport Injuries: An Overview of Psychological Perspectives

Chapter 2
Pain in Sport: A Biopsychological Perspective
John Heil

Chapter 3
Ethical and Legal Issues for Sport Professionals
Counseling Injured Athletes

Chapter 4
Psychological and Emotional Response to Athletic Injury:
Measurement Issues
Lynne Evans

SECTION 2: PSYCHOLOGICAL PERSPECTIVES ON ATHLETIC INJURY

SECTION 3: COUNSELING ATHLETES WHO ARE INJURED

SECTION 5: APPLICATIONS: CASE STUDIES

Contributing Authors

Theresa Bianco received her master's degree from the University of Ottawa and is completing her doctorate in the Department of Human Movement and Exercise Science at The University of Western Australia. Her research focuses on the role of social support in recovery from sport injuries, with a particular interest in coach support for injured athletes. Theresa has conducted workshops on the psychology of sport injury for Sports Medicine Australia and is currently involved in developing motivational programs for rehabilitation.

Britton W. Brewer, Ph.D., is an associate professor of psychology at Springfield College in Springfield, Massachusetts, where he teaches undergraduate and graduate psychology courses, conducts research on psychological aspects of sport injury, and coaches the men's cross-country team. He is listed in the United States Olympic Committee Sport Psychology Registry, 1996–2000, and is a Certified Consultant, AAASP.

Kevin L. Burke is an assistant professor and Director of the Sport Psychology Laboratory in the Department of Health and Kinesiology at Georgia Southern University. He received his Ph.D. in sport psychology form Florida State University. He received his M.A. in social/organizational psychology from East Carolina University and his B.A. in psychology and recreational studies, with a minor in sociology, from Belmont Abbey College. A charter member and past secretary-treasurer of the Association for the Advancement of Applied Sport Psychology (AAASP), Kevin also served on AAASP's original Executive Board as the first student representative. He has presented and published through local, state, regional, national, and international channels. Kevin has assisted professional, college, high school, and recreational athletes as a sport psychology consultant and is a Certified Consultant, AAASP. His current research interests are in optimism, momentum, humor, sport officials, and the effectiveness of intervention techniques in sport and exercise. Kevin has assisted many athletes with their psychological rehabilitation of sport injuries.

R. Kelly Crace is a staff psychologist at the Counseling Center of the College of William & Mary. Kelly received his M.A. in sport psychology and his Ph.D. in counseling psychology from the University of North Carolina at Chapel Hill. His psychology internship was at Duke University. He has published and presented nationally on topics such as performance enhancement, team development, social influence processes, career development, and stress management. He is a Certified Consultant, AAASP; is listed in the USOC Sport Psychology Registry; and has worked with athletes from the entry to elite levels for the past 10 years. In regard to sport injury, he has conducted research on the psychological aspects of career-ending injuries, provided individual counseling to injured athletes, and facilitated support groups for athletes dealing with the stress of injury. Kelly is co-inventor of a United States Patented Interactive Sport Simulator System designed for scientific and entertainment application. He is a member of numerous sport psychology and counseling psychology organizations and served as business manager of AAASP from 1986 to 1987. He was the 1995 recipient of the Chambers-Reid Award for professional excellence at William & Mary.

Edward F. Etzel is a licensed psychologist with the West Virginia University Counseling and Psychological Services Center, where he serves as psychologist for the Department of Intercollegiate Athletics. He is also an assistant professor within the School of Physical Education, where he teaches applied sport psychology and research methods. Ed is a 1984 Olympic Gold Medalist in Shooting. He was also coach of the five-time NCAA Champion WVU Rifle Team.

Lynne Evans is a senior lecturer at the University of Wales Institute Cardiff, contributing to undergraduate and postgraduate courses in sport psychology. She has been employed there since 1991. She graduated with a master's degree in coaching theory from Lakehead University, Ontario, Canada, in 1986 and is in the process of completing her doctoral studies in the psychological and emotional responses of injured athletes. Lynne is a British Association of Sport and Exercise Sport (BASES) accredited sport psychologist. She works with athletes from a range of sports in a psychological support capacity, with a particular interest in athletes rehabilitating from injury.

A. P. Ferrante is the psychologist for athletics at The Ohio State University. He is a Diplomate in counseling psychology of the American Board of Professional Psychology and is listed on the U.S. Olympic Committee's Registry for the Psychology of Sport. He served as sport psychologist for the U.S. Olympic Team in Seoul, Korea.

Perry G. Fine is an associate professor of anesthesiology at the University of Utah School of Medicine. He is an attending physician in the University Pain Management Center. He serves as a sports medicine consultant to the University Athletic Department with special interest in pain management and head injury assessment.

Frances A. Flint has been a faculty member at York University in the Department of Physical Education, Recreation, and Athletics since 1977. She obtained her master's degree and Ph.D. from the University of Oregon. Her doctoral work involved an integration of sport psychology and sports medicine and focused on the injured athlete. After her coaching career, she earned certification as an Athletic Trainer (NATA) and continues her work with injured athletes at York University. She has developed a sports therapy certificate program at York University for the training of future therapists in sport.

Lance B. Green is currently an assistant professor in the Exercise and Sport Sciences Department of Tulane University. His particular interests include the application of imagery to exercise and sport settings as well as the psychosocial context within which individuals pursue physical activity. He received his doctorate from the University of Hawaii–Hilo, where he taught and coached baseball.

J. Robert Grove received his master's degree from Southern Methodist University and his Ph.D. from Florida State University. He is currently an associate professor in the Department of Human Movement and Exercise Science at The University of Western Australia. He is editor of the Sport Psychologist's Digest for the *Journal of Sport and Exercise Psychology,* associate editor (social psychology) for the *Journal of Applied Sport Psychology,* and a member of the editorial board for the International *Journal of Sport Psychology.* Dr. Grove has published widely in the areas of coping processes and injury rehabilitation.

Charles J. Hardy is professor and chair of the Department of Health and Kinesiology at Georgia Southern University. He received his Ph.D. in sport psychology from Louisiana State University and completed a postdoctoral fellowship at the University of North Carolina at Chapel Hill. He received his M.S. from the University of Tennessee and his B.S. from East Carolina University. His research interests are in social influence processes within exercise and sport. In regard to sport injury, he has conducted research examining life stress, social support and the emotional response of athletes to injury. Along with R. Kelly Crace, he has conducted injury support groups to assist athletes in dealing with the stress of injury. He is a Certified Consultant, AAASP, and has consulted with athletes and coaches from the entry to the elite levels. He is a member of numerous sport psychology organizations, a Fellow in the Research Consortium of AAHPERD, and served as president of AAASP. He has been a visiting sport psychologist at the United States Olympic Training Center and a visiting principal fellow at the University of Wollongong, Australia.

Lew Hardy obtained a B.A. in pure mathematics from the University College of North Wales (UCNW) in 1970, completed his M.A. in 1971 and then his Ph.D. in 1973. He later obtained a postgraduate teaching qualification in physical education from Liverpool University in 1975. He has 9 research publications in pure mathematics and over 100 in sport and health psychology. He has been the psychological consultant to the British Amateur Gymnastics Association since 1983 and is currently serving his 3rd four-year cycle as chairman of the British Olympic Association's Psychology Steering Group. He has been both the secretary and the chairperson of the psychology section of the British Association of Sport and Exercise Sciences and currently sits on the editorial board of the *Journal of Applied Sport Psychology, The Sport Psychologist,* and the *Journal of Sports Sciences.* In 1992, he was invited by the British Psychological Society to become a Chartered Psychologist. In 1994, he was made a fellow of the British Association of Sport and Exercise Sciences, and in 1996, he was made the inaugural Distinguished International Scholar of AAASP and a fellow of the European College of Sports Science.

John Heil is a psychologist with Lewis-Gale Clinic in Roanoke, Virginia, who specializes in sport psychology, pain, and behavioral medicine. He is Coordinator of Psychological Services for the Lewis-Gale Hospital Pain Center. He serves on the United States Fencing Association Sportsmedicine Committee and the ASTM Committee on Sports Equipment and Facilities. Dr. Heil is also Director of Sportsmedicine for the Commonwealth Games of Virginia.

Jane Henderson teaches physical education at John Abbott College in Ste. Anne de Bellevue, Quebec, Canada. She received the M.S. from Southern Illinois University and a Ph.D. in sport psychology from Florida State University. Among her research interests are physiological manifestations of psychological stress. She has served as assistant trainer to the Canadian Judo Team and competes as a distance and marathon runner.

Keith P. Henschen is a professor at the University of Utah in the Department of Exercise and Sports Science, where he teaches courses in the psychosocial aspects of sports. He is a member of the American Psychological Association (APA); the American Alliance of Health, Physical Education, Recreation and Dance (AAHPERD); and is on the United States Olympic Committee (USOC) Sport Psychology Registry. Dr. Henschen has worked with two Olympic governing bodies, numerous professional and collegiate teams, and consulted for a variety of world-class athletes.

Lydia Ievleva is a sport psychologist whose practice has spanned three countries over the past 9 years, beginning in Canada and the United States; she is currently affiliated with the University of New South Wales, Sydney, Australia.

She has consulted with hundreds of athletes—from developmental and collegiate to world-class, Olympic, and professional athletes. Ievleva also conducts stress management and peak performance seminars for clients in the corporate sector. Ievleva is a certified AAASP consultant, as well as a registered psychologist in New South Wales, Australia.

Lou M. Makarowski is a licensed psychologist, author, and consultant who has been in full-time private practice since 1976 in Pensacola, Florida. He frequently consults on stress-related issues with elite and professional athletes, families, physicians, and other health care professionals. Dr. Makarowski received his Ph.D. specializing in pediatric, school, and clinical psychology from the University of Iowa. Dr. Makarowski is a member of the United States Olympic Committee Sport Psychology Registry, AAASP, and the Council for the National Register of Health Service Providers in Psychology and is a Registered Traumatologist with the Green Cross Project. He has written approximately 400 sport psychology columns for the popular media and his book, *How to Keep Your COOL with Your Kids* (Perigee, 1996), is scheduled for release in Taiwan and Mexico during 1998–99.

R. Renee Newcomer is a doctoral student in the sport psychology program at West Virginia University. She received her master's degree from the University of North Carolina at Chapel Hill. Ms. Newcomer's master's thesis focused on the psychological impact of athletic injury on college student-athletes.

Bruce C. Ogilvie is professor emeritus in the Department of Psychology at San Jose State University. Dr. Ogilvie is a world-renowned pioneer in applied sport psychology. He has researched, consulted, and published on performance and the high-performance person since 1955. He has contributed over 140 publications on issues ranging from children in sport, identification of psychological factors that contribute to performance success, and development of performance-enhancing strategies. Dr. Ogilvie has served as a team psychological consultant for numerous U.S. Olympic teams, as well as professional football, baseball, hockey, and soccer teams. He has also been a private consultant for elite athletes from various sports.

Terry Orlick is an internationally recognized mental training consultant and researcher in applied sport psychology as well as other performance-related fields. He is a professor in the School of Human Kinetics at the University of Ottawa and has been working in the field of applied sport psychology for over 20 years. Orlick is a consultant to numerous Olympic teams, as well as many others pursuing personal excellence in a variety of domains including medicine, professional and amateur sport, music, law, aerospace mission control, the military, sales, children, and parenting. He is the current president of the

International Society for Mental Training and the author of numerous articles and 15 books including most recently the second edition of *Pursuit of Excellence* and *Nice on My Feelings*.

Frank Perna is a licensed psychologist and an assistant professor in the sport psychology department at West Virginia University. Dr. Perna is an AAASP Certified Consultant and is listed on the U.S. Olympic Committee's Sport Psychology Registry. He has served as a psychologist at the U.S. Olympic Training Center in Colorado Springs, Colorado, and as a clinical health psychology research fellow at the University of Miami's behavioral medicine research center.

David H. Perrin is associate professor and director of graduate athletic training education and research in the Curry School of Education at the University of Virginia. He is editor of the *Journal of Sport Rehabilitation* and serves on the editorial board of three additional sports medicine periodicals. He has authored one textbook and has written chapters in several others. His research focuses on the assessment of human muscular performance and the treatment and rehabilitation of athletic injuries. He is a practicing athletic trainer at the University of Virginia, where he cares for the men's lacrosse team.

Albert J. Petitpas, Ed.D., is a professor of psychology at Springfield College in Springfield, Massachusetts, where he directs the graduate training program in athletic counseling. He is a fellow and Certified Consultant of AAASP. He has provided consulting services to a wide range of sport organizations, including the National Collegiate Athletic Association's Youth Education Through Sport Program, the United States Olympic Committee's Career Assistance Program for Athletes, the Ladies Professional Golf Association's Transitional Golf Program, and the United States Ski Jumping and Nordic Combined teams. His research and applied work focus on assisting athletes in coping with injury and other sport and career transitions.

Robert J. Rotella has recently retired as associate professor and director of sport psychology in the Department of Health and Physical Education at the University of Virginia. His research writings have focused on stress, anxiety, self-confidence, performance enhancement, and the psychology of injury rehabilitation. In addition, Dr. Rotella has co-authored six books and numerous chapters in sport psychology and sport medicine texts. Throughout his career Dr. Rotella has emphasized the application of sport psychology to enhance the lives and performances of highly committed athletes.

Michael L. Sachs is an associate professor in the Department of Physical Education, College of HPERD, specializing in exercise and sport psychology. He has been at Temple University since Fall 1989. He received his Ph.D. in sport psychology from Florida State University in 1980 and was an assistant professor at the University of Quebec at Trois-Rivières from 1980 to 1983. From 1983 to 1989 he served as a research project coordinator in the Applied Research and Evaluation Unit in the Department of Pediatrics, University of Maryland School of Medicine. He has an extensive list of publications and presentations, including authorship as associate editor of *Psychology of Running* (Michael Sacks & Michael Sachs, Human Kinetics Publishers, 1981) and co-editor of *Running as Therapy: An Integrated Approach* (Michael Sachs & Gary Buffone, University of Nebraska Press, 1984). He is a licensed psychologist in Maryland, as well as a Certified Consultant, Association for the Advancement of Applied Sport Psychology. Dr. Sachs currently serves as the president of the Association for the Advancement of Applied Sport Psychology (1991–92).

Gerry Schwille is the head athletic trainer in the Department of Intercollegiate Athletics at Temple University. He was the Director of the Valley Hospital Sports Institute, Ridgewood, New Jersey, and Head Athletic Manager for the New Jersey Generals of the United States Football League. He received his master's degree in physical education/sports medicine from Oklahoma State University and his Ph.D. in the Sports Administration Department at Temple University. He is a member of the American College of Sports Medicine, a Certified Athletic Trainer of the National Athletic Trainers' Association, and a Licensed Athletic Trainer in Pennsylvania and New Jersey.

Gregory A. Shelley is an assistant professor in the Department of Exercise and Sport Sciences at Ithaca College. He teaches classes in applied sport psychology, sport counseling, sport sociology, and history of sport and the Olympics. He has made over 20 presentations at both the regional and national levels, as well as conducted performance enhancement workshops for coaches and athletes. He has also presented seminars for parents of athletes in the area of parental support for children's success. He has spent the last several years consulting athletes and coaches across a variety of sports at the youth, high school, and collegiate levels and is currently the applied sport psychology consultant for Ithaca College athletics. He is one of three authors of a sport psychology text, as well as the author or co-author of several performance-enhancement and coaching articles, including two book chapters and three brochures detailing the mental aspects of athletic injury. His current research interests include qualitatively examining athletic injury, sport termination, group dynamics and cohesion, and Christianity in sport.

Michael R. Sitler is an assistant professor in the Department of Physical Education, Temple University, specializing in athletic training/sports medicine.

He received his Ed. D. in sports medicine from New York University. Prior to his arrival at Temple University, he was an assistant professor at the United States Military Academy, West Point, New York, for 6 years. He is a certified member of the National Athletic Trainers' Association (NATA) and is currently the Program Director of the NATA-approved undergraduate Athletic Training Education program at Temple University. One of his primary research interests is injury intervention in athletics, and his work in prophylactic ankle and knee bracing is recognized both nationally and internationally. Dr. Sitler is currently serving as the Chair of the Pennsylvania Athletic Trainers' Society Research Committee and is a member of the Eastern Athletic Trainers' Association Research Committee.

Aynsley M. Smith is a nurse counselor in sport psychology at the Sports Medicine Center of the Mayo Clinic in Rochester, Minnesota. She holds MA and R.N. degrees, and is currently completing her Ph.D. in kinesiology at the University of Minnesota–Twin Cities. Ms. Smith has published in journals such as the *Mayo Clinic Proceedings* and *Sports Medicine;* her research is primarily focused on the postinjury emotional responses of athletes and on the epidemiology of injury in ice hockey. As principal investigator, she has been awarded grants from the Mayo Clinic Institutional Review Board for her collaborative research with numerous sports medicine physicians at the Mayo Clinic and with Dr. Wiese-Bjornstal. Her applied work centers on counseling interventions with injured athletes.

Bruce W. Tuckman is a professor in the School of Educational Policy and Leadership and director of the Academic Learning Lab at The Ohio State University. He has written numerous textbooks, including *Conducting Educational Research* and *Theories and Applications of Educational Psychology.* He has published widely and was the first researcher to demonstrate a link between exercise and creativity. He has also authored a novel about running entitled *Long Road to Boston.* He currently does research on student motivation.

Eileen Udry, Ph.D., is an associate professor of sport and exercise psychology at Indiana University Purdue University Indianapolis (IUPUI). She received her M.S. degree from Miami University and her Ph.D. from the University of North Carolina–Greensboro. Dr. Udry has been involved in a number of research and applied projects that center on the psychology of athletic injuries, including work with the U.S. ski team and consultation with various sports medicine facilities. Dr. Udry's interests in injuries emanates from her own experience with injuries as a competitive, and now recreational, athlete/exerciser.

Judy L. Van Raalte, Ph.D., is an associate professor of psychology at Springfield College in Springfield, Massachusetts, where she teaches undergraduate and graduate psychology courses and conducts research on cognitive factors and sport performance. She is listed in the United States Olympic Committee Sport Psychology Registry, 1996–2000, and is a Certified Consultant, AAASP.

Diane M. Wiese-Bjornstal is an assistant professor in the Division of Kinesiology at the University of Minnesota–Twin Cities, where she teaches undergraduate and graduate courses in sport psychology. She received her Ph.D. in physical education, with emphases in the social psychology of sport and biomechanics, from the University of Oregon. Dr. Wiese-Bjornstal has published in a variety of journals such as *The Sport Psychologist, Journal of Sport and Exercise Psychology, Research Quarterly for Exercise and Sport,* and *Sports Medicine.* Her primary research interests in the sport injury area center on the role of athletic trainers and coaches in the injury recovery process and, in collaboration with Ms Aynsley M. Smith, the development of a theoretical model of postinjury psychological response and recovery.

Foreword

The need for a book on sport injury from a purely psychological perspective is strong and clear. Those who work with physically traumatized athletes recognize the existence of many psychological correlates or causal connections to injury. Simply put, injury on the field of play is a common consequence of athlete behavior. The athlete may or may not have executed a movement as prescribed, or another competitor may have behaved in such a fashion that could not be anticipated or prevented by the injured athlete. That is, someone did or did not do something right, and therefore, what is of essence is behavior. Whether this behavior, or failure to act, is essentially due to poor problem solving, weak learning of physical or mental skills, failure to attend to appropriate cues, improper communication with other participants and coaches, or pain, psychological variables are implicated. Psychology is, after all, the science of behavior, and it is this science that is brought to bear upon sport injury in this book. To better understand, prevent, and treat the physical and mental trauma that results from sport injury in the field, gymnasium, court, diamond, or pool, responsible sport leadership utilizes psychological principles, models, and theories.

This book attempts to integrate a wide variety of psychological theory and applied considerations into a unified perspective on sport-related injury. Considerable effort is also made to enlighten readers about ways in which injured athletes may optimize their rehabilitative efforts. Various psychological considerations such as social support, imagery, education, and modeling techniques are presented. Successful rehabilitation programs predicated upon the average are suggested and described in detail.

In addition to this more traditional coverage, the book also includes several chapters that cover unique areas. For example, one chapter deals with malingering in sport—a condition that has received very little attention in the sport psychology literature, but which is problematic from assessment, ethical, and preventive management perspectives. One unusual chapter discusses suicide among athletes, and yet another addresses ethical issues that persons who work with injured athletes should consider.

A variety of professionals, including athletic trainers, physical therapists, psychological consultants, coaches, and physicians, as well as athletes themselves, should benefit from reading this book. Collectively, the chapters express the breadth and depth of the psychology of injury field. The contributing authors are among the most well-known and knowledgeable persons in the area of psychology and athletic injury. All have impressive backgrounds and experiences in working with injured athletes and have contributed their expertise to the preparation of a worthwhile volume.

Jean Williams
University of Arizona

Preface

Each of the 20 chapters in this book relates in some important way to the psychology of athletic injury. Most sport participants at all levels of performance are prime candidates for physical injury. Such is the nature of sport; it involves rigorous training and great physical effort often fueled by an assortment of intense feelings associated with competition. Ironically, those with a powerful urge to succeed in sport are often the ones who succumb to debilitating trauma. When incapacitated, they are forced to disengage from what they love, from teammates they wish to be with, and, in many cases, from a way of life that has been a pillar of their psychological infrastructure.

This edition, as was also the case with the first, addresses sport injury from two primary perspectives: (a) identification and analysis of psychological factors that may make an athlete susceptible to sport-related injury and (b) discussion of psychological-oriented interventions, strategies, and responses from professional healers, helpers, friends, and relatives of the injured athletes designed to facilitate a speedy and successful rehabilitation or, perhaps, an eventual return to full sport participation.

Athletic leaders have, for years, been dedicated to improving playing conditions and rules. Coaches and trainers have always understood the need to lead athletes to optimal levels of fitness and biomechanical correctness. In other words, injury prevention has historically been viewed as being structurally and functionally oriented. Conventional wisdom would have us believe that athletes who fully understand their roles and who have the skills to execute appropriate behaviors properly are not inclined to suffer injury. Here, in this volume, the psychological domain, with its affective, perceptual/cognitive, and personality components, is emphasized. In particular, rehabilitative considerations predicated upon sound theoretical foundations are advocated.

The book should be a valuable resource for a variety of professionals who work with athletes. It should prove especially helpful to sport psychologists, athletic trainers, and physical therapists.

Five new chapters have been added to this second edition. As was the case in the first edition, the contributing authors are persons of considerable professional experience. They are either psychologists or mental health professionals with clinical interests in sport-related behavior. Some are experts in sport psychology per se (many of whom have to their credit personal histories of athletic participation as athletes or coaches), and some are athletic trainers who have worked through the years with very large numbers of injured athletes. Although those in the latter category are primarily concerned with organic and structural damage and its repair, they also must deal with motivation for adherence and compliance to rehabilitation programs.

Many fine chapter contributions from the first edition have been retained—but with two exceptions, content has been modified, references added and updated, and some material removed. Some overlap among authors of separate chapters is inevitable in a volume such as this because many have obviously often consulted the same pool of related literature. No editorial effort was made to purge occasional duplication of literature resources. I believe that contributing authors should be given latitude to integrate conclusions from journal articles and other sources according to their personal insights.

This second edition contains five sections, each of which includes selections that are relevant to its respective theme. Thus, this volume has one more section as well as five more chapters than does its predecessor.

Section 1 contains four chapters and is introductory in nature. It includes foundational materials designed to set the stage for subsequent sections.

In section 2, psychological correlates of sport injury are discussed, although not necessarily with an eye toward injury prediction.

Section 3, the largest, presents various counseling and rehabilitation approaches recommended for injured athletes. The focus of section 4 is the same but directed at those with permanent disabilities. It includes a chapter that addresses an increasingly troublesome problem, heretofore not frequently discussed and not likely to be found in other treatises on sport injury, namely, suicide in sport.

The last section, 5, presents case studies of injured athletes and describes ways in which they received assistance with their rehabilitative efforts.

As was the case with the first edition, this second edition is dedicated to the needs and interests of counselors, therapists, trainers, and students in these professional areas who are preparing to work with injured athletes. The contributing authors, all of whom are very highly qualified professionals, bring their expertise and experience to bear upon this objective.

David Pargman
Tallahassee, Florida

Acknowledgment

I wish to express a large measure of gratitude to my graduate student Teresa Johnson for her many contributions to the completion of this second edition. Her efforts towards this end are too varied and numerous to list here. Suffice it to say that her diligence was very much appreciated.

SECTION 1

INJURY AND SPORT— THE PROBLEM: CONCEPTUAL AND PRACTICAL APPROACHES

Chapter 1
Sport Injuries: An Overview of Psychological Perspectives
David Pargman

Chapter 2
Pain in Sport: A Biopsychological Perspective
John Heil
Perry G. Fine

Chapter 3
Ethical and Legal Issues for Sport Professionals Counseling Injured Athletes
Lou M. Makarowski

Chapter 4
Psychological and Emotional Response to Athletic Injury: Measurement Issues
Lynne Evans
Lew Hardy

▼

The purpose of this section is to present important injury-related factors that are basic to chapters in the following four sections of the book. This section begins with an introductory chapter written by the book's editor, **David Pargman**, which, in effect, is a brief review of pertinent psychological factors believed to be related to sport injury. Most of these issues are also discussed in considerably greater detail in subsequent chapters.

The second chapter, by **John Heil** and **Perry G. Fine**, elucidates a perceptual experience that is all too often part of the injury experience, namely, pain. Their perspective is biopsychological.

The third chapter in this section, by **Lou M. Makarowski**, deals with ethical issues facing professionals who counsel and work with injured athletes. It raises a number of provocative issues that deserve to be considered by such individuals.

The final chapter, written by **Lynne Evans** and **Lew Hardy**, discusses issues related to theory testing. They argue that models that attempt to clarify various psychological aspects of sport injury must be properly appraised. They offer suggestions and criticism to this end.

▲

1

Sport Injuries: An Overview of Psychological Perspectives

David Pargman
Florida State University

This chapter briefly reviews selected psychological factors associated with athletic injury that are discussed in greater detail in the subsequent chapters. Among the variables addressed are personality traits, self-concept, and response to psychosocial stress stimuli in athletes. In addition, a number of basic terms and concepts are defined and clarified.

If there is anything redeeming about athletic injury, it is assuredly of a secondary or very indirect benefit, at least as far as most athletes are concerned. Certainly some unexpected benefits may accrue from physical debilitation. Victims may be compelled to reorder their lives and lifestyles or to develop creative and fulfilling logistical strategies to meet the demands of heretofore uncommon physical challenges. New and meaningful relationships may also be established with others whom the injured athlete may never have encountered were it not for the sport-related trauma. Nonetheless, physical injury is essentially a negative experience that athletes typically and fervently try to avoid, but the rigorous, physical, competitive nature of organized sport often makes avoidance difficult. It may be concluded that sport is clearly a breeding ground for physical injury (Vitenbroek, 1996).

What follows in this chapter is an overview of selected psychological factors hypothesized to be related to sport injury. Subsequent chapters will discuss these factors in greater depth. Included here are certain perceptual/cognitive, affective, and personological considerations that have received attention in the general psychological and sport psychological (in particular) literature. Thus, the contents of this chapter emphasize causes and consequences of sport injury other than those that are structural, organic, and physiological. The tendency for medical or paramedical personnel is to dwell upon an injury's physical dimensions, although they recognize the realities of compulsory withdrawal from sport, namely, financial and competitive consequences. Behavioral, cognitive, and emotional dimensions of sport injury, from both causal and rehabilitative points of view, are often overlooked or minimized. This chapter, then, deals specifically and pointedly with the psychological dimensions of athletic injury.

The intensity with which sport proceeds, the attractive incentives offered to its successful participants, and the dangerous terrain and burdensome climatic conditions under which it often occurs account for a high incidence of sport injury. Although various operational definitions of the term injury becloud descriptive statistics, published estimates for secondary and collegiate levels in the United States, alone, are close to 750,000 injuries per year (Bergandi, 1985). Other estimates are for more than 850,000 per year at the high school level (Noble, Porter, & Bachman, 1982; Wrenn & Ambrose, 1980). When sport injury is examined out of the secondary and collegiate context (recreational activities and professional sport), the incidence may be as high as 3 to 5 million annually (Kraus & Conroy, 1984). More recently, Heil (1993) estimated the incidence to be as high as 17 million. Ironically, these numbers are expected to rise despite advances in athletic equipment and rule changes (Tator & Edmonds, 1986). This may be due to an ever-increasing number of participants, greater societal interest in sport, and greater availability of leisure time. Despite the well-intentioned efforts of the amateur and professional sport establishments (improvements in equipment and facilities, rule changes, etc.), athletic injury continues to undermine the aspirations and achievements of some participants. For them, it is a bane.

Whereas the term *accident* suggests something unforeseen, as in a totally random occurrence (equipment failure, slippery playing surface, etc.), injury may involve aggressive behavior with an intent to do harm (to oneself or to another). Indeed, results of some older studies point to personality and social adjustment variables as underlying causal factors (T. D. Brown, 1976; Conger et al., 1959; Levine, McHugh, Lee, & Rahe, 1977; Shaffer, Towns, Schmidt, Fisher, & Zlotowitz, 1974; Shaffer, Schmidt, Zlotowitz, & Fisher, 1977; Tillman & Hobbs, 1949). Accordingly, sport injury may be, at least in part, a function of psychological predisposition that, in turn, may clarify the incidence, type, or intensity of athletic injury. A number of published papers include findings in support of the relationship between psychological factors and sport injury (Bergandi, 1985; Burckes, 1981; Gould, Weiss, & Weinberg, 1981; Kerr & Minden, 1988; Pargman, 1976; Pargman & Lunt, 1989; Valliant, 1981; Weiss & Troxell, 1986; Yukelson, 1986).

In addition, attempts to clarify "injury responses" in sport have been attempted with psychodynamic explanations (Sanderson, 1977). Burckes (1981) suggested that some athletes may facilitate their own injury by volitionally entering high-risk situations. In such instances, injury satisfies a need for sympathy that resides at low levels of consciousness. Guilt related to poor previous performance or a need to escape anxiety associated with competition may be additional motives that operate at low level of awareness. Deutsch (1985) presented case studies that supposedly reveal underlying symbolic representations of sport injury that he suggests correlate with basic needs in other aspects of life. Beisser (1967) also described injury-related problems that appear to have psychiatric bases. Early work in the area of psychology and injury focused on the athlete's personality.

Personality. Among the unusually large number of personality studies reported in the sport psychology literature are some that use trait inventories and other personality variables to assess injury frequency and intensity (R. Brown, 1971; Jackson et al., 1978; Kraus & Gullen, 1969; Pargman, 1976; Valliant, 1981). Results from some of these studies point to significant relationships between variables such as time missed from games or practice due to injury and scores on trait personality scales. However, such alleged links are, at best, tenuous and far from definitive. Unfortunately, this literature, although thought provoking, has not yet generated conclusions that coaches, athletes, and trainers may find useful.

Some personality factors, such as *explanatory style* (Peterson & Seligman, 1987), characterized by either pessimism or optimism with regard to explaining why an injury occurred; *dispositional optimism* (Scheier et al., 1989), defined as a general expectancy for good rather than bad outcomes; and *hardiness* (Hull, Van Treuren, & Virnelli, 1987; Kobasa, Maddi, & Kahn, 1982), may have applications to sport injury rehabilitation (Grove, 1993).

Andersen and Williams (1988) have suggested that some personality traits "may dispose one to be less susceptible to the effects of stressors" (p. 301). Thus, they suggest an association between psychology (particularly the stress variable) and sport injury. Their hypotheses have been supported in football, but not in many other sports. Their original model, similar to one proposed by

Smith (1986), emphasizes an integration of cognitive, physiological, attentional, behavioral, intrapersonal, social, and stress history variables that may yet permit some prediction of sport injury. The model suggests the role of moderator variables (e.g., personality and coping skills) that affect life stress. Williams and Andersen (1998) revised their original model to include bidirectional arrows between personality, history of stressors, and coping resources (see Figure 1). Although a considerable amount of research supporting the revised model has been published recently, additional research is needed. Blackwell and McCullagh (1990) observed greater incidence of sport injury in athletes with high competitive anxiety in comparison to those who were low in anxiety.

Compliance. Yet another dimension of the relationship between sport injury and human psychology is athlete compliance with rehabilitation programs. In view of remarks made in the beginning of this chapter about the large numbers of athletes injured annually, it may be assumed that many are also engaged in, or should be engaged in, physical rehabilitative efforts. However, little investigation has been done with regard to athlete adherence to such

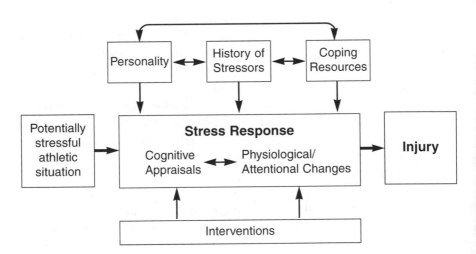

Figure 1. Revised Version of the Stress and Injury Model.
Note: The original model did not have the bidirectional arrows between personality, history of stressors, and coping resources.

From "Psychosocial Antecedents of Sport Injury: Review and Critique of the Stress and Injury Model," by J. M. Williams and M. B. Andersen, 1998, *Journal of Applied Sport Psychology, 10*, p. 7. Copyright 1998 by the Association for Advancement of Applied Sport Psychology. Reprinted with permission of the author.

programs (Fisher, Domm, & Wuest, 1988; Wiese & Weiss, 1987). This is an area in dire need of empirical investigation, as most of what has been reported to date is essentially anecdotal (e.g., Wiese & Weiss).

A few studies have examined adherence to exercise in relation to locus of control, which refers to a stylistic orientation rather than a personality trait in the true sense of the word. Dishman and Gettman (1980) found that when their subjects (not necessarily athletes) were informed about healthful benefits of exercise, a significant, positive relationship between internal locus of control and exercise adherence was observed. An internal locus of control suggests a tendency to attribute behavioral outcomes to personal causes, such as effort or ability. In contrast, those who are externally oriented tend to causally ascribe out-of-person factors (e.g., the weather, the facilities, or others in the environment). Because injury rehabilitation involves a high level of adherence (to exercise and physical activity), locus of control may be linked with injury recovery success. In this vein, Soenstrom and Walker (1973) found that persons who scored high on internal orientation reported significantly greater amounts of voluntary exercise, in contrast to other subjects. Self-motivation was found to be an important factor in rehabilitation program adherence (Duda, Smart, & Tappe, 1989; Fisher et al., 1988).

Self-concept. A number of studies have explored the relationship between injury and self-concept. For instance, Young and Cohen (1981) reported a significant difference in total self-concept score and four subscale scores between injured and noninjured female high school basketball players. Interestingly, the injured athletes demonstrated a more positive view of themselves (identity), their state of health, their physical appearance, their physical skills, and their personal worth than did the noninjured players. The overall self-concept of the injured group was also higher. These findings were interpreted by the authors as suggestive of greater physical risks being taken by the injured athletes during competition and practice because of the positive view held about themselves. Supposedly, this inclination resulted in greater vulnerability to injury. In contrast, the noninjured players expressed greater receptivity to mild derogatory statements included in the Tennessee Self-Concept Scale (TSCS). This may indicate lower self-confidence or esteem with regard to sport skill performance. Perhaps the noninjured players felt comparatively more inadequate than their injured counterparts and were, therefore, more receptive to criticism. Consequently, they may have behaved in a safer or more conservative way on the court.

This attractive speculation is, however, inconsistent with results from a previous study conducted by the same researchers. Young and Cohen (1979) used female college tournament basketball players as subjects. No differences were observed between injured and noninjured athletes with regard to total self-concept or other subscale scores.

Results reported by Lamb (1986) suggest an inverse relationship between self-concept and injury in college female varsity field hockey players as measured by the TSCS. Lamb concluded that a low self-concept level was related to a high frequency of injury.

Relationships between self-concept and sport injury should be investigated further. Additional findings from multivariate research designs with larger subject samples in a wider variety of sport areas may ultimately yield findings that are of practical application to athletic trainers, physical therapists, and coaches. Unlike personality traits, self-concept is a psychological variable that may fluctuate within short time frames and is, therefore, amenable to strategic manipulations. This may have important implications for injury prevention and rehabilitation.

Social factors. The direct or indirect interaction with others in the environment may exert both negative and positive influences upon athletes (Hardy, Richman, & Rosenfeld, 1991). For instance, an argument with a teammate or coach prior to or during competition may arouse an athlete to the extent that he or she is impeded in attentional or cognitive functions, thereby inhibiting performance and causing movement to be mechanically incorrect. The intensity and frequency of social stressors may thus have an impact upon vulnerability to sport injury (Wiese-Bjornstal, Smith, Shaffer, & Morrey, 1998).

Bramwell, Minoru, Wagner, and Holmes (1975) administered the Social and Athletic Readjustment Rating Scale (SARRS), consisting of 57 events likely to occur in an athlete's life, to 82 collegiate football players. Some of the events, such as making a serious mistake in a game or having "trouble with the coach," are sport-related. Others are unrelated to sport. The responses are indicative of the psychosocial disturbances in an athlete's life. Bramwell et al. observed that subjects with low Life Events scores had the lowest injury rates (35%); those with medium scores showed an injury rate of 44%; and those whose Life Event scores were high had an overwhelming injury rate of 72%. Coddington and Troxell (1980) modified the SARRS to make it appropriate to high school football players. Using 114 subjects, they concluded that subjects with emotional conditions associated with high scores on family instability and parental divorce or death incurred more "significant" injuries than did those whose scores were not elevated. These conclusions were also supported by subsequent work done by Cryan and Alles (1983), who used college football players.

Total life stress, competitive anxiety, and coping resources have been shown to be related to occurrence and severity of athletic injury (Blackwell &

McCullagh, 1990). Athletes high in life stress were more likely to be injured than those with low levels. Moreover, those with "adequate" coping abilities were less likely to incur sport injuries.

However, evidence contrary to the above findings is also available. Passer and Seese's (1983) work casts a shadow of doubt on the relationship between psychological factors and sport injury. In working with two different collegiate football teams, they observed a meaningful relationship between these variables in only one of the groups. Williams, Tonyman, and Wadsworth (1986) also failed to observe support for this association in male and female college volleyball players. Perhaps the interaction of attentional, cognitive/perceptual, and personality demands of certain sports, in combination with psychological attributes of individual athletes, should be carefully incorporated in future research designs in order to dispel uncertainty about the relationship between psychosocial factors and sport injury.

It seems appropriate to conclude by saying that additional well-conceived research will undoubtedly decrease conflicts and shortcomings in the existing literature related to the psychological bases of athletic injury. However, current available findings strongly suggest that injury prevention and the development of rehabilitation programs for injured athletes should be approached from psychological directions as well as anatomical, mechanical, and biological directions. Those who work professionally with athletes of all skill levels should strive to acquire insight into the emotional, perceptual, personological, and social psychological factors suggested in this chapter as potentially related to sport injury.

References

Andersen, M. B., & Williams, J. M. (1988). A model of stress and athletic injury: Prediction and prevention. *Journal of Sport and Exercise Psychology, 10,* 299–306.

Beisser, A. R. (1967). *The madness in sport.* New York: Appleton-Century-Crofts.

Bergandi, T. A. (1985). Psychological variables relating to the incidence of athletic injury. *International Journal of Sport Psychology, 16,* 141–149.

Blackwell, B., & McCullagh, P. (1990). The relationship of athletic injury to life stress, competitive anxiety and coping resources. *Athletic Training, 25,* 23–27.

Bramwell, S. T., Minoru, M., Wagner, N. N., & Holmes, T. H. (1975). Psychosocial factors in athletic injuries. *Journal of Human Stress, 1*(2), 6–20.

Brown, R. (1971). Personality characteristics related to injury in football. *Research Quarterly, 42,* 133–138.

Brown, T. D. (1976). Personality traits and their relationship to traffic violations. *Perceptual and Motor Skills, 42,* 467–470.

Burckes, M. E. (1981). The injury-prone athlete. *Scholastic Coach, 6*(3), 47–48.

Coddington, R., & Troxell, J. R. (1980). The effect of emotional factors on football injury rates: A pilot study. *Journal of Human Stress, 6*(4), 3–5.

Conger, J. J., Gaskill, H. S., Glad, D., Hassell, L., Rainey, R. V., & Sawrey, W. L. (1959). Psychological and psychophysiological factors in motor vehicle accidents. *Journal of the American Medical Association, 169,* 1581–1587.

Cryan, P. D., & Alles, W. F. (1983). The relationship between stress and college football injuries. *Journal of Sports Medicine and Physical Fitness, 23,* 52–58.

Deutsch, R. E. (1985). The psychological implications of sports related injuries. *International Journal of Sport Psychology, 16,* 232–237.

Dishman, R. K., & Gettman, L. R. (1980). Psychobiologic influences on exercise adherence. *Journal of Sport Psychology, 2,* 295–310.

Duda, J. L., Smart, A. E., & Tappe, M. K. (1989). Predictors of adherence in the rehabilitation of athletic injuries: An application of personal investment theory. *Journal of Sport and Exercise Psychology, 11,* 367–381.

Fisher, A. C., Domm, M. A., & Wuest, D. A. (1988). Adherence to sports injury rehabilitation programs. *The Physician and Sportsmedicine, 16,* 47–52.

Gould, D., Weiss, M., & Weinberg, R. (1981). Psychological characteristics of Big Ten wrestlers. *Journal of Sport Psychology, 3,* 69–81.

Grove, J. R. (1993). Personality and injury rehabilitation among sport performers. In D. Pargman (Ed.), *Psychological bases of sport injuries* (1st ed., pp. 90–120). Morgantown, WV: Fitness Information Technology.

Hardy, C. J., Richman, J. M., & Rosenfeld, L. B. (1991). The role of social support in the life stress/injury relationship. *The Sport Psychologist, 5,* 128–139.

Heil, J. (1993). *Psychology of sport injury.* Champaign, IL: Human Kinetics.

Hull, J. G., Van Treuren, R. R., & Virnelli, S. (1987). Hardiness and health: A critique and alternative approach. *Journal of Personality and Social Psychology, 53,* 518–530.

Jackson, D. W., Jarrett, H., Bailey, D., Kausek, J., Swanson, J. J., & Powell, J. W. (1978). Injury prediction in the young athlete: A preliminary report. *American Journal of Sports Medicine, 6*(1), 6–14.

Kerr, G., & Minden, H. (1988). Psychological factors related to the occurrence of athletic injuries. *Journal of Sport and Exercise Psychology, 10,* 167–173.

Kobasa, S. C., Maddi, S. R., & Kahn, S. (1982). Hardiness and health: A prospective study. *Journal of Personality and Social Psychology, 42,* 168–177.

Kraus, J. F., & Conroy, C. (1984). Mortality and morbidity from injury in sports and recreation. *Annual Review of Public Health, 5,* 163–192.

Kraus, J. F., & Gullen, W. H. (1969). An epidemiological investigation of predictor variables associated with intramural touch football injuries. *American Journal of Public Health, 59*(12), 2144–2156.

Lamb, M. (1986). Self-concept and injury frequency among female college field hockey players. *Athletic Training, 21,* 220–224.

Levine, J. G., McHugh, W. B., Lee, J. O., & Rahe, R. H. (1977). Recent life changes and accidents aboard an attack carrier. *Military Medicine, 27,* 469–471.

Noble, H. B, Porter, M., & Bachman, D. C. (1982). Athletic trainers: Their place in the health care system. *Illinois Medical Journal, 162,* 41–44.

Pargman, D. (1976). Visual disembedding and injury in college football players. *Perceptual and Motor Skills, 42,* 762.

Pargman, D., & Lunt, S. (1989). The relationship of self-concept and locus of control to the severity of injury in comparatively lower ability collegiate football players. *Sports Training, Medicine and Rehabilitation, 1,* 1–6.

Passer, M. W., & Seese, M. D. (1983). Life stress and athletic injury: Examination of positive versus negative events and three moderator variables. *Journal of Human Stress, 9*(4), 11–16.

Peterson, C., & Seligman, M. E. P. (1987). Explanatory style and illness. *Journal of Personality, 55,* 237–266.

Sanderson, F. H. (1977). The psychology of the injury-prone athlete. *British Journal of Sports Medicine, 11*(1), 56–57.

Scheier, M. F., Mathews, K. A., Owens, J. F., Magovern, G. J., Lefebvre, R. C., Abbott, R. A., & Carver, C. S. (1989). Dispositional optimism and recovery from surgery: The beneficial effects on physical and psychological well-being. *Journal of Personality and Social Psychology, 57,* 1024–1040.

Shaffer, J. W., Schmidt, C. W., Zlotowitz, H. I., & Fisher, R. S. (1977). Social adjustment profiles of female drivers involved in fatal and nonfatal accidents. *American Journal of Psychiatry, 134,* 801–804.

Shaffer, J. W., Towns, W., Schmidt, C. W., Fisher, R. S., & Zlotowitz, H. I. (1974). Social adjustment profiles of fatally injured drivers: A replication and extension. *Archives of General Psychiatry, 30,* 508–511.

Smith, R. E. (1986). Toward a cognitive-affective model of athletic burnout. *Sport Psychology, 8,* 36–50.

Soenstrom, R. S., & Walker, M. I. (1973). Relationship of attitude and locus of control to exercise and physical fitness. *Perceptual and Motor Skills, 36,* 1031–1034.

Tator, C. H., & Edmonds, V. E. (1986). Sports and recreation are a rising cause of spinal cord injury. *The Physician and Sportsmedicine, 14,* 157–167.

Tillman, W., & Hobbs, G. (1949). The accident-prone automobile driver: A study of psychiatric background. *American Journal of Psychiatry, 106,* 321–331.

Valliant, P. M. (1981). Personality and injury in competitive runners. *Perceptual and Motor Skills, 53,* 251–253.

Vitenbroek, D. G. (1996). Sports, exercise and other causes of injuries: Results of a population survey. *Research Quarterly for Exercise and Sport, 67,* 380–385.

Weiss, M. R., & Troxell, R. K. (1986). Psychology of the injured athlete. *Athletic Training, 21,* 104–109.

Wiese, D. M., & Weiss, M. R. (1987). Psychological rehabilitation and physical injury: Implications for the sports medicine team. *The Sport Psychologist, 1,* 318–330.

Wiese-Bjornstal, D. M., Smith, A. M., Shaffer, S. M., & Morrey, M. A. (1998). An integrated model of response to sport injury: Psychological and sociological dynamics. *Journal of Applied Sport Psychology, 10,* 46–69.

Williams, J. M., & Andersen, M. B. (1998). Psychological antecedents of sport injury: Review and critique of the stress and injury model. *Journal of Applied Sport Psychology, 10,* 5–25.

Williams, J. M., Tonyman, P., & Wadsworth, W. A. (1986). Relationship of life stress to injury in intercollegiate volleyball. *Journal of Human Stress, 12,* 38–43.

Wrenn, J. P., & Ambrose, D. (1980). An investigation of health care practices for high school athletes in Maryland. *Athletic Training, 15,* 85–92.

Young, M. L., & Cohen, D. A. (1979). Self-concept and injuries among female college tournament basketball players. *American Corrective Therapy Journal, 33*(5), 139–142.

Young, M. L., & Cohen, D. A. (1981). Self-concept and injuries among female high school basketball players. *Journal of Sports Medicine, 21,* 5–11.

Yukelson, D. (1986). Psychology of sport and the injured athlete. In D. B. Bernhart (Ed.), *Clinics in physical therapy* (pp. 175–195). New York: Churchill Livingstone.

2

Pain in Sport: A Biopsychological Perspective

John Heil
Lewis–Gale Clinic

Perry G. Fine
University of Utah

Pain is a complex and ever-present challenge to the athlete. How effectively pain is managed influences sport performance, injury risk, and injury rehabilitation and, hence, athletic success. All members of the sports medicine team play important roles in pain and injury management. Effective rehabilitation requires a thorough understanding of the dual, interacting psychological and biological influences that occur with pain and injury. Treatment is facilitated by careful comprehensive assessment, sensitivity to the "meaning" of pain to the athlete, and a psychologically minded treatment approach.

Introduction

The conquest of pain is a many-sided challenge to the athlete. There is routine performance pain, the nuisance of minor aches and soreness, the intense pain of sudden severe injury, the grind of rehabilitation, and the uncertainty of chronic injury. In sum, there are high expectations that athletes will tolerate pain across a broad range of circumstances. In pain, mind and body interact in complex ways that defy simple understanding. Consider the experience of the late NASCAR racer Neil Bonnett, who suggested, "A lot of times people confuse pain with fear . . . you get all excited when you get hurt . . . you almost overreact . . . jumping to conclusions." Describing his reaction to an accident in a Winston Cup race in which he fractured his sternum, he commented,

> When I wrecked I knew I was hurt . . . if that would have been the first wreck that I had ever had in a car I would have been jumping up and down, scared to death and going crazy . . . when the crew got to the car I said, "Just take it easy . . .." [Then] they were joking with me. I got to the hospital and they told me my heart rate was normal. (quoted in Heil, 1993, p. 41)

All sports medicine professionals have an important role to play in helping the athlete cope with routine performance and pain and the pain associated with injury and, most important, in helping the athlete understand the difference between the two. This, in turn, relies on a thorough understanding of the nature of the biological and psychological substrates of pain, the culture of sport, and the related pressures and expectations placed on the athlete.

This chapter provides sports medicine specialists with an appreciation of pain as a biopsychological phenomenon as well as an understanding of its potential impact upon sport performance, injury, and injury rehabilitation. Initial sections identify the biological and psychological substrates of pain. A brief look at routine performance pain is followed by a detailed review of pain assessment and management in injury. The chapter concludes with a theory-based look at remarkable feats of pain tolerance.

The Biopsychology of Pain

The biopsychological nature of pain is clearly reflected in the definition offered by the International Association for the Study of Pain (Merskey, 1986) in which pain is described as a "sensory and emotional" experience (p. 226). In spite of such unequivocal statements, there is a strong tendency in the medical and sport communities to try to define pain as either physical or mental, that is, as real or in one's head. This overly simplified and misleading conceptualization of a complex process is clearly a disservice to athletes.

Herein, pain refers to a perception that is an end product of a stimulus that is received and mediated by a complex biological system. The process of perception further elicits attempts to find the meaning of the pain and to guide one's behavior accordingly.

Biological Factors

The sensation, transmission, and perception of pain are the function of a distinct division of the nervous system, the *nociceptive system*. Nociception is a multistage process built on complex anatomic networks and chemical mediators that constitute the fundamental substrates of the pain experience. Table 1 provides definitions for the processing components of nociception.

Table 1. Processing Components of Nociception

TRANSDUCTION — noxious stimuli are translated into electrical activity at the sensory ending of nerves.

TRANSMISSION — transduced electrical impulses are propagated throughout the sensory nervous system.

MODULATION — nociceptive transmission is modified by a number of neural influences, including central cortical and peripheral sensory inputs.

PERCEPTION — transmission, transduction, and modulation culminate in the cognitive-emotional experience of pain.

Pain is triggered by the activation of two identifiable sets of receptors, high threshold mechanoreceptors and polymodal receptors. High threshold mechanoreceptors respond to strong mechanical stimuli transmitting pain signals with relative speed. In contrast, polymodal nociceptors respond to thermal, chemical, and mechanical stimuli, and are relatively slow in transmission. This latter group of receptors continues to fire for a time after the cessation of the pain-provoking stimulus. In addition, these receptors have a lower threshold of response when subsequently exposed to similar stimuli. This process, known as a sensitization, may cause higher sensitivity to pain-producing stimuli and also to pain in response to ordinarily nonpainful stimuli.

Sensitization is most likely to occur when there is repeated exposure to severe pain over days and weeks. Persistent pain syndromes such as myofascial pain and sympathetically maintained pain appear to have roots in this process. Myofascial pain syndrome is a musculoskeletal dysfunction with points of tenderness that when activated, trigger referred pain (Fine & Petty, 1986). Sympathetically maintained pain most commonly occurs in the arm or leg. This syndrome is characterized by hypersensitivity of the skin and spontaneous burning pain that appears to be reflexively driven by sympathetic nervous system activity (Roberts, 1986). In essence, these syndromes evolve as a nociceptive system comes to behave in a new way to old or otherwise ongoing pain stimuli. These syndromes often go unrecognized and as such are the cause of suffering and diminished performance. For more information, see Fine (1993).

Pain stimuli are transmitted via peripheral nerves to the spinal cord, which functions as a neurosensory switching station. Here pain and other sensory stimuli from the periphery, as well as information received centrally (via descending tracts) from the brain, converge upon common neurosensory pathways. The investigation of these interactions led Melzack and Wall (1965) to propose the *gate control theory* of pain. It holds that processing centers in the spinal cord may either decrease or increase the intensity of pain as a neuro-electric phenomenon and so result in the perception of relatively lesser or greater pain than that initially signaled. Subsequent research suggests that a similar process of modulation potentially occurs at other locations in the nociceptive system. The gate control theory has been used to explain the efficacy of pain control of various therapeutic modalities ranging from cryotherapy to ultrasound to acupuncture.

Modulated pain signals then ascend to the brain along any of several pathways. These transmit information with varying speed and directness to higher cortical centers, conveying a sensory as well as an emotional-reactive component of pain. The final perception of pain is based upon a summation of inputs from multiple brain centers including those that serve emotion and memory. As a consequence, even at its initial awareness, pain gains some of its meaning from prior experience and present state of mind. Once registered as perception, pain inputs also set off a cascade of electromechanical events via feedback loops within the nociceptive and autonomic nervous system that influence subsequent pain transmission and psychological status. This feedback system is directly triggered by the onset of pain-inducing stimuli.

Although firmly rooted in physiology, this system has a potentially wide range of psychological sequelae. Phenomena ranging from enhanced mood following exercise to "runner's high," as well as remarkable feats of pain tolerance during sport and the placebo response to treatment, have been explained via the action of this feedback system. Why such effects may be profound under some circumstances and absent under others remains a mystery.

The important role of naturally occurring opioids, known as endorphins, in pain inhibition is well accepted. However, as pathways and mediators of the pain system are more fully elucidated, the complexity of the interactions of these substrates only becomes more evident (Pasternak, 1988). For the sake of true understanding, any temptation toward oversimplification needs to be resisted. For instance, endorphins represent only one class of the many neurotransmitters that are involved in pain modulation. Serotonin, which also influences emotion and sleep, is a prominent pain-processing intermediary. Like serotonin, the endorphins also subserve a variety of other neuroendocrine functions.

The characteristics of the nociceptive system—sensitization, spinal gating, and pain as a summative perception (of multiple physiological factors)—underscore the complexity of the biology of pain. To arrive at a better understanding of the actual experience of pain, the interplay and integration of psychological influences upon these characteristics must be explored.

Psychological Factors

At the instant of perception, pain emerges as a more distinctly psychological phenomenon with intrapsychic and social components. Perception sets off a psychologically driven chain of reactive events (in contrast to the biologically driven events of nociception proper), the goal of which is to give meaning to pain. This complex process, subserved by multiple brain centers, yields an interpretation that is influenced by prior experience and current context, and that has cognitive and affective components. Pain is essentially a private intrapsychic experience and can remain so—although it seldom does. When pain becomes social communications (in the form of pain report or nonverbal display), it takes on an added dimension. An additional element of meaning arises as significant others (teammates, coaches, friends, health providers) react to the athlete's expression of pain. The importance of the social component in pain has led some to characterize pain as a biopsycho*social* phenomenon (Fordyce, 1988).

Pain is most simply understood in terms of location, intensity, and sensory type. Pain comes to have meaning as this basic information is evaluated in light of functional limits on physical ability, memory of similarly painful events, and assessment of the impact of injury on current and future activity. The single most important element of meaning is the assumed status of pain as benign, or alternately, as a sign of injury. A simultaneously evolving emotional understanding incorporates cognitive evaluative information and leads to response on a continuum ranging from relief ("No problem! This is routine pain") to distress ("Oh no! I'm really hurt"). In the latter case, some degree of negative emotion in the form of fear, anxiety, or sense of loss is likely to follow.

Out of this cognitive-emotional understanding of pain comes action. Intrapsychically, this understanding triggers psychological coping. Actions in the form of reports of pain and demonstrated limits in functional activity also carry pain into the social sphere. The way an athlete displays pain is an important determinant of the way others respond. However, this is ultimately influenced by a host of factors ranging from cultural differences to the specific expectations of a given sport environment. In the case of injury, this influences the promptness and the type of care that will be given. More protracted response to the athlete's pain may be helpful or harmful. Such attention may be useful in the form of ongoing social support that functions as a buffer against the psychological sequelae of injury. Conversely, overattention by significant others may elicit guilt or fear of reinjury, or potentially lead to maladaptive secondary gain.

As pain gains meaning, it also gains complexity as social and psychological factors build upon the nociceptive imprint that is the basis of pain. In the end, pain may be experienced in its most useful form as a transient phenomenon heralding a self-limited relatively inconsequential event. Alternatively, it may take a pathological form leading to a highly disruptive life-altering disease process of indeterminable proportions.

Sport Performance

Understanding the ability of athletes to tolerate pain rests in turn on an appreciation of the mind-set of the committed athlete and how it is cultivated in the competitive sport environment. The mind-set is reflective of the sport's specific culture, which creates expectations regarding pain tolerance and risk taking, and of the system of mental training, which complements physical conditioning and technical training. Pragmatically, awareness of pain elicits a multilayered decision-making process: Is pain routine and best ignored? Does pain indicate a need to adjust pace (e.g., in a marathon run) or to modify technique to avoid injury (e.g., in fencing)? Does pain signal an injury is in the making? If so, can the athlete persevere until competition concludes, or is immediate medical attention needed?

Sport as Culture

It is useful to think of sport as a subculture in which behavior is guided by a unique set of principles, which are implicitly observed and fundamental to success. This idea is reflected in subtleties of language and in expectations for behavior. Special privileges and recognition are accorded to the elite competitor. The path to elite status involves "survival of the fittest." Through youth sport, high school, and college-level competition, as well as different degrees of professional involvement, the challenges become more and more formidable. Fewer and fewer athletes remain, and pain management skills significantly influence this survival. The unsubstantiated allegation "no pain, no gain, no fame" still prevails within athletic circles, and athletes are encouraged to play with pain, to give 110%, and to be mentally tough. The expectation for high performance and maximal effort permeates the world of sport. Fans and media professionals often join the athlete and coach in evaluating performance by these standards. As a consequence, the athlete is encouraged to tolerate pain and to take risks that potentially influence both physical and mental well-being.

Mental Training

Mental training is the systematic use of self-regulation methods to modulate psychophysiological intensity and to direct attention to specific sport-relevant cues in complex training and competitive environments. This means maintaining an appropriate mental state despite distractions internally (cognitions, for example, pain) and externally (irrelevant sport cues, for example, crowd noise). Although regarded as a contemporary phenomenon, mental training has roots in the ancient meditative martial arts traditions (Heil, 1984). To meet the simultaneous challenges of pain control and highly skilled sport performance, formidable mental skills are required of the athlete. A series of studies have examined the cognitive strategies used by distance runners to cope with the discomfort of pain, fatigue, and exertion (Masters & Lambert, 1989; Morgan, 1978; Peterson, Durtschi, & Murphy, 1990; Schomer, 1986, 1987). This research has characterized the successful distance runner as having the ability to shift attention according to the demands of the sport from a dissociative, distractive mode to an associative, focusing mode and the ability to tune into performance cues as needed despite pain. Mental training helps the athlete move to an ideal performing state, in pain or in its absence.

Pain Tolerance Illustrated

Loeser (1982) has been credited with the creation of a graphic model of pain as a biopsychological phenomenon. This describes the electrochemical process of nociception that produces a subjective perception of pain, which in turn gains meaning as personal suffering, which ultimately gives rise to idiosyncratic actions and pain-driven behaviors. Generic adaptations of this model are presented in the figures below, whereby perception gives way to personal meaning with actions following accordingly. Figure 1 depicts the basic structure for this model of pain. The scenarios that follow are examples for application of the model and are depicted in Figures 2, 3, and 4.

Scenario #1. Consider a distance runner who has the *perception* of a burning feeling in her legs as she climbs a hill. Evaluating this perception in comparison to prior experiences, she determines that the *meaning* of this burning feeling is routine performance pain. The likely *action* to follow is to continue running. Research by Peterson et al. (1990) revealed that many elite runners relabel pain as exertion when describing the sensations associated with a maximum running effort and thus evaluate this perception as a positive sign

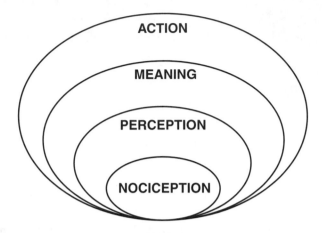

Figure 1. A Conceptual Model of Pain

From "A Multifaceted Model of the Components of Pain," by J. Loeser, 1982, found in *Chronic Low Back Pain* (p. 146), by M. Stanton-Hicks and R. A. Boas, New York: Raven Press. Adapted with permission by the author.

of good effort. The situation is summarized in Figure 2.

Scenario #2. Following *perception* of a burning feeling in his shoulder, an athlete concludes that an injury is developing (*meaning*). Should the activity be stopped, or is some alternate course of *action* acceptable? To a swimmer, this pain might mean an overuse injury is in the making, which can be cor-

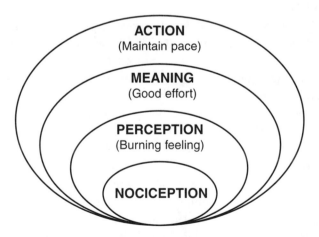

Figure 2. Scenario #1 Applied to Pain Model

From "A Multifaceted Model of the Components of Pain," by J. Loeser, 1982, found in *Chronic Low Back Pain* (p. 146), by M. Stanton-Hicks and R. A. Boas, New York: Raven Press. Adapted with permission by the author.

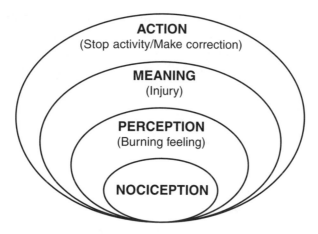

Figure 3. Scenario #2 Applied to Pain Model

From "A Multifaceted Model of the Components of Pain," by J. Loeser, 1982, found in *Chronic Low Back Pain* (p. 146), by M. Stanton-Hicks and R. A. Boas, New York: Raven Press. Adapted with permission by the author.

rected by a change in stroke mechanics. Alternately, a power lifter preparing for a maximum lift in practice might determine that additional conditioning is needed before attempting the lift. A basketball player in the middle of a game may decide to wait until the next time-out to take himself out of a game and be evaluated by a physician. Figure 3 illustrates this scenario.

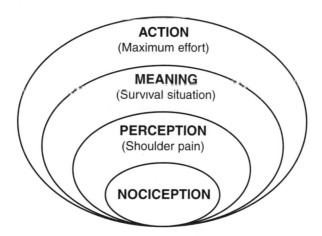

Figure 4. Scenarios #3 and #4 Applied to Pain Model

From "A Multifaceted Model of the Components of Pain," by J. Loeser, 1982, found in *Chronic Low Back Pain* (p. 146), by M. Stanton-Hicks and R. A. Boas, New York: Raven Press. Adapted with permission by the author.

Scenario #3. The swimmer in Scenario #2 takes time off from practice in order to allow his shoulder to recover. He goes fishing. His boat is capsized some distance offshore, requiring him to swim to safety. As he is cautiously making his way to shore (protecting his injured shoulder), he notices that sharks are approaching. The need to escape and survive takes precedence over pain, and he abandons his conservative style of swimming and makes an enormous effort to swim as rapidly as possible to reach the shore (see Figure 4).

Scenario #4. Pain due to an acute shoulder injury has limited the swimmer's practice (Scenarios #2 and #3) immediately prior to the Olympic trials. He is favored to win a medal in the Olympics, but must compete successfully in the trial to qualify. His goals and aspirations are to be tested. In a sense, his survival as an elite competitive swimmer is at stake. He decides to race in the trials and is successful. He is surprised by the very low level of pain that he feels. Figure 4 also applies to this scenario.

Injury and Rehabilitation

Pain Assessment

Because pain is a complex, multidimensional phenomenon, its assessment should acknowledge the circumstances surrounding the injury with which it is associated as well as the athlete's response to it. The more complex and distressing the injury, the more important is the comprehensive approach to assessment. In their edited volume, Turk and Melzack (1992) have included detailed aspects of this comprehensive approach. Among these are the athlete's subjective report of pain intensity (e.g., rated on a 0 to 10 scale) and the quality (e.g., burning, stabbing, electric, aching, etc.) of the pain. A self-report 0 to 10 scale is quite versatile and allows pain to be assessed across a variety of situations. Measures of "average daily pain," pain at its "worst," and pain at its "least" may also be obtained. In addition, it is useful to identify those specific factors or situations that lead to an increase or decrease in pain (e.g., specific movements or postures). This line of inquiry provides insight into the challenges the athlete faces in sport, rehabilitation, and activities of daily living. It also offers a perspective on the athlete's coping methods and how effectively they are working.

It is of paramount importance to understand the meaning the athlete attaches to pain and how this influences his or her behavior. Consider the situation where an athlete fears that pain experienced during muscular rehabilitation is a sign of reinjury (when in fact it is benign, non-tissue-damaging pain). As a consequence, the athlete may unwittingly erect a serious barrier to rehabilitation (e.g., he may not appear for a scheduled rehabilitation appointment).

Thus, a cycle may ensue that undermines the rehabilitation process. Self-confidence in the ability to recover effectively and trust in the ability of treatment providers to safely direct rehabilitation may be inhibited. Compliance problems may then follow and be interpreted by treatment providers as a lack of motivation. This common, fairly simple, misunderstanding of pain may also trigger a variety of other difficulties.

An altogether different problem may arise when the athlete fails to heed pain messages that do in fact signal reinjury. In this situation, rehabilitation can be marred by treatment setbacks. The more severe or enduring the pain, the progressively greater becomes the role played by factors such as attention, expectation, autonomic arousal, and muscle tension. With chronicity also comes greater suffering (Fordyce, 1988). Over time, complaints of pain are increasingly likely to reflect an overall "distress quotient," a measure of suffering that combines pain and distress about the pain.

Where inconsistency is noted in athlete behavior and reports of pain, care providers may question the athlete's sincerity or even challenge complaints of pain. ("Doesn't he want to get better?" "Maybe she is not a serious competitor.") There is relatively little to be gained, and potentially much to be lost, in adopting such a strategy, especially in regard to treatment rapport and trust. As pain persists, it becomes increasingly situation specific. It can be triggered by circumstances that elicit fear, anxiety, or lack of confidence, independent of tissue injury. In this situation, it is recommended that the athlete's complaints of pain be accepted as legitimate and that a vigorous effort be made to understand the full scope of the pain as a biopsychological problem (Rotella & Heil, 1991).

Often the source of such pain problems arises from implicitly held distorted "cognitive schema" (Heil, 1993). These are essentially misinterpretations of injury that are rooted in a poor understanding of pain and the recovery process. Difficulties arise when the perspectives of athlete and treatment provider diverge. For example, the athlete may interpret continuing pain as a sign of unresolved injury, whereas the treatment provider assumes that objective signs of recovery mean there is no basis for pain. Assessment of the injured athlete begins with an understanding of pain as a normative consequence of injury; however, it is useful to supplement this perspective with a secondary focus on adjusting to persistent pain or nonhealing injury.

Pain Management

There is a wide variety of pain management treatments commonly used by athletic trainers and therapists (e.g., ice, ultrasound, TENS, diathermy, electrical stimulation, acupressure, massage). However, injury-related pain may be associated with psychological sequelae that require the athlete to mobilize coping resources. Although the athlete's individual efforts are usually sufficient, the athletic trainer or therapist who adopts a psychologically minded approach to rehabilitation will facilitate recovery and pain management.

There are four pillars of psychological rehabilitation that enhance speed of recovery and maximize the athlete's sense of well-being. These are education, goal setting, social support, and mental training. The first three of these fall within the purview of the athletic trainer or other sports medicine specialist. On the other hand, mental training techniques more often fall within the province of the psychological expert. These techniques are typically directed toward pain control, as well as stress management and mental readiness for return to play. Ideally, the psychologist and athletic trainer collaborate in order to optimize their effectiveness.

A variety of self-directed pain management techniques have been devised for use in general medical settings (Turk, Meichenbaum, & Genest, 1983). These are most effective when the athlete is at rest. Their utility in an action-oriented athletic setting is generally limited. Research on the mental strategies by distance runners during training and competition (e.g., Morgan, 1978; Schomer, 1987) offers insight into pain management approaches that are suitable for athletic performance. However, their utility in injury management situations is limited. The work of these two management techniques is integrated and extended to an action-oriented injury management strategy in the pain-sport attentional matrix (Heil, 1993). This conceptual scheme identifies four broad classes of pain-coping methods. These are defined by whether the athlete "focuses on" or "focuses away from" both pain and sport simultaneously—or whether there is a separation of attention between sport and pain (e.g., "focus on" sport while dissociating from pain). For more on mental training in pain management, see Heil (1993, 1995).

The primary responsibility of the athletic trainer is to differentiate benign pain from pain associated with reinjury and to determine a relatively safe level of physical activity. At the time of injury, it is important to create a sense of calm and security in the midst of the pain and fear of further injury. Once rehabilitation commences, the trainer or specialist should emphasize an educational approach wherein the nature of the injury as well as rehabilitative strategies is delineated. This is particularly true in the event of setbacks whereby progress in rehabilitation halts or there occurs regression to a lower level of recuperation, or both. If and when the athlete is unable to return to play, his or her disappointment (and distress) should be acknowledged and treatments adjusted. In case of chronically failed rehabilitation, sport medicine specialists should strive to maintain athlete trust and confidence. Table 2 offers a brief summary of recommendations for pain management across differing rehabilitation situations. For a more detailed treatment of approaches to chronically failed rehabilitation, see Fordyce (1976) and Sternbach (1987).

Table 2. Guidelines for the Psychological Management of Pain

Situation: At the occurrence of injury (especially if severe or psychologically traumatic),
◆ establish rapport and create positive, realistic expectations.
◆ shift focus from pain to thoughts of a positive outcome or to the next necessary step in injury management.

Situation: During otherwise uncomplicated rehabilitation,
◆ educate the athlete regarding the mechanisms of injury and treatment.
◆ identify pain as a routine aspect of rehabilitation.

Situation: With treatment plateaus or setbacks,
◆ clarify treatment goals and encourage conscientious adherence.
◆ reassure athlete of the benign status of pain.

Situation: At failed return to play,
◆ acknowledge discouragement and provide support.
◆ differentiate routine pain from dangerous pain (which signals reinjury).

Situation: With chronically failed rehabilitation,
◆ treat pain complaints as real even if inconsistent.
◆ review the rehabilitation program with respect to all factors identified above, searching for mitigating or sabotaging factors.

Remarkable Feats of Pain Tolerance

Remarkable feats of pain tolerance are frequently observed in sport and have long been noted in the pain medicine literature (e.g., Beecher, 1946, 1956; Janal, Colt, Clark, & Glusman, 1984). During World War II, military surgeon Lieutenant Colonel Henry Beecher (1946) observed that soldiers wounded in combat needed fewer narcotics for relief of pain than did civilians who suffered similar injuries. In subsequent research, Beecher (1956) revised this observation and concluded that there was not a dependable relationship between severity of a wound and the pain experienced. The degree of suffering is a reflection of the meaning of pain to the patient. In his work, Beecher comments on the similar ability of athletes to tolerate the severe pain of acute injury.

This section presents a psychological model of acute pain tolerance specific to athlete performance—broadly defined to include sport and other activity requiring performance of physical skill under demanding conditions (such as by soldiers in combat and police or firefighters in the line of hazardous duty) (Heil, 1998). This model is pretheoretical and speculative. It draws on the sport psychology literature and on anecdotal reports of pain tolerance. This model also reflects the personal experiences and professional perspectives of the authors as pain and sports medicine specialists and as athletes. This psychological model assumes physiological correlates. The stress-induced analgesia literature supports this assumption (Kelly, 1986).

Remarkable feats of pain tolerance are typically associated with the following elements:

- the expectation that pain can and will be tolerated;
- a strong goal orientation;
- absorption in the "work in progress," that is, a focus on sport over pain;
- a survival context (literal or metaphorical);
- the assumption of limited pain duration.

Expectations that athletes will tolerate pain related to performance and injury permeate sport. The time-honored nature of these expectations is reflected in the story of an ancient warrior whose conquest of performance over pain is recognized in modern sport. The Greek soldier Pheidippides allegedly ran from the site of a battle on the Plains of Marathon to the city of Athens to announce a critical victory over an invasion force—then collapsed and died. His efforts today are honored in the marathon, which extends the 26 miles and 385 yards he covered in his run.

The importance of goal orientation is deeply rooted in coaching theory and practice. It is ingrained in the athlete through repeated training, often over years' time. Goal setting helps the athlete remain committed to performance and orients the athlete to effective action. Overlearning associated with almost countless repetitions automizes sport skills and facilitates their execution under a wide variety of circumstances. Goal orientation is typically strongest during competition. Where there is close proximity to important sport goals, the goals are most compelling.

A predominant focus on sport-related perceptual inputs (i.e., the sights, sounds, and "feel" of competition) is made possible by the great importance the athlete places on competitive success. Absorption in the sport experience fosters keen concentration and focused psychophysiological intensity. This enables the athlete to hold sport at the center of his or her awareness. Other inputs (including pain) are thereby held out of awareness. This ability rests on skills in attention control and in the modulation of intensity, which are cultivated through sport performance and enhanced by mental training. The athlete comes to instinctively seek an ideal performing state that facilitates sport behavior.

Many examples of remarkable pain tolerance are seen in a survival context, that is, in life-threatening conditions. Examples include soldiers in combat, firefighters and police in line-of-duty actions, and individuals in wilderness survival situations. The adaptive value of pain is lost when the threat of danger to the entire organism is greater than the threat of pain. Although sport is seldom a true life or death situation, the personal investment in success and the personal cost of failure can be tremendous. In certain competitions (e.g., Olympic trials), the athlete's survival at sport is dependent upon a successful outcome.

Most notable feats of pain tolerance are typically of relatively brief duration. Concentration is more easily sustained and pain control more easily attained when there is an end in sight. In the competitive context, the athlete is able to look ahead to a time when the event will be over and pain will cease. In contrast, the outcome (success or failure) of competition endures indefinitely.

Summary

Pain is a complex biopsychological phenomenon. The goal of this chapter is to enhance the sport psychologist's and other sports medicine specialist's knowledge of pain and to broaden skills in pain assessment and intervention. An understanding of pain is based on knowledge of the anatomic and chemical elements of the pain-processing nociceptive system, and of the interplay of biological and psychological factors. Pain signals are subject to modulation by the nervous system. Pain intensity may be reduced by mechanisms described in the gate control theory or enhanced by factors such as attention, expectation, autonomic arousal, and muscle tension. The perception of pain sets off a psychologically driven chain of events by which behavior is modified according to the meaning assigned to pain. The ability to differentiate routine performance pain from injury is critically important to the athlete. The psychological sequelae of pain in injury will be most readily recognized and effectively managed with a team-based, psychologically minded approach to rehabilitation. Understanding remarkable feats of pain tolerance requires insight into both the biopsychology of pain and the culture of sport.

References

Beecher, H. K. (1946). Pain in men wounded in battle. *Annals of Surgery, 123*(1), 96–105.

Beecher, H. K. (1956). Relationship of significance of wound to pain experienced. *Journal of the American Medical Association, 161*(17), 1609–1613.

Fine, P. G. (1993). The biology of pain. In J. Heil (Ed.), *The psychology of sport injury* (pp. 269–280). Champaign, IL: Human Kinetics.

Fine, P. G., & Petty, W. C. (1986). Myofascial trigger point pain: Diagnosis and treatment. *Current Reviews in Clinical Anesthesia, 7,* 34–39.

Fordyce, W. E. (1976). *Behavioral methods for chronic pain and illness.* St. Louis: Mosby.

Fordyce, W. E. (1988). Pain and suffering: A reappraisal. *American Psychologist, 43*(4), 276–283.

Heil, J. (1984). Imagery for sport: Theory, research and practice. In W. F. Straub & J. M. Williams (Eds.), *Cognitive sport psychology* (pp. 245–252). Lansing, NY: Sport Science Associates.

Heil, J. (1993) . *The psychology of sport injury.* Champaign, IL: Human Kinetics.

Heil, J. (1998, July). *Remarkable feats: Of pain tolerance, injury, rehabilitation, and coping with adversity.* Keynote presentation at the 2nd International Meeting of Psychology Applied to Sport and Exercise, Braga, Portugal.

Heil, J. (1995). Pain management: What price the gain? *Performance Edge, 5*(2), 3–8.

Janal, M. N., Colt, E. W. D., Clark, W. C., & Glusman, M. (1984). Pain sensitivity, mood, and plasma endocrine levels in man following long-distance running: Effects of naloxone. *Pain, 19,* 13–25.

Kelly, D. D. (1986). Stress-induced analgesia [special issue]. *Annals of the New York Academy of Sciences, 467.*

Loeser, J. (1982). A multifaceted model of the components of pain. In M. Stanton-Hicks & R. A. Boas (Eds.), *Chronic low back pain* (p. 146). New York: Raven Press.

Masters, K. S., & Lambert, N. J. (1989). The relationship between cognitive coping strategies, reasons for running, injury, and performance of marathon runners. *Journal of Sport and Exercise Psychology, 11*(2), 161–170.

Melzack, R., & Wall, P. D. (1965). Pain mechanisms: A new theory. *Science, 150,* 971–979.

Merskey, H. (1986). Classification of chronic pain: Descriptions of chronic pain syndromes and definitions of pain terms. *Pain, Suppl. 3,* 226.

Morgan, W. P. (1978, April). The mind of the marathoner. *Psychology Today,* pp. 38–40, 43, 45–46, 49.

Pasternak, G. W. (1988). Multiple morphine and enkepathlin receptors and the relief of pain. *Journal of the American Medical Association, 259,* 1462–1367.

Peterson, K., Durtschi, S., & Murphy, S. (1990, September). *Cognitive patterns and conceptual schemes of elite distance runners during submaximum and maximum running effort.* Paper presented at the annual meeting of the Association for the Advancement of Applied Sports Psychology, San Antonio, TX.

Roberts, W. J. (1986). A hypothesis on the physiological basis for causalgia and related pains. *Pain, 24,* 297–311.

Rotella, R. J., & Heil, J. (1991). Psychological aspects of sports medicine. In B. Reider (Ed.), *Sports medicine: The school-age athlete* (pp. 105–117). Philadelphia: W. B. Saunders.

Schomer, H. H. (1986). Mental strategies and perception of effort of marathon runners. *International Journal of Sports Psychology, 17,* 41–49.

Schomer, H. H. (1987). Mental strategy training programme for marathon runners. *International Journal of Sports Psychology, 18,* 133–151.

Sternbach, R. A. (1987). *Mastering pain: A 12 step program for coping with chronic pain.* New York: Putnam.

Turk, D. C., Meichenbaum, D., & Genest, M. (1983). *Pain and behavior medicine: A cognitive behavioral perspective.* New York: Guilford Press.

Turk, D. C., & Melzack, R. (Eds.). (1992). *Handbook of pain assessment.* New York: Guilford.

3

Ethical and Legal Issues for Sport Professionals Counseling Injured Athletes

Lou M. Makarowski
Achievement Place, Pensacola, Florida

This chapter examines some of the ethical and legal issues relevant to sport professionals who counsel injured athletes. Particular emphasis will be given to issues and scenarios that are pertinent to trainers and other sport medicine specialists who have not received extensive training in counseling theory and techniques. Value decision-making guidelines are described. Codes and their derivation that are routinely used by professional counselors to guide them when confronted with ethically challenging situations are described as well.

Introduction

What you do with information you acquire from those in your charge has important implications for individual and team levels of performance as well as your ethical stress level and liability exposure. Trainers and team physicians are the front line of health care in sports. As a health care provider, your service to the athlete should be guided by professional, moral, ethical, and legal directives.

As a professional, you will follow a code of ethical conduct, but as an employee of an organization, your job description may conflict with ethical requirements of your profession (Ungerleider & Golding, 1992; Voy, 1991). Ethical principles are only part of the picture. As a sport health professional, you can be held legally accountable for the way you carry out your counseling responsibilities.

The American Medical Association now recognizes athletic trainers as allied health providers. Twenty-six states license athletic trainers at the A.T.C. (athletic trainer, certified) level. The scope of the legislation varies from state to state, but the trend toward licensure is very likely to continue. With increasing professional status comes increased vulnerability to lawsuits. Tortuous activity of all types will increase as trainers are held accountable legally for increasingly higher levels of knowledge.

The fact that licensed athletic trainers may now open free-standing clinics is another indication that athletic trainers are now expected to know more. Malpractice insurance costs for trainers have increased significantly. This increase in costs is based upon insurers' projections of increased monetary awards paid to plaintiffs who sue trainers for damages. As public knowledge of sports' inner sanctums grows, so will the creativity of lawyers who seek to protect athletes from exploitation, and to protect the public from incompetent or unethical sport professionals (Voy, 1991).

In team sports, you may wear several hats. You may be a trainer, assistant coach, psychological counselor, and representative of the employing organization or entity. Wearing different hats can increase opportunities for ethical conflicts. Ethical conflicts are a major source of stress and anxiety. Ethical responsibilities are different for a psychologist than they are for a coach, university professor, health club employee, or professional boxing promoter.

Ethical stress occurs when a trainer's personal philosophy of right and wrong differs from that of the client, employer, profession, or employing organization. Ethical stress can produce anxiety or worry. Ethical anxiety may lie dormant until trainers find themselves confronted with some ethical dilemma or legal proceeding. Trainers confront ethical stressors regularly. Sport professionals can minimize ethical stress by developing a strong personal ethical philosophy and a system that guides their personal decision making.

Value Decision-Making Guidelines

In order to make decisions based on your value system, you have to know yourself. To counsel ethically, a clear understanding of your personal value system is crucial. Knowledge of your personal value system will help you to understand yourself and others. You will also be in a better position to communicate value-laden information in a way that you recognize and the athletes you counsel will accept.

Your personal value system can create ethical stressors if it is in conflict with the decisions you make. Your value system also creates emotional blind spots that incline you to give the benefit of the doubt. Blind spots may also cause you to be overly scrupulous. Trainers who are emotionally close to their athletes will counsel more effectively and ethically if they learn to recognize their own personal value system as well as the personal value systems of the athletes they counsel. Ask yourself these questions when making decisions that are of value importance:

1. Is my decision/action compatible with my goals, values, and expectations?
2. Does it feel right?
3. Where does my action/decision ultimately lead?
4. What is the track record of others when making a similar decision? What is my track record when making a similar decision?
5. By doing this, what am I saying about myself?

When struggling to evaluate your decision-making process, a matrix for examining your decisions may prove helpful. These guidelines and systems based on the work of Simon, Howe, and Kirschenbaum (1974) and Raths, Merrill, and Simon (1966) can help you maintain consistency and clarity in your thinking when counseling athletes.

For example, if you are struggling with a decision of whether or not to work for a prominent coach who insists that steroids be a part of the training regimen, list "steroids" on the first line of the matrix (see Table 1). If you are troubled by the method chosen to help junior athletes "make weight," list "weight loss" in the matrix. If sex is being exchanged for playing time and you are struggling to decide just how badly you want to play, include "sexual barter" in the matrix. Other areas of value concern complete the matrix.

Table 1. Decision-Making Matrix

DECISIONS	1	2	3	4	5	6	7
STEROIDS	7	6	5	6	7	7	5
WEIGHT LOSS							
SEXUAL BARTER							
BLOOD DOPING							
ABUSIVE RELATIONSHIPS							
CHEAT OR NOT TO CHEAT							
PAIN KILLERS							

For each decision/situation included in the matrix above, circle the number below that best describes YOU in the decision process, and enter the number on the horizontal axis of the box. Your responses will be selected from a continuum numbered 1 to 7; selection of "1" indicates a definite "yes" answer to the question, whereas selection of "7" indicates a definite "no" answer to the question. All other responses (i.e., 2–6) indicate varying degrees of agreement.

1. Freely made the decision?	YES 1 - 2 - 3 - 4 - 5 - 6 - 7 NO
2. Like the position taken?	YES 1 - 2 - 3 - 4 - 5 - 6 - 7 NO
3. Looked at the pros & cons?	YES 1 - 2 - 3 - 4 - 5 - 6 - 7 NO
4. Examined outcomes?	YES 1 - 2 - 3 - 4 - 5 - 6 - 7 NO
5. In accordance with my values, attitudes, beliefs?	YES 1 - 2 - 3 - 4 - 5 - 6 - 7 NO
6. Stand up for my actions?	YES 1 - 2 - 3 - 4 - 5 - 6 - 7 NO
7. Made a personal commitment?	YES 1 - 2 - 3 - 4 - 5 - 6 - 7 NO

Answering Scale
1–4, decision is consistent with your values.
5–7, decision is inconsistent with your values.

Now, what does the matrix tell you about your decision? If the decision you are considering has the answering scale values that mostly lie between 1 and 4, then you are probably making decisions that will promote a healthy lifestyle with less stress and less risk of injury. If your answering scale values mostly lie between 5 and 7, as in the first one (Steroids), you are probably making decisions that will promote an unhealthy lifestyle, add greater stress, and increase the risk of injury.

Ethical/Legal Issues

Personal morality is certainly an important aspect of an individual's ethical philosophy, but counselors/trainers who set themselves the task of being "Morals Police" may unnecessarily limit their contribution to the athlete/patient and to the employing organization. When psychologists counsel, they must make every effort to work within the value system of the client. The psychologist who is unable to listen empathically and nonjudgmentally has an ethical duty, as well as a professional obligation, to help the client identify a more impartial confidant. The professional psychologist must not breach the client's right to confidential, competent treatment in the referral process or in the transition to a more appropriate counselor. A trainer who counsels should do likewise.

The penalty for a psychologist who violates the client's right to confidentiality could be extreme. The results of breaching such rights might include being found guilty of malpractice by the legal system with penalties that could include substantial monetary damages. Loss of license may occur in case of conviction of violation of professional statutory proscriptions. For lesser ethical breaches, which do not involve civil or criminal misconduct, the penalties for psychologists might range from censure to expulsion from professional organizations.

Ethical decision making greatly reduces the likelihood of any form of criminal, civil, or malpractice violation. Ethical codes for counselors routinely define ethical practice as practicing within the limits of the law. Conduct that violates legal mandates will almost always be clearly unethical. Your value decision-making tools will help you make decisions that are clearly within the legal codes and most likely to result in a healthy lifestyle.

A trainer who counsels athletes in areas that provoke ethical concerns has a right to refer that athlete to a professional who does not have that conflict. Risk is always present in the sports environment. Sport participants at every level are attracted to risk. They see it as a challenge. Mastery of risk is a thrill that makes sport exciting (Tricker & Cook, 1990). In a highly competitive environment, it is easy for athletes and support staff to get caught up in a "win at any cost" mentality. When ends justify means, risks of cheating may be emotionally denied or considered part of the excitement, a necessary evil, or even a demonstration of willingness to pay the price of success.

Sport professionals working with elite athletes will regularly be confronted with evidence of illegal or unethical practices designed to enhance performance (Ungerleider & Golding, 1992; Voy, 1991). An athlete quoted by Ungerleider and Golding (1992) reported anonymously:

> My belief is that if I had to take an estimate, about sixty-five percent of the top five, let's say top ten in the world in every event, are doing something illegal. That basically is the growth hormones in the ballistic events and blood doping for the distance events. I think all of the major distance runners that have run really incredible times are blood doping. I think middle distance runners are using a combination of blood doping and steroids. (quoted p. 119)

Director of the Olympic drug testing lab in Seoul, Dr. Park Jong Sei stated that "as many as 20 athletes at the games turned up positive, but were not disqualified" (quoted in Ungerleider & Golding, 1992, p. 119). If these claims are true, one must question the ethics of these sport physicians and administrators. Some coaches have been known to refuse to train athletes who wanted to compete clean (Voy, 1991). Sport professionals who counsel have obviously chosen to ignore these facts for a long time. With respect to performance enhancement, they may look away because they sincerely believe the athlete who does not cheat will not be able to compete.

Athletic leadership represents an extremely important, yet underestimated factor influencing unethical behavior. Coaches, trainers, and even athletic directors may fit into the following categories (McGuire, 1990):

1. Leaders who INSTRUCT drug usage,
2. Leaders who ALLOW drug usage,
3. Leaders who COVER drug usage,
4. Leaders who are the PROVIDERS of the "CAINES." (p. 10)

Sport professionals, physicians, or administrators who can rationalize instructing, allowing, covering, or providing drugs obviously value winning above societal codes designed to promote a healthy lifestyle or avoid exploitation.

Competition is Americana. Cheating has always been a part of sport competition. America's silent majority has always idealized fair competition. Elite athletes and university presidents are not the silent majority. What values do they endorse? Who are the beneficiaries of the practices that have unethical roots? Unethical practices profit all who are a part of the sport food chain. Coaches get victories. Athletes get—choose one of the following—

1. rich and famous
2. exploited
3. opportunity.

Academics and lay writers get publication credits, and maybe even money, for work publishers sell for profit. Pharmaceutical companies, sport gurus, and drug dealers get rich. Bankers have money to lend, the economy prospers, and lawyers, of course, get a cut of it all.

Clearly, other areas of unethical behavior are commonplace in sports. Manipulating academic eligibility requirements is unethical. Unethical behavior may also include overt child abuse, unethical weight-loss practices, or sexual barter (Rotella & Connelly, 1984). In the case of moral issues, boundary violations, illegal activity, or abusive relationships, the motivation for condoning such practices may also be justified by the belief that everyone is doing it.

Recognizing abuse can be difficult in the competitive environment. Personal criteria of abuse are culture laden and highly subjective. Legal criteria are clear. In the sport environment, abusive behavior is disguised, tolerated, and, at times, celebrated. The need for aggression in the world of sport can lead one to accept abusive coaching or parenting activities that are designed to increase aggressive behavior at game time. Abusive behavior may be publicly abhorred, but privately condoned when it leads to success.

Abusive behaviors may be justified in a sports family the same as they are justified in other abusive families. Fear of being rejected typically leads family members to see no evil, hear no evil, speak no evil. There may be an unspoken conspiracy of silence resulting from a fear of job loss or a glorification of the coach, athlete, or abusive sport professional. Many believe the risks from the questionable sport procedures are far less dangerous to the athlete than other likely alternatives. Sometimes, they are correct.

Fear of violating a sports family's value system is a powerful motivator, especially if you consider the intensity of the desire some athletes have to succeed. "*Sports Illustrated* reported the results of a survey which asked athletes whether they would take a drug that guaranteed them a gold medal but would kill them within a week after winning, and 50% responded affirmatively" (Ungerleider & Golding, 1992, p. 123).

All achievers have dues to pay, but when sport professionals step outside ethical codes and exercise their right to risk, they are on shaky ground. Without a well-developed value-based decision system to guide their counsel, they are skating on thin ice. Risk may entail experiencing censure by professional or employing organizations even if the ethical violation is not criminal in nature. Criminal penalties or civil suits may follow ethical breaches that violate statute law as well.

Ethical Standards

The National Athletic Trainers' Association completed a role-delineation validation study for the entry-level athletic trainers' certification examination in 1990. "One of the major functions of a certification program is the protection of the public from the practice of the incompetent professional" (National Athletic Trainers' Association [NATA], 1990, p. 4).

NATA considered six major domains as essential components for competent functioning at the entry level. These are (NATA, 1990)

1. Prevention
2. Recognition and Evaluation
3. Management/Treatment
4. Rehabilitation
5. Organization and Administration
6. Education and Counseling (p. 5)

That education and counseling skills are viewed as critically important competencies for entry-level certified athletic trainers is not at all surprising. The advising of athletes and coaches, as well as others interested in athletic endeavor, is clearly within the purview of the work of a trainer.

A sport professional's academic training may be adequate for counseling a cooperative individual who is seeking noncontroversial information. Situations such as those do not normally pose ethical or legal issues for the sport professional. The more emotionally charged issues, however, involving fear, insecurity, depression, anger, drugs, dependency, deceit, boundary violations, sexuality, and secrets, tend to be much more taxing ethically and emotionally for the trainer and the athlete.

Each of us confronts life situations every day that call for thought, opinion formation, decision making, and action (Simon et al., 1972). Sport professionals recognize that frequently they must make decisions regarding what might be the best course of action for the athlete (Rotella & Connelly, 1984). If one agrees with this position, it becomes imperative that the course selected be guided by ethics based not only in codes, but also in a workable system for clarifying values trainers and athletes cannot find in codes. All good people who have power over others, even just a little power, and even for a little while, need access to an ethic that can guide their use of that power (Thompson, 1983). Although ethical codes establish restrictions, restrictions imposed by responsible professions are more desirable than those imposed by external forces (Van Hoose & Kottler, 1988).

Some sport professionals are all too well aware of the limitations their academic training provides for the challenges they face in counseling athletes. Others express a willingness to counsel on virtually any topic. For these reasons it might be useful to review some of the ethical guidelines that have been imposed upon psychologists by The American Psychological Association. The ethical guidelines discussed in this chapter are drawn from a draft of the Revised Code of Ethical Principles of The American Psychological Association, 1991.

Six general principles state the aspirational norms that guide psychologists toward the highest ideals of psychology:

1. Competence
2. Integrity
3. Professional and Scientific Responsibility
4. Respect for People's Rights and Dignity
5. Concern for Others' Welfare
6. Social Responsibility

This code represents a dynamic set of ethical standards for work-related conduct that requires "a personal commitment to a lifelong effort to act ethically, to encourage ethical behavior by students, supervisees, employees, and colleagues as appropriate, and to consult with others as needed concerning ethical problems" (American Psychological Association [APA], 1991, p. 4).

Psychologists are expected to supplement, but not violate, the ethical code values and rules based on guidance drawn from personal values, culture, and experience. This ethic has implications for other sport professionals as well.

Counselor's Role

As a trainer counseling the injured athlete, you must identify as early as possible what service it is that you are expected to perform. Clarify for the athlete the limits of your competencies and identify any duality of roles. Let the athlete know. Are you acting as faculty member, coach, or owner? The role you are taking may limit your ability to protect the athlete's confidentiality. It may also conflict with his interests.

Boundary and role delineation aspects of the sport consultant's job are other issues inherent in the nature of the job itself. A sport consultant may spend a great deal of time with a team or with an individual athlete during conditioning, practice, travel, and competition. When you eat, sleep, sweat, mourn, and celebrate together, it is easy for boundaries, particularly in matters of a personal nature, to become blurred. The sport professional should be sensitive to the need to keep the athlete informed, at all times, of the nature of the relationship and of changes in the relationship that may occur as a result of changes in the trainer's responsibility. Changes in the nature of information that surfaces as result of the increasing willingness of the athlete to confide in the trainer requires trainers to be in tune with their value blind spots as well as guiding ethical codes.

Another issue of ethical significance when counseling athletes pertains to the dangers of developing an overly dependent relationship as opposed to encouraging independent behavior. Van Hoose and Kottler (1985) warned that failure to set and hold to time guidelines when counseling may reinforce dependent behavior on the part of clients and encourage them to renege on their responsibility for self-direction. The authors point out that fostering excessive dependency in response to your intervention would not only be destructive to the client, but could also be ethically questionable.

Contractual obligations pose ethical dilemmas for the sport consultant who provides ongoing personal counseling. Sport psychologists or trainers with a counseling degree should be aware of their contractual obligation to the client. A client may quit the counseling at any time for any reason; however, a psychologist or sports professional who terminates a counseling relationship without sufficient notice may be liable for malpractice if the client sustains damages of a type recognized by law. In other words, when functioning in the role of a counselor, trainers might be held legally accountable if they depart from the standard of care that a jury might consider appropriate for that particular relationship. Obviously, individuals who misrepresent themselves as psychologists are subject to sanction by the state for such misconduct. All professionals, in and outside of sport, counsel in a variety of ways. Coaches frequently consider helping to mold young people's values as the most important and rewarding part of their job. Certainly, they do not consider themselves as providers of psychotherapy (Zeigler, 1987).

Consider the case of the athlete who may deliberately injure himself as a face-saving way to avoid competitive stress (Kane, 1984). NATA would emphasize the importance of recognizing the problem and referring such an athlete to an appropriate professional therapist. When the sports professional uses referral and informal counseling techniques, athletes may leave competition or compete at a reduced level and still maintain their dignity. This type of intervention is not only ethically appropriate, but is also consistent with NATA recommendations for both competent functioning in the counseling as well as injury prevention domains. You should be sure to complete the transfer process with follow-up, if you believe there is danger to an athlete or another person.

Mentors and counselors need to be mindful that they provide services that are within the boundaries of their own competence. Trainers, coaches, and other sport professionals who counsel athletes do help them as many of us can attest. You can be even more helpful when counseling ethically. The serious personal or interpersonal problems that athletes experience can result in anxiety, depression, acting out, or abuse of substances. Trainers will be more effective when they recognize the minimal level of training required of a licensed psychologist who counsels for a living.

A psychologist licensed to provide diagnostic and therapeutic services typically has completed a 4-year undergraduate degree in psychology or a related field. An additional 3 to 4 years of advanced study in behavioral science, abnormal behavior, and tools of intervention lead to the required doctoral degree. A requirement of 2 years of supervised practice of these skills under the supervision of a licensed psychologist is the minimum required to take the licensing exam in most states. Once licensed, the psychologist may begin independent practice.

Sport professionals who find themselves questioning their competency to deal with serious psychological situations should be applauded. Being scrupulous may be the best liability insurance. Trainers who feel uneasy should review their value decision-making procedures. Use your option to refer liberally. Inform the client of the seriousness of the matter and remind her or him that a high level of training is ordinarily required to provide the athlete minimal assurance of access to competent help with this type of problem. Tell the athlete that psychologists, psychiatrists, and other therapists who are more qualified are readily available. To direct the athlete to such services is consistent with NATA and APA guidelines.

Knowledge of referral procedures and community resources is specifically referenced as a minimum competency for Certified Athletic Trainers by NATA. In fact, TASK 3 under NATA's Education and Counseling Domain specifically addresses this issue.

TASK 3: Directs the athlete to professionals in order to receive consultation for social and/or personal problems by the establishment of referral procedures. NATA further delineates knowledge required to accomplish TASK 3 as the following:

1. Knowledge of situations requiring consultation with professionals regarding the athletes' social and/or personal problems.
2. Knowledge of available professionals for consultation regarding the athletes' social and personal problems.
3. Knowledge of required referral procedures for consultation with professionals for the athletes' social and/or personal problems.

NATA's panel of experts identified specific skills necessary in order to implement the TASK 3 KNOWLEDGES as

1. Skill in recognizing an athlete's need for professional consultation for social and/or personal problems.
2. Skill in communicating to the athlete the purpose or need for professional consultation for social and/or personal problems.
3. Skill in establishing referral procedures regarding social and/or personal problems.
4. Skill in interacting with allied health care professionals.
5. Skill in assisting in intervention as directed by the appropriate allied health care professionals. (NATA, 1990, p. 62)

Trainers who engage in counseling athletes with social and/or personal problems would be considered incompetent by the standards of NATA were they to exceed the boundaries of their competence to counsel.

This directive from NATA can be a strong tool when directing athletes to professionals more appropriately suited to deal with such problems. The ethic would appear identical, then, both for the psychologist to counsel and deliver psychological services within his or her level of competence and also the trainer as directed by NATA. There is no other mention in the entire domain of counseling and education competencies for trainers that deals with ongoing personal counseling relationships.

Trainers are expected to have knowledge in the area of psychological readiness for the return to activity and should have skill in evaluating the athlete's present physical and psychological status as it pertains to sports participation. The trainer is also expected to have knowledge of implications of unhealthy personal situations (e.g., substance abuse, eating disorders, victims of assault, abuse, etc.). Lastly, the trainer is expected to have skill in recognizing the athlete's need for information regarding personal and/or community health topics. Trainers should also be skilled with instructional methods as well as information dissemination procedures regarding personal and/or community health topics (NATA, 1990). Clearly, the intent of the counseling mission of the Certified Athletic Trainer is directed toward education, recognition, and referral of athletes for appropriate services in the area of personal, social or mental health problems.

Conflicting Interests

Sport consultants who function as trainers may risk the appearance of conflict of interest. This appearance can be problematic, imposing unnecessary hardship on the athlete and the counselor. The proposed APA Ethical Standard 1.21 offers sound guidance:

> When a psychologist agrees to provide services to a person or entity at the request of a third party, the psychologist clarifies to the extent feasible, at the outset of the service, the nature of the relationship with each party. This clarification includes the role of the psychologist (such as therapist, organizational consultant, diagnostician, or expert witness) and the probable uses of the services provided or the information obtained.
>
> If there is a foreseeable risk of the psychologist's being called upon to perform conflicting roles because of the involvement of a third party, the psychologist clarifies the nature and direction of his or her responsibilities, keeps all parties appropriately informed as matters develop, and resolves the situation in accordance with this Ethics Code. (APA, 1991, p. 11)

By following these ethical guidelines, it is clear who the trainer is actually working for. Trainers have an obligation to their employers, but they also have a responsibility to the athletes whom they counsel. In performance-enhancement settings, it is possible to maintain a very positive relationship with both management and athlete.

Make it clear, early on, that what the athletes tell you in confidence will stay in confidence unless it is a matter of life and death to them or someone else. For psychologists, working in a counseling role, this is a standard requirement.

There are times, however, where this requirement is not the rule, such as in the case of military psychologists or certain organizational or forensic work. The military psychologist must inform his clients of his duty to follow the chain of command. Information is not confidential.

Most employers understand it would be difficult for one to gain an athlete's trust without such an understanding and therefore readily consent to it. When things are going well, there will be few problems. In bad times, when injuries take their toll and pressure to win builds, coaches, owners, or parents, for that matter, may lose sight of the ethical issues involved. In the heat of competition, a coach might ask you, "What's the matter with Brown? How come he's not putting out in practice?" At this point, with a solid understanding in place from the beginning, the trainer can remind whoever asks that Brown is working on it. If pressed for more detail, consider the value decision-making system before disclosing any more information. If disclosure gets Brown eliminated from the opportunity to compete, the violation of Brown's privilege of confidentiality could cause problems for you.

Begin every new personal counseling relationship by reviewing the limits to which information discussed can ethically be kept confidential. It is critically important that you not mislead yourself or the athlete. A psychotherapist's records may be subpoenaed and admitted into evidence in some jurisdictions even where the psychologist-patient privilege is recognized. Most, if not all jurisdictions recognize, at a minimum, the priest-penitent and psychologist-patient relation as confidentially protected.

Too Much, Too Soon

Communication is good. Confession may be good for the soul, and catharsis can alleviate energy-sapping stress, but too much self-disclosure, too soon, can be harmful (Derlega & Chaikin, 1975) Many times, clients will begin talking about stressful situations. Before long, they may blurt out a series of thoughts and feelings that have been on their mind for some time. Beware of clients who seem to say too much, too soon, particularly if they are new clients. Listen attentively, but be mindful of the fact that sometimes a client who tells too much too soon may feel violated later.

Self-reliant, emotionally stable, independent people with a streak of cynicism can become overwhelmed, stressed out, and depressed like anybody else. Nine times out of ten, just talking will be good medicine. Players will appreciate your willingness to listen, and may call on you from time to time as they feel the need.

Occasionally, an athlete who is obviously agitated and under pressure will come to a trainer. If the player is highly emotional or anxious, reassure him or her of your availability to help or to assist in finding someone else who can help. The athlete does not need to say everything in one meeting. A trainer sometimes needs to put the brakes on self-disclosure. Be sure the athletes are making an informed decision when they attempt to tell all. You have a duty to inform them if their confidential revelations are not legally exempt from discovery by the legal system in the jurisdiction in which you work.

Athletes raised with an aggressive, competitive, racist, or "macho" mentality may feel compromised if they are encouraged to reveal too much of themselves in a moment of weakness. Later, they may feel uncomfortable. Feeling that they have been robbed of their dignity or taken advantage of in their moment of weakness, they may even resent the counselor. This reaction is not typical, but it does occur. With awareness, catharsis can be kept helpful. A confident manner will project a reassuring sense of optimism that a solution will be found. By the counselor's being there to help, a referral, if needed, can be easily made.

It is a counselor's responsibility to have a clearly established protocol when counseling. With internal consistency between personal morality, ethical principles, and legal responsibilities, making ethically and legally correct decisions will be more comfortable.

Potential Traps

What do you do in a situation where the athlete says, "I have to tell you something, but you must promise not to tell"? You may have many options here. I would recommend that you tell the athlete, "It is my role to listen. I will be happy to listen to what you have to say, if you trust me to use what you tell me in your best interests." Statements such as this allow the athlete to make the decision on the level of risk and relieve trainers of the burden of getting involved in a bargain they may not be able to keep.

By telling the client, "I'd like you to tell me anything you trust me to use in your best interest," you are offering the opportunity to be of professional assistance without having your hands tied. This approach will be adequate with youngsters, but adults may press for higher levels of secrecy. At that point you must explain the limits of their privilege of confidentiality. You must also explain at that point any role conflicts such a contract may involve.

Clients will almost always continue speaking. If athletes balk and are unwilling to tell their secret under that contract, you should offer assurance that if they change their mind, you will be happy to listen. At this point, you may also offer athletes the option of speaking to someone else regarding the matter. You could indicate to the client that there are many people trained and willing to help—personal physicians, clergy, mental health professionals, and even anonymous crisis call-in services. In this way, you are not leaving the athlete without the option of help; you are providing the athlete an opportunity to make an informed choice among a variety of options.

Triangles

Triangles can be particularly challenging to many helping professionals. In such a situation a client will share some information about a second party. You are put in a position of trying to help someone solve a problem involving someone else without permission to involve that third party. Here again, the best course of action is to be a reflective listener. Avoid the temptation to rescue the athlete from the problem. Do nothing, assuming, that is, that the athlete is not psychotic, suicidal, or homicidal.

Triangle situations ask you to be accountable for solving a problem without the power or authority to do so. This is a losing proposition. Remember, it is not your job as a counselor to solve problems. You are a facilitator who assists athletes to find their own solution. An exception to the facilitator role occurs when you are asked for help by someone who is clearly in danger and who lacks access to a power base adequate to cope with the danger. Children and teenagers who are abused are cases in point. Adult victims of crime also fit this category.

Victims of abuse require immediate action by a counselor of any type. You are to report the abuse to an investigative agent. You are not to investigate yourself. The cornerstone of helping victims of abuse is to stop the abuse. Your ethical and legal duty to report abuse offers the best chance to halt abuse.

Misuse of Influence

Trainers who coach and counsel on personal matters should also be aware of Ethics Standard 1.15. Misuse of Psychologists' Influence: "Because psychologists' scientific and professional judgments and actions may affect the lives of others, they are alert to and guard against personal, financial, social, organizational, or political factors that might lead to misuse of their influence" (APA, 1991, p. 9). This standard might apply to any competitive environment. In highly competitive situations, the perception of value to the cause is of paramount significance. The depth-chart composition is a direct function of such perceptions. Emotional factors influence such perceptions. To use one's influence, gained through personal counseling, to discourage an athlete from questioning access to playing time could be ethically questionable. The same could be said of those who would influence a player to return to competition prematurely following injury.

Cultural Values and Ethical Counseling

Racial bias can prove ethically challenging for those who are counseling athletes. Widespread cultural stereotyping by media, coaches, fans, and athletes has led to a general acceptance of racial stacking in many sports ("Shake," 1991). Trainers who counsel need to be prepared to confront ethical values that involve discrimination. Minorities are advancing to management positions, albeit slowly. Allegations of discrimination will reemerge; whites attempting to gain a larger market share will reenter sports currently dominated by minorities and will complain of prejudice.

Opportunities for value conflicts will increase. Racism sells. Media will continue to pay attention to stories with racial overtones. Racism will continue to be a significant issue with implications for team harmony as the world of sport continues its journey toward the ethical ideal of color-blind sports with equal opportunity for all. The opportunity "haves" and opportunity "have-nots" will continue to struggle. The struggle may be confounded with minorities' attempts to solidify racial identity and majority attempts to get a piece of that ever-growing financial pie they have ignored for the past 20 years. Turf battles to protect lucrative sport colonies will create subtle, as well as not so subtle, pressures for all whose counsel has an impact on motivation, playing time, and depth-chart status.

Racial, or for that matter any personal, values that would conflict with your ability to provide unbiased consultation are considered reasons to refer the client to someone else. If referral is not practical, make the client aware of values you hold that may be influential in subconsciously slanting your counsel.

Gender identity issues have ethical implications for personal counseling. Homophobia is a factor that may lead to ethical conflicts when sexual preference differs for counselor and client. Homophobic beliefs create anxieties that subconsciously or consciously guide statements, as well as nonverbal communication. Sexual nepotism, or favoring individuals of one's sexual preference, is increasingly discussed as a problem among psychologists who counsel and offer services to female sport teams. The ethical warning to avoid misuse of power when counseling holds true for homosexual as well as heterosexual coaches, trainers, and sport psychologists.

Sexual harassment, discrimination, and lack of respect for the values and human differences among those you counsel is clearly unethical and to be avoided. Exploitative relationships are unethical. Sexual relations between counselor and client are considered exploitative, unethical, and are the leading reason for malpractice awards against professional counselors.

Documentation of Your Work

Ethical and legal considerations require that you keep records and document services performed. This is particularly important in the private sector, although institutional and organizational policies may be similar. If policy doesn't require such record-keeping, prudence does.

When dealing with sensitive personal information, it is critical to have minimum entries in your confidential file of personal meetings. The notes do not need to be exhaustive, but should include a minimum of a date, who was present, problem addressed, recommendations made, estimates of progress, and your plans for the future. By keeping notes, you will be able to document positions that you have taken should you be ordered to appear in court. You need not keep records for each conversation about every ankle that you tape, but in cases where you develop an ongoing confidential relationship, it is important to keep records. This is particularly true in cases where you see athletes in crises dealing with significant areas of abuse or emotional disturbance, such as depression or suicidal ideation.

It is also quite important to document things that were said and done during rehabilitation of sport injuries. Such documentation may help protect you from litigation. When you are sued, deposed, or brought into court as an expert witness, you will present a much more professional impression if you can cite documents to support your statements. By keeping appropriate records you will be sending a message to the athletes as well. They will know that you have documentation. If they should grow angry with you at some point in the future, they might be more willing to be reasonable knowing that you have taken notes. Malpractice situations are not pleasant for anyone. When professionals are sued for malpractice, it is much easier to defend their conduct if they have records. Malpractice and lawsuits may seem to be a long way from the training table, but serious injuries and death of athletes do result in lawsuits. Lawsuits are sometimes brought in revenge for real or imagined slights or offenses. Suing coaches, high schools, universities, and even youth sport associations has become more widespread (Ball, Robinson, & Narol, 1991).

Consider the case of Len Bias, an outstanding collegiate basketball player. According to press releases, a problem with cocaine killed him. Alleging that the university was in some way responsible for his death, the Bias family went on to sue his university. In such a case, a sport psychologist or athletic trainer who counseled Bias might conceivably be called into court and find it necessary to defend against allegations of professional negligence. The process is extremely draining. You, your family, and, in some cases, the entire team suffer. Having documentation for what you said and why you said it can lessen the stress you personally will experience in such a case and, most important, may provide your best defense.

I don't want to sound too negative, but it is important to realize that the amicable relationship that you enjoy with the athletes with whom you are working will not survive the adversity intrinsic to a lawsuit for damages. The late Pappy Gault, Olympic boxing coach, had a favorite saying in matters such as this: "Money makes people funny." The saying is not particularly scholarly, but it is to the point. The lawyers you will face in a courtroom when you are a defendant are your adversaries. The family of the dead or injured players will not be friendly. You may face witnesses in a courtroom, you may not even know and may never see again. They will not like you. The attorneys will try to discredit you and to get money for their client. Having notes to back up your testimony will support your professionalism and, although not a guarantee, will go a long way toward making your day in court a more comfortable one. APA Standard 1.23 may be useful at this point:

Documentation of Professional and Scientific Work

a) Psychologists appropriately document their professional and scientific work in order to facilitate provision of services later by the psychologist or other professionals, to ensure accountability, and to meet other requirements of institutions or the law.

b) When psychologists know that records of their services are likely to be used in legal proceedings involving recipients of or participants in their work, they create and maintain such documentation consistent with the standards generally applied in such proceedings. (APA, 1991, p. 11)

When counseling or referring, be sure to note the problem or issue, your estimate of the client's mental state at time of consultation—lucid, clear versus desperate, despondent. Note your recommendation or action, especially if referral was made. The notes do not have to be extensive. They need only include enough information so that another professional might evaluate the scope of the problem and the appropriateness of your recommendations. This may be enough to convince an adversarial party's attorney and expert that there is no likelihood of deviation from the standard of care.

It is important to recognize that the burden of a plaintiff's proof is not always easy. A tort is a civil wrong. The requirements of proof for a plaintiff in tort are four in number. The first is duty. This means that there must have been a duty of the defendant to the plaintiff, that duty arising from the particular relationship that they had, for instance, a doctor-patient relationship. Second, there must have been a breach of that duty by either an overt act or the failure to act by the person who owes the duty. Third, there must be damages proven that are recognized by law. Last, there must be proof that the act or non-act must have resulted proximately in the damages accrued (Jay Williams, M.D., J.D., personal communication, April, 1992).

Summary

Ethical guidelines of the American Psychological Association and virtually all human relations ethics codes affirm the dignity of the client. Virtually all codes ban discrimination, sexual harassment, or other types of harassment, and encourage respect for the rights and diverse values and opinions of the people served. Beyond ethics, it is helpful to realize that we are privileged that our clients choose to share information with us. The act of sharing particularly sensitive personal information involves considerable risk on the part of the athlete. It is hoped that by increasing your awareness of values, your work with athletes will be more rewarding to them as well as to yourself.

References

American Psychological Association. (October 3, 1991). *Ethical principles revision draft*. Washington, DC: Author.

Ball, R. T., Robinson, R., & Narol, M. S. (1991). *Legal aspects* [Audio Recording No. 5A, B]. Orlando, FL: National Youth Sports Coaches Association.

Derlega, V., & Chaikin, A. (1975). *Sharing intimacy*. Englewood Cliffs, NJ: Prentice-Hall.

Kane, B. (1984). Trainer counseling to avoid three face-saving maneuvers. *Athletic Training, 19*(3), 171–174.

McGuire, R. (1990). History and evolution of drugs in sport. In R. Tricker & D. L. Cook (Eds.), *Athletes at risk: Drugs and sport* (p. 10). Dubuque, IA: Wm. C. Brown.

National Athletic Trainers' Association. (1990). *Role delineation validation study for the entry-level athletic trainers' certification examination*. NATA Board of Certification.

Raths, L., Merrill, H., & Simon, S. (1966). *Values and teaching*. Columbus, OH: Charles E. Merrill.

Rotella, R. J., & Connelly, D. (1984). Individual ethics in the application of cognitive sport psychology. In W. F. Straub & J. M. Williams (Eds.), *Cognitive sport psychology* (pp. 102–112). Lansing, NY: Sport Science Associates.

Shake racial stereotypes. (1991, December 19). *USA Today*, p. 12A.

Simon, S. B., Howe, L. W., & Kirschenbaum, H. (1974). *Value clarification*. New York: Hart.

Thompson, A. (1983). *Ethical concerns in psychotherapy and their legal ramifications*. Lanham, MD: University Press of America.

Tricker, R., & Cook, D. L. (Eds.). (1990). *Athletes at risk: Drugs and sport*. Dubuque, IA: Wm. C. Brown.

Ungerleider, S., & Golding, J. M. (1992). *Beyond strength*. Dubuque, IA: Wm. C. Brown.

Van Hoose, W. H., & Kottler, J. A. (1985). *Ethical and legal issues in counseling and psychotherapy* (2nd ed.). San Francisco: Jossey-Bass.

Voy, R. (1991). *Drugs, sport, and politics*. Champaign, IL: Leisure Press.

Zeigler, E. F. (1987). Rationale and suggested dimensions for a code of ethics for sport psychologists. *The Sport Psychologist, 1*, 138–150.

4

Psychological and Emotional Response to Athletic Injury: Measurement Issues

Lynne Evans
University of Wales Institute, Cardiff

Lew Hardy
University of Wales, Bangor

Theory development and theory testing are fundamental to sound research in any discipline or subdiscipline, including applied sport psychology. The purpose of this chapter is to discuss these elements as they pertain to the psychology of injury response from measurement as well as practical perspectives. Of particular interest here are the grief models and stress-based cognitive appraisal models typically employed in efforts to clarify cognitive and affective responses to sport injury. This chapter is divided into four sections. The first section reviews some of the more current and important research findings relative to psychological response to injury, with emphasis upon measurement considerations. The second section provides a discussion of grief and cognitive appraisal models, and in the third section an attempt is made to integrate both of these into a unitary model of injury response. The fourth and final section of this chapter presents implications and conclusions intended to facilitate future research efforts as well as assist those who work directly with injured athletes.

Introduction

The importance of theory development and theory testing has been widely acknowledged within applied sport psychology research in general (Brawley, 1993, Hardy, Jones, & Gould, 1996; Singer, Murphey, & Tennant, 1993) and, in particular, in research dealing with the psychological response to injury (Brewer, 1994; Evans & Hardy, 1995). Practitioners concerned about the relationship between theory and practice in the application of sport psychology to sport performance might find Lewin's (1951) comments reassuring:

> Many psychologists working today in an applied field are keenly aware of the need for close cooperation between theoretical and applied psychology. This can be accomplished . . . if the applied psychologist realizes that there is nothing so practical as a good theory. (p. 169)

Hardy et al. (1996) illustrate the importance of theory in applied sport psychology in their classification of characteristics of good research. They do this in the context of the performance-enhancement literature, and studies that they consider have had a major impact on the field. They identify three characteristics: (a) *asking important questions*—significant studies ask high-impact questions from a theoretical/practical perspective; (b) *systematic lines of research*—learning is enhanced more by systematic lines of research answering important questions than by isolated studies; and (c) *theoretically based research*—significant studies "strive to go beyond specific findings and data patterns to develop explanations that help us better understand" a major goal being theory development, be this testing a specific theory or developing a new one (p. 274).

Brawley (1993) also identifies a number of characteristics of good theories within the context of intervention research. According to Brawley, good theories (a) focus on processes susceptible to social change, (b) adequately describe the relationship between key sets of variables so that they can be targets of change, (c) have an associated set of assessments of the theoretical variables so that change can accurately be measured, (d) have a substantive research base that indicates the theory's validity, (e) offer concepts that can be translated into operational manipulations thought to affect cognitive and/or behavioral change, and (f) clarify why an intervention failed to produce change. Brawley concludes, however, that "for all the practicality offered by good theories, there continues to be an apparent resistance to adopting theory to practice (and the reciprocal) despite the continued encouragement of various well known psychologists" (p. 100).

Current Research:
Measurement and Applied Issues

In an effort to design scientifically rigorous and meaningful research, a number of conceptual and practical issues must be addressed. On a conceptual level these issues are focused upon the why, how, and when of measurement, whereas related practical considerations relate to the implementation of the research design or its procedural concerns. Practical issues such as gaining access to homogenous populations of injured performers present enormous challenges to researchers.

Moderating variables such as injury severity, level of participation, and social support and mediating variables such as coping strategies must be identified and accounted for. Researchers are also obliged to deal with issues related to validity and reliability in an area still acknowledged to be in its infancy (Smith, 1996).

However, one of the most substantive concerns for those who conduct research into psychological response to sport injury is the development and testing of theoretical models. A review of some of the most recent research in sport injury research illustrates this point.

Empirical findings suggest that compared to their noninjured counterparts, injured athletes experience heightened levels of tension (Chan & Grossman, 1988; Pearson & Jones, 1992; Smith, Scott, O'Fallon & Young, 1990), anger (Gordon & Lindgren, 1990; McDonald & Hardy, 1990; Pearson & Jones, 1992; Smith et al., 1990; Smith et al., 1993), depression (Chan & Grossman, 1988; Gordon & Lindgren, 1990; Leddy, Lambert & Ogles, 1994; McDonald & Hardy, 1990; Pearson & Jones, 1992; Smith et al., 1990), confusion (Chan & Grossman, 1988; McDonald & Hardy, 1990; Pearson & Jones, 1992; Smith et al., 1990), fatigue (Pearson & Jones, 1992; Smith et al., 1990), and lower levels of vigor (Pearson & Jones, 1992; Smith et al., 1990), and self-esteem (Chan & Grossman, 1988; Leddy et al., 1994). Comparisons of athletes pre- and postinjury have demonstrated increased levels of depression (Leddy et al., 1994; Smith et al., 1993), anger (Smith et al., 1993), and state anxiety (Leddy et al., 1994), and decreased vigor (Smith et al., 1993). Findings with regard to self-esteem pre- to postinjury are equivocal (Leddy et al., 1994; McGowan, Pierce, & Eastman, 1994; Smith et al., 1993).

Although most of these findings appear to be relatively consistent, many of the studies from which they derive employed the Profile of Mood States (POMS) as the primary measurement tool. Other instruments that measure anxiety, self-esteem, and depression have also been frequently used. However, a central issue in measurement is validity, and although the variables assessed by the POMS may in part be applicable to the population of injured performers, the POMS was not developed in conjunction with, or for specific application for, any psychological model of injury. Of concern is not what POMS *does* measure (and the way in which it measures it), but what it *does not* measure. Do the findings from studies that have incorporated the POMS adequately represent the psychological and emotional responses that result from injury? Moreover, are the most appropriate psychological variables related to athletic injury being measured? If not, then conclusions from many of the above-cited studies may be inappropriate. They may be misleading the well-intentioned practitioners who work with injured performers.

A key feature of emotions and psychological responses is their transient nature. The relevance of this to athletic injury research has been acknowledged (Evans & Hardy, 1995; McDonald & Hardy, 1990; Quackenbush & Crossman, 1994; Smith et al., 1990), however, to a limited extent. Generally, the temporal pattern of psychological responses has proceeded from a negative to positive affect over time (McDonald & Hardy, 1990; McGowan et al., 1994; Smith et al., 1990; Smith et al., 1993; Uemukai, 1993). Some researchers have even suggested that a number of injured athletes' mood states may be elevated simultaneously (Brewer, Linder, & Phelps, 1995; Smith et al., 1990). There has been less support for oscillation between highs and lows during the rehabilitation period (Pearson & Jones, 1992). However, these findings must be viewed in terms of each study's research design. To date, the time intervals used in the studies have ranged from twice weekly (McDonald & Hardy, 1990) to twice monthly (Smith et al., 1990). Equally variable has been the proximity of the first data-collection point relative to injury occurrence. The rigor with which researchers are able to explore the temporal pattern of psychological responses to injury is confounded by factors such as access to homogenous samples. In cross-sectional designs, stratified sampling of the various phases of the injury period, although essential, is not easy to achieve. Allowing for such difficulties, the continued variability in the procedures for sampling the injury period is far from satisfactory. Sampling of distinct time phases within the injury period is crucial in exploring the way athletes' psychological and emotional responses change over time. If injury severity could be accounted for, resultant insights might be further enhanced. Brewer et al. (1995) conducted one of the few studies where no temporal pattern was found to exist. This finding, they suggested, may be due to athletes in this study being more seriously injured than were athletes in other studies where temporal patterns have been observed. However, for inclusion in this cross-sectional study athletes were required to be injured for a minimum of one day, with a further one day's preclusion from sports participation up to a maximum of 120 days. The argument for the absence of a temporal pattern from a sample that includes athletes with an injury duration of 2 days and utilizes one data collection is unsustainable. However, it does raise the question of sample characteristics with regard to injury severity in emotional response research, generally, and in cross-sectional research, specifically. Arguably, within psychological response research there needs to be a minimum requirement of injury severity, for example, 2 to 3 weeks. Cross-sectional research has much to offer. However, unless the sampling procedure is stratified to account for different points in time across individuals (relative to onset and duration of injury), it has limited capacity to infer the presence, or absence, of a temporal pattern.

A number of models have been proposed within the injury literature as a means of explaining athletes' psychological responses to injury. The most frequently cited of these include the grief model and stress-based cognitive appraisal model. Other recently proposed models include Heil's (1993) injury recovery model, and Rose and Jevne's (1993) risks model. The current chapter will restrict its focus to grief models and cognitive appraisal models, exclusively addressed below.

Recently, a noticeable trend among researchers has been to dismiss grief models that attempt to clarify the emotional responses to sport injury in favor of cognitive appraisal-based models. The alleged inadequacy of grief models has been based on (a) the inappropriateness of the populations from which they are derived—Kübler-Ross's (1969) stage model was derived from her work with terminally ill patients (Brewer, 1994; Rose & Jevne, 1993; Smith et al., 1990); (b) their inability to account for individual differences in injury response (Brewer, 1994; Smith et al., 1990); (c) the absence of denial as a consistent feature of emotional response to injury research (Quackenbush & Crossman, 1994, Smith et al., 1990); and (d) the rigidity with which athletes would have to sequentially experience each stage (Brewer et al., 1994). (The validity of these criticisms will be discussed in the next section.)

Cognitive appraisal models (which largely emanate from the stress and coping literature) have evolved from the injury prediction model proposed by Anderson and Williams (1988). The basis of these models is that one's interpretation (appraisal) of an injury will determine the psychological response (Weiss & Troxel, 1986). Much of the support for cognitive appraisal models is predicated on their ability to account for individual differences in psychological responses to injury. This is due mainly to the proposed interaction between personal and situational factors, and the subsequent appraisal of these factors. Although within the injury literature there has been a limited attempt to test the validity of cognitive appraisal models (Brewer et al., 1995; Daly, Brewer, Van

Raalte, Petitpas, & Sklar, 1995), there is support for the relationship between emotional response to injury and a number of situational variables. These include injury severity (Leddy et al., 1994; Smith et al., 1990; Smith et al., 1993), injury duration (McDonald & Hardy, 1990; Smith et al., 1990; Uemukai, 1993), injury history (Johnson, 1996), social support for rehabilitation (Brewer et al., 1995), physician-rated current injury status, and impairment of sports performance (Brewer et al., 1995). Personal factors found to be associated with athletes' emotional responses include age (Brewer et al., 1995) and self-esteem (Chan & Grossman, 1988; Leddy et al., 1994). Nonetheless, genuine person-by-situation interactions have rarely been assessed.

The Conceptual Basis of Models of Grief and Cognitive Appraisal

Grief

Although research into the grief response was first conducted in the 1920s, work in this area is ongoing, the focus of which is its application to a variety of different types of perceived loss. Examples of these are bereavement, job loss, marital separation, loss of a pet, loss of a limb, and injury. Within the clinical psychology literature, grief is defined as "an intense emotional suffering set off by a loss" (Simos, 1977, p. 337). The significance of the loss is determined by the individual's value system. According to Archer and Rhodes (1987), grief theory, as currently considered, views grief as an active process that changes over time through different stages. They also maintain that grief entails a number of components, some of which are episodic whereas others constitute a pattern of background stress responses (p. 212). Although there is some debate among authorities as to how much of the grief response is active or adaptive for those who experience it, most attention has focused on its stages. Stage theorists propose that certain features of grief are sufficiently uniform to permit a judgment that healing is taking place. These theorists suggest that between three and six stages most adequately account for the grief response but that it is not true that each grieving person "goes through every stage, in this exact sequence, at some predictable pace" (Kübler-Ross, 1975, p. 10).

On the other hand, critics of the stage approach contend that the existence of individual differences in grief experiences detracts from the usefulness of grief models (Bugen, 1977; Rosenblatt, 1988). They further suggest that attempts to systematically test the existence of the proposed stages have been inadequately investigated. Moreover, the critics argue that support for stage models has largely resulted from limited qualitative research approaches (Archer & Rhodes,

1993; Rosenblatt, 1988; Wortman & Silver, 1989). Such criticisms also undermine the application of grief models to the broader area of psychological response to injury. However, grief models per se have not been categorically rejected by their critics. In fact, even those who are critical of stage approaches have been supportive of so-called components of grief. They do, none the less, take to task the notion of prescribed sequential arrangement of these components. These episodic experiences comprise features such as (a) preoccupation, pining, and searching; (b) anger and guilt; (c) feelings of internal loss of self; (d) identification phenomena; and (e) mitigating defenses. General background components constitute (a) emotional stress response, (b) inhibition of other activities, and (c) feelings of dejection and despair (Archer & Rhodes, 1993). Psychological responses to grief generally include phases of shock and disbelief, despondency and depression, and recovery or adaptation (Averill, 1968). Shock and disbelief represent an initial reaction, commonly reported to be followed by a phase of despondency and depression. In this context depression is considered to represent a number of psychological response variables that include despair, apathy, irritability, isolation, withdrawal, and in some instances, hostility, anger, denial, anxiety, and guilt. Other characteristics include a feeling of loss of self, searching for meaning, inability to concentrate, and physiological symptoms such as fatigue, insomnia, and hyperactivity. Extinction of established, highly motivated and goal- directed behavior is thought to underlie these responses. There is also considerable support for moderating and mediating variables in the grief process, including personality variables (e.g., age, sex, coping capacity), the nature of the loss, social isolation (following the loss), historical antecedents (previous experience of loss), and the relationship with the lost object / person (Archer & Rhodes, 1993; Ben-Sira, 1983; Engel, 1964; Parkes, 1986; Worden, 1991).

A number of similarities in the response characteristics described above and those described within the injury literature are apparent. Also, grief models in an injury context are supported by Kübler-Ross's (1975) suggestion that grief can " . . . if used in a flexible, insight-producing way, be a valuable tool in understanding why a patient may be behaving as he does" (p. 10). This is not to ignore the criticisms aimed at the idea of stages of grief, but rather to urge additional study of its role.

Cognitive Appraisal

The roots of cognitive appraisal models are to found in various theories that deal with stress, coping, and emotional responsivity. Stress is best understood as a relationship between the person and the environment, appraised as taxing or exceeding resources (Folkman, Lazarus, Dunkel-Schetter, DeLongis, &

Gruen, 1986). Cognitive appraisal plays a central role in many stress models in that it is viewed as a process through which a particular situation is evaluated as stressful and, if so, to what extent.

Coping is defined as the person's ever-changing efforts to manage circumstances that are appraised as stressful (Lazarus & Folkman, 1984). This process is termed one of transaction because it proposes a bidirectional transaction between the person and environment. In other words, coping is thought to vary within individuals, depending on the circumstances, and in turn, circumstances depending upon individual differences. Three major categories of coping have been proposed: problem-focused coping, emotion-focused coping, and avoidance (Cox & Ferguson, 1991). Cognitive appraisal or an individual's subjective interpretation of a situation takes two forms, primary appraisal and secondary appraisal (Lazarus & Folkman, 1984). Primary appraisal involves an assessment of what is at stake; secondary appraisal involves an assessment of the coping options available. Appraisal in turn determines emotional response, which serves a number of functions: (a) The quality and intensity of the response indicate the importance of ongoing relationship between the person and environment; (b) the response tells us what is important in a given situation; (c) the response provides insight into a person's beliefs about "self and world"; and (d) the response reveals how a person has appraised a situation with respect to its significance for well-being (Lazarus, 1991, p. 22). Emotion in this context is a reaction to meaning.

Although the essence of appraisal models is change, all too often appraisal and coping have been treated as static and unchanging (Aldwin, 1994). Clearly, the main way of assessing change and the factors that contribute to it is to assess and compare the same person's response repeatedly. Such comparisons, made at different times or under different conditions, represent an *intraindividual approach,* in contrast to an *interindividual* approach involving comparisons of one person with another person or persons. Unfortunately, interindividual comparisons fail in essence to answer questions about the interactions between coping and emotions (Aldwin, 1994). Intraindividual research involving the application of time-phased assessment points across individuals would enable interindividual comparisons over time to form the basis for developing normative adaptational response patterns. Such longitudinal research would also provide far more powerful explanations of the influence of mediating variables that are not adequately addressed by correlational studies (Lazarus & Folkman, 1984). Thus, intraindividual designs are essential for the study of transaction, process, and adaptation.

Cognitive appraisal models provide a valuable framework for understanding the process athletes may experience in response to injury. They also emphasize the importance of the appraisal of the injury, as opposed to the injury per se, in determining an athlete's psychological responses. Appraisal largely accounts for individual differences in response characteristics and provides a basis for understanding why athletes may be experiencing certain emotions and thus behave in certain ways. Models of cognitive appraisal do not preclude the application of models of grief to injury.

A Rationale for Incorporating Grief and Cognitive Appraisal Into a Model of Injury Response

Having provided an overview of models of cognitive appraisal and grief, it is our intention now to propose a model of injury response that includes both models. Brawley's (1993) discussion on the practicality of social psychology provides a useful rationale. According to Brawley, "one research practice that may be delaying attempts to apply theory may be the approach to theory testing itself" (p.100). A common approach is to pit one theory against another, in order to discard variables or models that may be less appropriate in clarifying behavior. This invariably prevents consideration of similarities at conceptual, operational, and measurement levels (Brawley, 1993). According to Brawley, this approach contributes to the fragmentation of knowledge and limited potential for application. It clearly has been a deterrent to research in the area of psychological response to sport injury.

Although infrequently studied, many commonalities exist between models of grief and cognitive appraisal. Both are adaptational models and therefore influence situational, as well as personal response, to perceived threat (cognitive appraisal) or loss (grief). These include the significance or threat of loss, previous experience of the loss or stressor, perceived social support, and the psychological and emotional response characteristics.

Perception about the significance of loss is central to grief models and is also a determinant of the emotional response. An equally important role is attributed to threat of harm in cognitive appraisal models, for example, threat to ego. Within the injury literature, severity of injury is consistently identified as a determinant of emotional response. Controllability and anticipatory loss are examples of two variables that may form part of the appraisal of significance of loss. Controllability is certainly a feature of grief, and within the cognitive appraisal literature, life events appraised as uncontrollable are more strongly associated with depression than are events appraised as controllable (Vitaliano, DeWolfe, Maiuro, Russo, & Katon, 1990). Responses of confusion, helplessness, and the need to rationalize, reported in a number of injury response studies (McDonald & Hardy, 1990; Pearson & Jones, 1992), are consistent with strategies of emotion-focused coping in situations appraised as uncontrollable. Both appraisal and grief models acknowledge the anticipatory function of loss and harm. Reminders of mortality are ever present, and certain types of loss are inevitable. Injury is a dramatic reminder of these. An example would be developmental loss characterized by loss of range of movement due to injury.

A person's previous experience with stressors in the appraisal process, notably his or her psychological and emotional responses, is important in both cognitive appraisal and grief model research. As a moderating variable, social support is assigned a key role in the both clinical and injury literature. However, in situations where athletes need to initially withdraw (as may be the case in injury because of the threat to self-esteem and self-confidence) and as a result become isolated, the role of social support is not clear.

The intensity and duration of psychological and emotional responses as predicted by models of appraisal and grief are difficult to study. One of the features of grief that has received much criticism is the affiliated emotional responses predicted by the models. Such criticisms have not been directed at cognitive appraisal models ostensibly because their included variables that predict psychological and emotional responses are not described in comparable detail. In an injury context, cognitive appraisal models have tended to focus on the process of appraisal as opposed to the responses that result from this process. In order to enhance understanding of the psychological responses of athletes to injury, appraisal models must provide testable predictions both in relation to process (appraisal) and outcome (response) variables.

As suggested previously, both models of grief and appraisal propose that at any one time several different emotions might occur in response to loss/stress (grief models have been criticized for this). Indeed, it has been suggested that some emotions may fluctuate to such an extent that they may last only hours or days. Grief models generally predict an initial phase of shock and disbelief, followed by a phase (or phases) that involve depressive symptoms such as despair, despondency, preoccupation, searching for meaning, and in some instances anxiety, anger, and hostility. Behavioral responses include withdrawal and isolation, with such behavior frequently not being conducive to adaptation and recovery. The latter two responses characterize a final phase during which a strong effort is made to return to normal functioning (Averill, 1968). As with appraisal models, these responses are considered to be a direct result of what appraisal models term goal incongruence, wherein goal-directed behavior is seriously disrupted. According to cognitive appraisal models, responses to an appraised stressor include shock, anger, guilt, anxiety, depression, helplessness, apathy, frustration, problem-solving cognitions, and behaviors such as isolation and withdrawal. Although these are rarely placed within a temporal pattern, some researchers have suggested stages within the context of the coping process. For example, Shontz (1975) has suggested stages of shock, encounter, and retreat or reality testing. The apparent overlap in the response characteristics described is hardly surprising when one considers that the stressor in appraisal frequently results in an actual or perceived loss, the basis of grief models.

The above discussion provides a strong rationale for a model of injury response that encompasses cognitive appraisal and grief. This model is illustrated below (Figure 1).

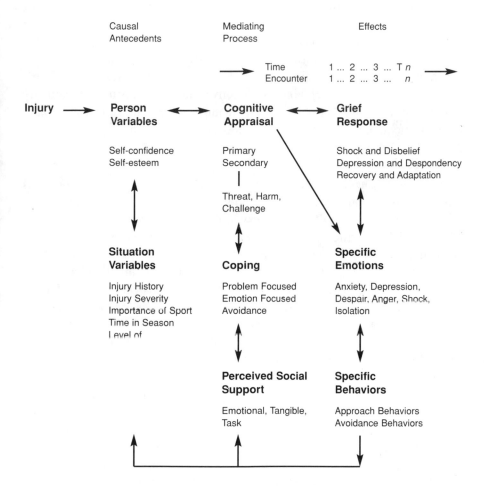

Figure 1. Psychological Model of Injury Response

From *Stress, Appraisal and Coping* (p. 305), by R. S. Lazarus and S. Folkman, 1984, New York: Springer. Copyright 1984. Adapted with permission.

The model proposed differs from previous appraisal models in as much as it acknowledges grief as a response to loss through injury. The model does not prescribe that all individuals will experience grief, rather that appraisal will determine whether the emotions and behaviors elicited characterize a grief response. This distinction should enable the investigation of responses to injury within an appraisal framework that accounts for the potential of a grief-like response. In addition, practitioners may find this approach helpful as they attempt to understand the various ways in which individual and situational differences affect the response of injured athletes. In this context a performer who responds with grief will not simply be viewed as maladaptive, but rather as someone requiring greater understanding and help in resolving his or her circumstances. This approach emphasizes the perceived significance of the loss and thus may determine the nature of the psychological and emotional responses to injury. A critical feature of the model is that it acknowledges the process of appraisal and response as adaptive and dynamic, one that explicitly changes over time. It is hoped that this feature will encourage research to address the temporal pattern, central to models of adaptation.

Practical Implications

A number of issues have been identified in this chapter that have implications for researchers and practitioners. In addition, measurement tools frequently used in the assessment of athletes' psychological and emotional responses to injury have been criticized. Clearly, better measures are needed in order to enable injury models to achieve optimal levels of predictive accuracy. Although some preliminary steps have been taken in this direction, highly reliable measures do not currently exist. In the absence of alternative measures, and in the context of the current knowledge base, interim strategies are herewith identified that apply to both qualitative and quantitative research. For instance, simple Likert scales could be used to enable athletes to report the intensity of their emotions, behaviors, and cognitions. This would enable a more complete picture of the various emotional responses to athletic injury and would be far more helpful than the current practice of adopting existing clinical measures that may have little relevance in the context of injury. Such measures would also provide a useful means of monitoring changes in an athlete's response to injury over time.

What, then, are some practical implications of the above discussion for designing rehabilitation regimens for injured athletes? It appears that the effectiveness of popular sport psychology interventions such as goal setting, cognitive restructuring, and positive self-talk should be enhanced by application of grief and appraisal models. Responses to loss in both models of grief and appraisal result from the disruption of goal-directed behavior. The use of goal setting during injury rehabilitation may help to restore goal-directed behavior and enhance motivation and adherence to rehabilitation programs. This may counteract feelings of apathy, a characteristic response predicted by models of grief. Goal setting should also have a positive effect on levels of self-confidence. Within the clinical literature, reduced levels of self-confidence have been identified as a function of loss.

Irrational and self-defeating thoughts are considered to be a characteristic of the depressive symptoms predicted by models of grief and appraisal. Although measurement tools have not been sensitive to the presence of such cognitions, cognitive restructuring would seem to be beneficial. The grief model may be particularly useful in this respect and, if presented in an appropriate manner, could be used to help athletes understand the adaptive nature of irrational and self-defeating thoughts. Positive self-talk may help in this adaptive process, and at the same time reinforce positive aspects of injury rehabilitation such as rehabilitation progress. The adaptive nature of models of appraisal and grief makes the role imagery may play, particularly in the early stages of injury, less clear. If, as such models predict, the early stages of injury are characterized by depressive symptoms associated with the perceived loss, athletes may be too emotionally linked with past performances (loss) for imagery to be of help. However, athletes who possess good imagery skills may utilize imagery to reinforce rehabilitation activities and the "form" with which these activities need to be executed. Imagery may be most beneficial when athletes are returning to sport via processes of mentally rehearsing skills and enhancing self-confidence. Empirical research that examines the temporal pattern of injured athletes' responses would be required to assess the validity of these observations.

Coaches and support sport psychology specialists have a number of distinct advantages when working with injured performers. An understanding of the factors predicted by the model of injury response proposed herein in conduction with knowledge and understanding of how performers normally respond in stressful situations might enable intervention administrators to identify athletes who are likely to experience exacerbated problems with injury. For example, grief models suggest athletes who show prolonged depressive symptoms may require additional support in overcoming the frustrations of injury (loss). The need for any model of injury to adequately account for individual differences has received a great deal of support. Therefore, it is essential that those who organize rehabilitation regimens for injured athletes be sensitive to individual differences in athletes. Some performers may require and seek social support. Others may need to withdraw from the sporting environment for a period of time. It is important that social support be made available whether the athlete initially requests it or not. In order to prevent further isolation of the injured performer, where possible, injured athletes should be kept as involved in team activities as possible. The athlete should be encouraged to feel that coaches, staff, and team members care about his or her condition.

Of particular relevance to coaches and support staff is the return of injured performers to sport. The model of injury response outlined in this chapter makes explicit the adaptive nature of response to loss and injury. However, it does not emphasize the relationship between physical and psychological adaptation. It is often assumed that when athletes are physically ready to return to practice and competition, they are also psychologically ready. Self-confidence may be of particular relevance here. Although self-confidence has received limited attention in injury research, it has been identified as an important factor within models of grief and appraisal. In the context of injury, self-confidence may play an important role in an athlete's psychological readiness to return to sport. Indeed, it may also be a factor in the potential for reinjury in athletes who prematurely return to sport. Despite pressures that may exist in high-level sport to return as quickly as possible following injury, those who work with injured athletes should provide them with opportunities to regain levels of self-confidence through practice games and lower level competition, prior to their return to full competition. Although psychological factors may be assumed to play a more significant role in more severe injuries, this may not always be the case. The significance of any loss is determined by an athlete's own value system and by an interplay of personal and situational factors. Coaches and others should be sensitive to individual differences and circumstances as they relate to each athlete.

The purpose of this chapter has been to propose a theoretically derived model of injury response that embraces cognitive appraisal and grief (Figure 1). In doing so, a number of measurement issues have been identified and discussed.

References

Aldwin, C. M. (1994). *Stress, coping, and development: An integrative perspective*. New York: Guilford.

Anderson, M. B., & Williams, J. M. (1988). A model of stress and athletic injury: Prediction and prevention. *Journal of Sport and Exercise Psychology, 10*, 294–306.

Archer, J., & Rhodes, V. (1987). Bereavement and reactions to job loss: A comparative review. *British Journal of Social Psychology, 26*, 211–224.

Archer, J., & Rhodes, V. (1993). The grief process and job loss: A cross-sectional study. *British Journal of Psychology, 8*, 395–410.

Averill, J. A. (1968). Grief: Its nature and significance. *Psychological Bulletin, 70,* 721–748.

Ben-Sira, Z. (1983). Loss, stress and readjustment: The structure of coping with bereavement and disability. *Social Science and Medicine, 17,* 1619–1632.

Brawley, L. R. (1993). The practicality of using social psychological theories for exercise and health research and intervention. *Journal of Applied Sport Psychology, 5,* 99–115.

Brewer, B. W. (1994). Review and critique of models of psychological adjustment to athletic injury. *Journal of Applied Sport Psychology, 6,* 87–100.

Brewer, B. W., Linder, D. E., & Phelps, D. O. (1995). Situational correlates of emotional adjustment to athletic injury. *Clinical Journal of Sport Medicine, 5,* 241–245.

Bugen, L. A. (1977). Human grief: A model for prediction and prevention. *American Journal of Orthopsychiatry, 47,* 196–206.

Chan, C. S., & Grossman, H. Y. (1988). Psychological effects of running loss on consistent runners. *Perceptual and Motor Skills, 66,* 875–883.

Cox, T., & Ferguson, E. (1991). Individual differences, stress and coping. In C. L. Cooper & R. Payne (Eds.), *Personality and stress: Individual differences in the stress process* (pp. 7–30). Chichester: Wiley.

Daly, J. M., Brewer, B. W., Van Raalte, J. L., Petitpas, A.J., & Sklar, J.H. (1995). Cognitive appraisal, emotional adjustment, and adherence to rehabilitation following knee surgery. *Journal of Sport Rehabilitation, 4,* 23–30.

Engel, G. L. (1964). Grief and grieving. *American Journal of Nursing, 64,* 93–98.

Evans, L., & Hardy, L. (1995). Sport injury and grief responses: A review. *Journal of Sport and Exercise Psychology, 17,* 227–245.

Folkman, S., Lazarus, R. S., Dunkel-Schetter, C., DeLongis, A., & Gruen, R. J. (1986). Dynamics of a stressful encounter: Cognitive appraisal, coping, and encounter outcomes. *Journal of Personality and Social Psychology, 50,* 992–1003.

Gordon, S., & Lindgren, S. (1990). Psycho-physical rehabilitation from a serious sport injury: A case study of an elite fast bowler. *The Australian Journal of Science and Medicine in Sport, 22*(3), 71–76.

Hardy, L., Jones, G., & Gould, D. (1996). *Understanding psychological preparation for sport: Theory and practice of elite performers.* Chichester: Wiley.

Heil, J. (1993). *Psychology of sport injury.* Champaign, IL: Human Kinetics.

Johnson, U. (1996). The multiply injured versus the first-time-injured athlete during rehabilitation: A comparison of nonphysical characteristics. *Journal of Sport Rehabilitation, 5,* 293–304.

Kübler-Ross, E. (1969). *On death and dying.* London: Tavistock.

Kübler-Ross, E. (1975). *Death: The final stage of growth.* London: Tavistock.

Lazarus, R. S. (1991). *Emotion and adaptation.* New York: Oxford Press

Lazarus, R. S., & Folkman, S. (1984). *Stress, appraisal and coping.* New York: Springer.

Leddy, M. H., Lambert, M. J., & Ogles, B. M. (1994). Psychological consequences of athletic injury among high-level competitors. *Research Quarterly for Exercise and Sport, 65,* 347–354.

Lewin, K. (1951). *Field theory in social science: Selected theoretical papers.* New York: Harper.

McDonald, S. A., & Hardy, C. J. (1990). Affective response patterns of the injured athlete: An exploratory analysis. *The Sport Psychologist, 4,* 261–274.

McGowan, R. W., Pierce, E. F., & Eastman, N. W. (1994). Athletic injury and self-diminution. *Journal of Sports Medicine and Physical Fitness, 34,* 299–304.

Parkes, C. M. (1986). *Bereavement: Studies of grief in adult life* (2nd ed.). London: Tavistock.

Pearson, L., & Jones, G. (1992). Emotional effects of sports injuries: Implications for physiotherapists. *Physiotherapy, 78,* 762–770.

Quackenbush, N., & Crossman, J. (1994). Injured athletes: A study of emotional responses. *Journal of Sport Behaviour, 17,* 178–187.

Rose, J., & Jevne, R. F. J. (1993). Psychosocial processes associated with athletic injuries. *The Sport Psychologist, 7,* 309–328.

Rosenblatt, P. C. (1988). Grief: The social context of private feelings. *Journal of Social Issues, 44*(3), 67–78.

Shontz, F.C. (1975). *The psychological effects of disability and physical illness and disability.* New York: Macmillan

Singer, R. N., Murphey, M., & Tennant, L. K. (1993). *Handbook of research on sport psychology.* New York: Macmillan.

Simos, B. G. (1977). Grief therapy to facilitate healthy restitution. *Social Casework, 58,* 337–342.

Smith, A. M. (1996). Psychological impact of injuries in athletes. *Sports Medicine, 22,* 391–405.

Smith, A. M., Scott, S. G., O'Fallon, W. M., & Young, M. L. (1990). Emotional responses of athletes to injury. *Mayo Clinic Proceedings, 65,* 38–50.

Smith, A. M., Stuart, M. J., Wiese-Bjornstal, D. M., Milliner, E. K., O'Fallon, W. M., & Crowson, C. S. (1993). Competitive athletes: Preinjury and postinjury mood state and self-esteem. *Mayo Clinic Proceedings, 68,* 939–947.

Uemukai, K. (1993). Affective responses and the changes in athletes due to injury. *Proceedings of the Eighth World Sport Psychology Conference, Portugal* (pp. 500–503). Lisbon: International Society of Sport Psychology.

Vitaliano, P. P., DeWolfe, D. J., Maiuro, R. D., Russo, J., & Katon, W. (1990). Appraised change-ability of a stressor as a modifier of the relationship between coping and depression: A test of the hypothesis of fit. *Journal of Personality and Social Psychology, 59*(3), 582–592.

Weiss, M. R., & Troxel, R. K. (1986). Psychology of the injured athlete. *Athletic Training, 21,* 104–110.

Worden, W. (1991). *Grief counseling and grief therapy: A handbook for the mental health practitioner* (2nd ed.). London: Routledge.

Wortman, C. B., & Silver, R. C. (1989). The myths of coping with loss. *Journal of Consulting and Clinical Psychology, 57,* 349–357.

SECTION 2

PSYCHOLOGICAL PERSPECTIVES
ON ATHLETIC INJURY

Chapter 5

Assessing and Monitoring Injuries and Psychological Characteristics
in Intercollegiate Athletes: A Counseling/Prediction Model

Michael L. Sachs
Michael R. Sitler
Gerry Schwille

Chapter 6

The Paradox of Injuries: Unexpected Positive Consequences

Eileen Udry

Chapter 7

Personality Correlates of Psychological Processes
During Injury Rehabilitation

J. Robert Grove
Theresa Bianco

Chapter 8

The Malingering Athlete: Psychological Considerations

Robert J. Rotella
Bruce C. Ogilvie
David H. Perrin

Each of the four chapters in this section addresses some aspect(s) of athletic injury rehabilitation. Those whose primary interests are in the construction and implementation of rehabilitation programs will find value in this section.

In the first chapter, **Michael L. Sachs**, **Michael R. Sitler**, and **Gerry Schwille** discuss the role of life stress, mood, anxiety, and personal coping skills in understanding and predicting athletic injury. They provide a model that includes these factors, which they suggest is useful in the rehabilitation of injured collegiate athletes.

In the second chapter, **Eillen Udry** argues that despite the pain and turmoil induced by injury, athletes may also experience positive consequences that should be understood by professional helpers.

J. Robert Grove and **Theresa Bianco** write about personological aspects of sport injury rehabilitation in the third chapter of this section. They suggest that ideal rehabilitative approaches may vary according to personality dispositions.

The focus of this section's fourth chapter is the malingering athletes. **Robert J. Rotella**, **Bruce C. Ogilvie**, and **David H. Perrin** define and discuss the term *malingerer* and indicate that some athletes seek out and profit from the "injured" status. Suggestions are made for dealing with this type of athlete.

5

Assessing and Monitoring Injuries and Psychological Characteristics in Intercollegiate Athletes: A Counseling/Prediction Model

Michael L. Sachs
Michael R. Sitler
Gerry Schwille
Temple University

One of the consequences of participation in intercollegiate athletics for almost all athletes at some point during their careers is injuries. Although not all athletes are injured severely enough to miss practices and/or games, virtually all intercollegiate athletes sustain injuries at least one or more times during their careers to the extent that medical treatment is required. These injuries may be due to any number of factors, which include, but are not limited to, contact with another player or equipment, overuse, equipment failure, previous injury, exposure to injury, and conditioning. An additional important factor may be life stress, resulting from issues both within the athletic context and outside the athletic domain, which may negatively affect the person physically and psychologically. A counseling/prediction

model is discussed that incorporates the development of a database of key physical and psychological characteristics of the athlete to track changes in the athlete that might alert the sport psychologist to potential stress, as well as encompass periodic monitoring and referral as needed. The prediction of athletic injuries and adherence to rehabilitation regimens may also be an outcome of use of the model.

One area that has recently been examined more extensively is the effect of psychological factors on injuries. In particular, the area of life stress is one that applied sport psychologists find especially important. Although life stress may not lead directly to injuries in intercollegiate athletes, dealing with stress (or, more precisely, not dealing effectively with stress) may indirectly affect the athlete. Life stress resulting from factors both within the athletic context (concern about upcoming games, conflicts with teammates or coaches, pressure to perform, etc.) and, particularly, outside the athletic domain (family problems; difficulties with significant others—spouse, boyfriend/girlfriend; academic problems; etc.) may negatively affect the person physically (i.e., immune system responses, excessive fatigue) and psychologically (i.e., distraction—constant thinking about the problems faced).

A proactive approach to dealing with life stress would encompass periodic monitoring, through established psychological inventories, interviews, and other approaches, of the athlete's psychological well-being. Those athletes who offer evidence of some degree of psychological distress could be offered counseling to help them deal with the stress. Reducing/eliminating the stress would then facilitate restoration of psychological well-being and concomitant physical well-being, thereby reducing one key factor that may result in injuries. Although injuries will occur during participation in the sporting environment, the underlying, precipitating factor may lie in the stress experienced by the individual.

Given their regular interaction with many athletes and their frontline contact and responsibilities for the care and well-being of the athletes, athletic trainers are key individuals in the athletic environment. Although other medical professionals, such as doctors and nurses (Gregory & Van Valkenburgh, 1991), have roles to play with injured athletes, athletic trainers are, in many ways, potentially the staff most likely to hear about concerns of the athletes and/or spot physical and related mood changes in athletes. As part of a proactive model in dealing with stress, athletic trainers must be involved in a significant way. Recent work (Wiese, Weiss, & Yukelson, 1990) indicates that athletic trainers are aware of, and supportive of, the key role of sport psychology in athletics, particularly in the injury rehabilitation process.

Background

On first examination it appears reasonably clear from the literature that life stress has a significant impact on injuries in athletes. Kerr and Minden (1988) examined elite female gymnasts and found that stressful life events were significantly related to both frequency and severity of injuries. Hardy and Riehl (1988) found that total life change and negative life change significantly predicted frequency of athletic injury (although not severity) among noncontact sport participants. Similar results with football players were found by Blackwell and McCullagh (1990). Injured players had higher scores on life-stress factors and competitive anxiety, and lower scores on coping resources, than did uninjured players.

Recent work, however, suggests that the relationship of life stress to injuries may be more complicated than first thought. R. E. Smith, Smoll, and Ptacek (1990) found that, in considering the variables of life stress, social support, and coping skills, these factors must be considered together rather than separately. They describe this as conjunctive moderation, "in which multiple moderators must co-occur in a specific combination or pattern to maximize a relation between a predictor and an outcome variable" as opposed to disjunctive moderation, "in which any one of a number of moderators maximizes the predictor-criterion relation" (R. E. Smith et al., 1990, p. 360). The authors found that, for adolescent sport injuries, social support and psychological coping skills acted in a conjunctive manner—a significant relationship between stress and injury was found only for athletes low in both coping skills and social support.

In attempting to clarify the life stress, coping skills, and social support interaction, a model of stress and athletic injury may be helpful. Andersen and Williams (1988) developed a theoretical model of stress and athletic injury that includes cognitive, attentional, behavioral, physiological, intrapersonal, social, and stress history variables. A comprehensive view of the stress-injury relationship requires this type of multivariate approach. Previous studies (with the exception of R. E. Smith et al., 1990) have tended to examine only components of this model with comparatively small groups of athletes. Advancement in theory, research, and practice (i.e., potential application) in this area would be aided by examining an array of factors within the model with a much larger group of athletes, across a variety of sports, for an extended period of time.

Monitoring

A basic component of a counseling/prediction model would be the development of a database of key physical and psychological characteristics of the athlete to track changes in the athlete that might alert the sport psychologist to potential stress. The physical (including demographic) components would include a number of factors. These would encompass age, gender, height, weight, percent body fat, years and level of participation in sport, and previous history of injuries.

A battery of psychological inventories (see Table 1 and discussion in the section on psychological tests) dealing with a number of different psychological states and traits suggested in the model—life stress, mood, anxiety, coping skills, etc.—would, in this model, be administered to all intercollegiate athletes at a given university during the period set aside for physical examinations at the start of the school year. This could also be done, of course, with interscholastic athletes at a high school, members of a club team, etc. These results would provide baseline data from which to work with athletes during the school year. Some of the tests could be scheduled for administration several times during the semester. The complete battery could also be administered again prior to the start of the spring semester to increase the probability of detecting psychological problems that might have arisen since the earlier testing points.

The information obtained would be used in three ways. First, if the results indicated a clinically significant level of psychological distress on one of the inventories, the athlete would be counseled to seek assistance, either at the university counseling center or with one of the sport psychologists working with athletes at the university. Although this would potentially confound the research component of the study, it represents a proactive approach based on the desire to ensure maximum psychological mental health and well-being of the athlete and, concomitantly, readiness to practice and compete in intercollegiate athletics. In this case, ethical principles would suggest that applied concerns outweigh research considerations. Follow-up information would be obtained on each athlete to ascertain adherence to recommendations to seek counseling and readministration of appropriate psychological inventories to measure potential changes on the psychological measure of concern.

Second, the results could be used in a model to attempt to predict occurrence of athletic injuries during the course of the year. These injuries might be suffered as a result of practices or games, or in other settings (i.e., basketball players playing on their own before practice for the season can officially begin). This model might be useful at other universities as well or may be found to be specific to the university where testing takes place (e.g., perhaps due to peculiarities in environmental conditions).

Third, it is possible that some of the psychological factors measured may allow prediction of which athletes will return to practice and competition most quickly. Delineation of factors related to adherence to a rehabilitation regimen and a return to participation may be an added outcome of this model, although not a primary focus.

It is important to emphasize that all information obtained through the testing procedures would be kept confidential. The information is designed to be used in an individual, counseling/prediction approach by sport psychologists. Coaches and athletic administration personnel would not have access to the information unless written permission was obtained from the athlete. Indeed, one problem encountered is reluctance on the part of some athletes (and teams in general) to complete a battery of standardized inventories. One will most likely find that participation in the program will be considerably less than 100%. However, those motivated to participate will probably find the process useful, and this may "sell" the program to others who initially are hesitant to participate.

Injury Definition and Documentation/Guidelines

Important to psychological intervention studies in athletic settings is defining the term injury. It is from this most fundamental level that the incidence of injury can be determined and interpretation of findings and comparison of results between studies can be made more reliably.

The most basic elements in the establishment of an injury definition encompass the need for detail, explicitness, and ease of interpretation (Wallace & Clark, 1988). A set of inclusive and exclusive criteria are needed that allow for differentiation between those who have been injured and those who have not been injured. To date, however, no universally agreed-upon definition of what constitutes an injury has been established, although three generally accepted classification criteria include (a) time loss from participation, (b) anatomical tissue diagnosis, and (c) medical consultation. Each of the definitions available has its own strengths and weaknesses and, as such, varies in its ability to meet research objectives.

One way we have found most helpful is to define an injury as (a) being sports related, (b) resulting in a player's inability to participate one day after injury, and (c) requiring medical attention (university athletic training staff, physician, emergency room), including concussions, nerve injuries (regardless of their time loss), eye injuries, and dental care (Noyes, Lindefeld, & Marshall, 1988). This definition has the advantage of comprising a multidimensional approach and is relatively sensitive to the broad spectrum of injuries encountered in the athletic setting. This does not include, however, occurrences of the flu, colds, and other related illnesses that would not be seen as sports related per se but could still be due, in part, to psychologically induced stress/depression resulting in a weakened and potentially more susceptible bodily state. Recent work on psychoneuroimmunology supports this point of view and may lead to a change in how we define injury in the future.

Injury frequency is determined by the total number of occurrences encountered during the course of testing (e.g., a season, a year). Injury frequency can then be expressed as a function of the exposure to injury, resulting in determination of an injury rate. The injury rate (see Figure 1) comprises a numerator, the number of events (i.e., injuries) under study, and a denominator, the number of persons at risk of a specific occurrence or event, providing for a determination of risk. A useful way of expressing the denominator is to base it upon every 1,000 athlete-exposures. Athlete-exposures are defined as the frequency with which an athlete is exposed to the potential of injury, and every player at a practice or game is counted as one athlete-exposure. Although this determination involves a fair amount of record keeping, much of this information is already being kept by athletic training staff and may only require a systematic organization of the record-keeping process.

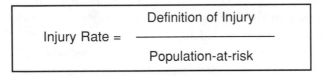

Figure 1. Injury Rate and Determination of Risk

Injury severity is defined by the significance of the injury sustained. Here again, no universal definition exists, although time-loss from activity has been used in several nationally based sports injury epidemiology studies (Alles, Powell, Buckley, & Hunt, 1979; Powell, 1988). The utility of a time-loss definition is that it is relatively easy to measure and is based on the functional consequences of participation (or not participating!) following the injury. When more objective criteria are needed, as is frequently necessary with ligamentous and muscle-related injuries, categorization in accordance with the injury severity index established by the American Medical Association's *Standard Nomenclature of Injuries* (1968) can be used.

Injury data can be prospectively collected by the medical staff assigned to the study. This includes the university's intercollegiate athletic training staff and student athletic trainers who are enrolled in the National Athletic Trainers' Association Approved Undergraduate Athletic Training Program.

Psychological Tests

There are numerous psychological inventories that can be administered to athletes. Ostrow (1996), for example, has a *Directory of Psychological Tests in the Sport and Exercise Sciences* with information on 314 psychological tests specifically related to sport and exercise. There are many inventories that could be used in a battery of tests, including ones on injury as well as self-efficacy, athletic identity, commitment to exercise, and so on. One suggestion for a set of inventories (see Table 1) that may be of particular interest in applying the counseling/prediction model is as follows:

Table 1. List of Psychological Inventories

Profile of Mood States (*POMS*) (McNair, Lorr, & Droppleman, 1971)
Brief Assessment of Mood States (*BAMS*) (Dean, Whelan, & Meyers, 1990)
Sport Anxiety Scale (*SAS*) (R. E. Smith, Smoll, & Schutz, 1990)
Eating Disorders Inventory-2 (*EDI-2*) (Garner, 1991)
Health Attribution Test (*HAT*) (Lawlis & Lawlis, 1990)
Coping Resources Inventory (*CRI*) (Hammer & Marting, 1988)
Life Experiences Survey—Athletes (*LES-A*) (Hardy, 1989)
The Exercise Salience Scale (*TESS*) (Morrow & Harvey, 1990)

Profile of Mood States (*POMS*). The *POMS* (McNair, Lorr, & Droppleman, 1971) is a 65-adjective rating scale, derived through factor analysis, that measures six dimensions of *mood states:* Tension-Anxiety, Depression-Dejection, Anger-Hostility, Vigor-Activity, Fatigue-Inertia, and Confusion-Bewilderment. The *POMS* has excellent psychometric properties (established validity and reliability). Instructions request respondents to indicate how they have been feeling during the past week, but the scale can be used to ask how respondents have been feeling for longer (i.e., past month) or shorter (i.e., daily) periods of time. Ideally, athletes would have comparatively high scores on Vigor-Activity and comparatively low scores on the other five factors, providing what has been termed an *iceberg profile* (Morgan & Pollock, 1977), with a peak of vigor and 'submerged' levels on the other factors.

The *POMS* is an excellent means of regularly measuring mood and is used frequently in applied and research contexts, but can become burdensome if administered too frequently, although 65 items is not a great number, too frequent administration may be undesirable. One way around this problem may be a "new" instrument termed the *Brief Assessment of Mood States* (Dean, Whelan, & Meyers, 1990), or *BAMS,* which has reduced the 65-item *POMS* to 6 items. Concurrent validity appears acceptable, and this instrument has been used effectively in athletic contexts (Fritts, 1992). One advantage found with administration of the *BAMS* on a regular basis is that respondents develop the habit of completing the form at a regular time in their schedule in a matter of only 10 to 15 seconds, placing little burden on their time and energy. However, we have also found that coaches are hesitant to have athletes complete even the *BAMS* on days when competition is scheduled, for fear of having the athletes focus too much on their mood states, particularly, of course, if the mood state is negative.

Sport Anxiety Scale (SAS). The *SAS* (Smith, Smoll, & Schutz, 1990) is a sport-specific measure of cognitive and somatic trait anxiety. Current thinking in sport psychology suggests the advisability of using sport-specific measures as well as instruments that address both cognitive and somatic components of anxiety, such as the *SAS.* Individual differences in somatic anxiety and two classes of cognitive anxiety—Worry and Concentration Disruption—are measured. The *SAS* has excellent psychometric properties.

Eating Disorders Inventory-2 (EDI-2). The *EDI-2* (Garner, 1991) is a 91–item self-report inventory that assesses an array of *factors related to anorexia nervosa and bulimia nervosa.* Eleven subscales make up the *EDI:* Drive for Thinness, Bulimia, Body Dissatisfaction, Ineffectiveness, Perfectionism, Interpersonal Distrust, Interoceptive Awareness, Maturity Fears, Impulse Regulation, Social Insecurity, and Asceticism. The *EDI-2* has excellent psychometric properties. A new symptom checklist provides additional information about the frequency and severity of symptoms important in considering a diagnosis of an eating disorder, a problem area particularly prevalent in some athletic populations (e.g., gymnasts, runners, divers, wrestlers).

Health Attribution Test (HAT). The *HAT* (Lawlis & Lawlis, 1990) is a 22-item test that evaluates an individual's *health locus of control.* Attributions for control of one's health may be made to internal factors, powerful others, and chance. The *HAT* has excellent psychometric properties. This scale provides an excellent measure for attempting to develop a predictive profile for recovery time for individuals who are injured.

Coping Resources Inventory (CRI). The *CRI* (Hammer & Marting, 1988) is a 60-item inventory that assesses one's *resources for coping with situations.* Coping resources can be defined as "those resources inherent in individuals that enable them to handle stressors more effectively, to experience fewer or less intense symptoms upon exposure to a stressor, or to recover faster from exposure" (Hammer & Marting, 1988, p. 2). The *CRI* measures resources in five domains: cognitive, social, emotional, spiritual/philosophical, and physical. Hammer and Marting identify seven uses for the *CRI,* two of which are particularly relevant to this study: "as a research instrument to investigate coping resources in various populations" and "as a tool for identifying individuals who might be at-risk, in need of counseling, or in need of medical intervention" (p. 2). The *CRI* has excellent psychometric properties.

Life Experiences Survey—Athletes (LES-A). The *LES-A* (Hardy, 1989) is an 80-item survey that attempts to determine if any of a variety of *life experiences* have occurred to the athlete within the past 12 months *and* the perceived impact of the event on the person at the time the event occurred. The survey provides a framework within which to potentially understand moderate to high levels of stress that athletes might be experiencing.

The Exercise Salience Scale (TESS). The *TESS* (Morrow & Harvey, 1990) measures a number of factors that determine dependence upon exercise. Athletes who are more dependent upon exercise may be more likely to persist in participating in athletics in spite of negative life stress. The *TESS* has strong psychometric properties.

It is important to emphasize that these are neither the only psychological inventories nor the only psychological constructs that can be used. Different researchers/practitioners have other areas, and other tests they have found meet their needs more effectively. For example, Bergandi and Wittig (1991) found that attentional style was related to frequency of athletic injury with some athletes (in one sport, women's softball), but not others. The Test of Attentional and Interpersonal Style (*TAIS*) (Nideffer, 1976) could, therefore, be used to measure this construct. Other approaches, looking at other variables (Nideffer, 1989), may prove attractive for different needs in different athletic settings.

Model Application

As noted earlier, the battery of inventories would be administered before the fall semester begins or before the first practice in the case of sports (i.e., football) that begin their season before school is in session. This initial baseline also provides an indication of psychological problems that may have arisen during the summer, when contact with athletes may have been minimal. Intervention can then occur if the sport psychologist feels that the test scores indicate this course of action.

Injury data are then collected throughout the course of the year, through the competitive season and practices, as well as recreational periods (i.e., basketball before the "official" practice date). Some inventories may be readministered on a regular basis to monitor potential changes. This is particularly important for those measures addressing issues that are state, rather than trait, in nature. Trait measures will tend to remain stable over time, and administering such measures twice a year may be sufficient. State measures, however, by definition, will change, even on a daily basis. Administering these measures, such as the *BAMS*, on a more frequent basis is, therefore, desirable. Of course, scoring of these inventories must be done quickly to ensure opportunities for intervention if this is so desired.

At the end of the year data from the psychological inventories and the injury data can be analyzed to assess potential relationships of theoretical and applied importance, as well as detect changes over time if this is an ongoing process. It is important to note that the process of administering the psychological inventories must have the cooperation of the coach and the athletes. As noted, there will be coaches and athletes who choose not to participate (and human subjects guidelines at universities require that this nonparticipation option be present), and this must be respected.

In applying the model, there are a number of potential uses, as noted earlier. Perhaps the most important, from a clinical/proactive perspective, is the case wherein the results indicate a clinically significant level of psychological distress on one of the inventories. For example, Jane Doe, athlete on Team Sport x, provides a *POMS* with a "negative" or inverted iceberg profile, with high scores on tension, depression, anger, fatigue, and confusion, and a low score on vigor. This suggests that something may be going on in Jane's life: This something could "simply" be overtraining (Morgan, Costill, Flynn, Raglin, & O'Connor, 1988) or could reflect some other problems, such as interpersonal relationships, academic difficulties, or family matters. The athlete would be counseled to seek assistance, either at the university counseling center or with one of the sport psychologists working with athletes at the university. Providing the athlete with a choice and maintaining confidentiality are important elements in this process.

In Jane's case, the *POMS*, as well as the *BAMS*, could be used to follow up progress in the weeks following the beginning of counseling. Some of the inventories, such as the *POMS*, may prove quite useful as well in working with athletes who are recovering from an injury (A. M. Smith, Scott, O'Fallon, & Young, 1990), and "facilitate the athlete's optimal rehabilitation and a safe return to participation in sports" (p. 38).

This approach provides for a unique partnership of the sport psychologist and athletic trainer. Both groups of individuals have the physical and psychological well-being of the athlete as their greatest concern. Interventions as described in the above model provide a means for facilitating the help we give our athletes in achieving their goals as individuals, students, and athletes.

Conclusion

Although injuries are a fact of life in intercollegiate athletics, it is extremely desirable to minimize injury frequency and severity. The impact of physical and psychological factors on the frequency and severity of injuries is critical and is worthy of in-depth investigation. A counseling/prediction model is proposed as an effective means of working with athletes and providing important information for theory and research in this critical area of study.

References

Alles, W., Powell, J., Buckley, H., & Hunt, E. (1979). The national athletic injury/illness reporting system: Three-year findings of high school and college football injuries. *Journal of Orthopedic and Sports Physical Therapy, 11,* 103–108.

American Medical Association. (1968). *Standard nomenclature of injuries.* Chicago, IL: American Medical Association.

Andersen, M. B., & Williams, J. M. (1988). A model of stress and athletic injury: Prediction and prevention. *Journal of Sport and Exercise Psychology, 10,* 294–306.

Bergandi, T. A., & Wittig, A. F. (1991). *Attentional style as a predictor of athletic injury.* Unpublished manuscript, Spalding University, Louisville, KY.

Blackwell, B., & McCullagh, P. (1990, Spring). The relationship of athletic injury to life stress, competitive anxiety and coping resources. *Athletic Training, 25,* 23–27.

Dean, J. E., Whelan, J. P., & Meyers, A. W. (1990, September). *An incredibly quick way to assess mood states: The Incredibly Short POMS.* Paper presented at the annual meeting of the Association for the Advancement of Applied Sport Psychology, San Antonio, TX.

Fritts, S. M. (1992). *Psychological factors that predispose athletes to injury.* Unpublished master's thesis, Temple University, Philadelphia, PA.

Garner, D. M. (1991). *Eating Disorder Inventory-2 manual.* Odessa, FL: Psychological Assessment Resources, Inc.

Gregory, B., & Van Valkenburgh, J. (1991). Psychology of the injured athlete. *Journal of Post Anesthesia Nursing, 6*(2), 108–110.

Hammer, A. L., & Marting, M. S. (1988). *Manual for the Coping Resources Inventory (research ed.).* Palo Alto, CA: Consulting Psychologists Press.

Hardy, C. J. (1989). *Life Experience Survey—Athletes.* Chapel Hill, NC: Department of Physical Education, University of North Carolina.

Hardy, C. J., & Riehl, R. E. (1988). An examination of the life stress-injury relationship among noncontact sport participants. *Behavioral Medicine, 14,* 113–118.

Kerr, G., & Minden, H. (1988). Psychological factors related to the occurrence of athletic injuries. *Journal of Sport and Exercise Psychology, 10,* 167–173.

Lawlis, J., & Lawlis, G. F. (1990). *Health Attribution Test manual.* Champaign, IL: Institute for Personality and Ability Testing.

McNair, D. M., Lorr, M., & Droppleman, L. F. (1971). *Manual: Profile of Mood States.* San Diego, CA: Educational and Industrial Testing Service.

Morgan, W. P., Costill, D. L., Flynn, M. G., Raglin, J. S., & O'Connor, P. H. (1988). Psychological monitoring of overtraining and performance. *British Journal of Sports Medicine, 21,* 107–114.

Morgan, W. P., & Pollock, M. L. (1977). Psychologic characterization of the elite distance runner. *Annals of the New York Academy of Sciences, 301,* 382–402.

Morrow, J., & Harvey, P. (1990). *The exercise salience scale.* Unpublished manuscript, New York, NY.

Nideffer, R. M. (1976). Test of Attentional and Interpersonal Style (TAIS). *Journal of Personality and Social Psychology, 34,* 397–404.

Nideffer, R. M. (1989). Psychological aspects of sports injuries: Issues in prevention and treatment. *International Journal of Sport Psychology, 20,* 241–255.

Noyes, R., Lindefeld, T., & Marshall, M. (1988). What determines an athletic injury (definition): Who determines an injury (occurrence)? *American Journal of Sports Medicine, 16* (supplement), 134–135.

Ostrow, A. C. (1996). *Directory of psychological tests in the sport and exercise sciences* (2nd ed.). Morgantown, WV: Fitness Information Technology, Inc.

Smith, A. M., Scott, S. G., O'Fallon, W. M., & Young, M. L. (1990). Emotional responses of athletes to injury. *Mayo Clinic Proceedings, 65,* 38–50.

Smith, R. E., Smoll, F. L., & Ptacek, J. T. (1990). Conjunctive moderator variables in vulnerability and resiliency research: Life stress, social support, and coping skills, and adolescent sport injuries. *Journal of Personality and Social Psychology, 58,* 360–370.

Smith, R. E., Smoll, F. L., & Schutz, R. W. (1990). Measurement and correlates of sport-specific cognitive and somatic trait anxiety: The sport anxiety scale. *Anxiety Research, 2,* 263–280.

Wallace, R., & Clark, W. (1988). The numerator, denominator, and the population-at-risk. *American Journal of Sports Medicine, 16*(supplement 1), 55–56.

Wiese, D. M., Weiss, M. R., & Yukelson, D. P. (1990). *Sport psychology in the training room: A survey of athletic trainers.* Paper presented at the annual meeting of the American Alliance for Health, Physical Education, Recreation, and Dance, New Orleans, LA.

6

The Paradox of Injuries: Unexpected Positive Consequences

Eileen Udry
Indiana University at Indianapolis

I had all these desperate feelings. I kept thinking "How will I ever play football again if I can't even get out of this bed?" I was an invalid. Football had given me everything: identity, money, confidence, friendships. I wondered what kind of man I would be without it. (quoted in Lieber, 1991, p. 38)

The above statement was made by Keith Millard, an NFL defensive tackle, after he sustained a season-ending knee injury. Millard's comments highlight the enormous emotional toll that athletic injuries may take on individuals who are physically active. Indeed, numerous studies have documented the negative psychological impact of sport injuries (e.g., Brewer, Linder, & Phelps, 1995; Brewer, Petitpas, Van Raalte, Sklar, & Ditmar, 1995; Crossman & Jamieson, 1985; Leddy, Lambert, & Ogles, 1994; Smith, Scott, O'Fallon, & Young, 1990; Udry, Gould, Bridges, & Beck, 1997). The stress associated with sport injuries may stem from a variety of sources including pain, loss of mobility, performance decrements, social isolation, threats to self-esteem and identity, and, in some instances, a loss of livelihood (Gould, Udry, Bridges, & Beck, 1997; Petitpas & Danish, 1994).

In short, the emotional distress of sport injuries is not disputed. However, consider the following statement also made by Millard as he reflected on his injury and the rehabilitation process:

> The injury made me a lot more mature. I have a better grasp of reality in life. I'm more patient and giving . . . I'm so much stronger emotionally. I've proven to myself that I can overcome the most dreaded injury in football. (quoted in Lieber, 1991, p. 44)

This statement suggests that Millard felt that he grew in significant and positive ways from his injury and raises some compelling questions. Are injured athletes able to garner long-term positive consequences or benefits from their injuries?[1] If so, what type of benefits? Are there ways to facilitate these positive consequences associated with athletic injuries? This chapter explores these questions. More specifically, the chapter begins with an overview of several conceptual models that address how individuals may respond to adversity and/or stress (e.g., injuries, loss of health). Second, research that has been conducted examining how individuals respond to adversity will be briefly discussed. Finally, recommendations for facilitating the development of long-term positive consequences from injuries are offered.

Conceptual Models of Adversity and Stress

Although the ways in which athletes respond to injury-related stress has been the focus of a considerable amount of recent research, researchers have had a long-standing interest in the more general question of how individuals cope with a variety of different types of stressors. Selye (1974), a pioneer in the area of stress theory and research, forwarded a model of stress adaptation termed General Adaptation Syndrome (GAS). Selye suggested that when individuals are first exposed to a stressor, their initial response is *alarm*. During this period it is thought that individuals' resistance to additional stressors is compromised. If the intensity and duration of the stressor continue (e.g., there is not adequate time to adapt), individuals may experience *exhaustion* and succumb to the stressor. However, if the strength of the stressor is such that individuals are not overwhelmed, they enter an *adaptation* phase. It is in this adaptation phase that individuals become stronger than they were initially.

---

1. Heil (1993) discusses the notion of what are termed "secondary gains" of injuries. Heil suggests that secondary gains *may* function to reinforce the "sick role" of an injured athlete and thereby increase the likelihood of a delayed rehabilitation. The use of the terms "positive consequences of" and "benefits from" injuries here is distinct from Heil's usage in that they do not refer to these undesirable behaviors.

Thus, according to Selye, under the right circumstances stressors act as catalysts for higher levels of functioning and adaptation.

From a developmental psychology perspective, Erikson (1959) theorized that normal personality growth occurred only when "developmental crises" were resolved. According to Erikson, if individuals successfully resolved problems from a previous stage, they were thought to be more likely to achieve lasting a solution to a present dilemma because the achievements from the previous situation were used as the building blocks (Turner & Avison, 1992). Hence, Erikson proposed that individuals emerged from developmental crises with new skills, confidence, or enabling self attitudes that added to their arsenal of coping responses (Turner & Avison).

More recently, Danish, Petitpas, and Hale (1995) have proposed a Life Development Model (LDM) for use with athletes. The LDM makes several assertions. First, the LDM proposes that individuals are continually growing and changing but not necessarily in a sequential manner. Thus, an event such as an injury might cause athletes to be temporarily thrust into a downward spiral relative to mental health functioning. However, this downward spiral is not necessarily permanent. Second, according to the LDM perspective, when individuals are faced with what are called "critical life events" or "turning points," they may respond in several ways. Specifically, critical life events can result in (a) debilitation or decreased functioning, (b) little change in individuals' lives, or (c) increased opportunities for growth. In summary, according to the LDM, individuals are capable of shaping rather than simply responding to the negative forces in their environment.

To summarize, conceptual models from diverse areas have suggested that stress and adversity may serve as an impetus for individuals' growth and development. When applying these models to injured athletes, one implication would be that, although not frequently discussed, there may be some positive consequences or benefits of sport injuries. In the following section, research that has examined positive consequences of stress will be discussed. Because a limited amount of research on this topic has been conducted specifically with injured athletes, information from the general and health psychology domains will be examined first.

Stress and Positive Consequences Research

During the 1950s and 1960s researchers often studied the effects of natural disasters, war and combat, and a host of personal forms of stress (Turner & Avison, 1992). These early researchers found, for example, that in certain parts of the country where extreme weather conditions occur, individuals who were routinely exposed to immoderate conditions tended to deal with them more effectively as compared to those who were not exposed to these conditions. In fact, not only did these individuals deal with the stressor better when they are exposed to it, but they also tended to engage in more preventative efforts to avoid the stressor (Turner & Avison).

Research has also revealed that finding meaning in life's adversity may be important in regaining or maintaining mental and physical health (Silver, Boon, & Stones, 1983). Weisman and Worden (1976) suggested that those cancer patients who were able to find something meaningful in their illness were least distressed by their condition. In a similar vein, Riessman (1990) conducted in-depth interviews with divorced individuals. Interestingly, despite the fact that both males and females who underwent divorce reported that they were more likely to drink in excess during and immediately after the divorce, they also described positive consequences that followed from their postdivorce adjustment.

As has been noted previously, there has been little research on what ways, if any, athletes may come to view their injuries in a positive manner. One exception to this has been the work of Udry et al. (1997), which involved retrospective interviews with elite injured athletes. Specifically, 21 athletes who had skied for the United States ski team were asked about their psychological reactions to season-ending injuries. Not surprisingly, athletes in this study reported in rich detail the negative affect that accompanied their injuries. This was reflected in statements such as "There was a lot of depression," "I just felt numb," "I was just really miserable." Thus, it was clear that for these athletes, who were highly invested in their sport, experiencing a season-ending injury was a distinct stumbling block. However, somewhat paradoxically, skiers in this study were also asked whether there were positive consequences associated with their injuries. Approximately 95% of the athletes reported one or more positive consequences from their injuries. When these athletes' comments regarding their injuries were content analyzed, it was found their responses coalesced into three general categories: personal growth, psychologically based performance enhancements, and physical-technical development.

The personal growth category was mentioned by approximately 80% of the athletes and included comments such as "I learned how to help other injured skiers" and "After I was hurt, I tried to be sure to write those girls (injured teammates) letters and faxes and whatever to be sure that they know I am thinking about them and can't wait for them to get better." Thus, athletes seemed to be saying they felt they were better people after their injury because their injury taught them how to be more empathetic toward other injured athletes. In addition, another salient idea that was captured within this category related to the idea of developing skills and interests outside of the skiing realm. This was reflected in comments such as "I developed different (non-ski) sides of self" and "I had time to go back to school." Hence, athletes felt their injuries provided them with compelling evidence of their physical vulnerability, and as a result, they began to seek out more experiences in non-physical settings.

The second category of positive consequences of mentioned by injured athletes was psychologically based performance enhancements, which was mentioned by approximately 80% of the athletes. This category captured comments such as "I became mentally tougher," "It (injury) gave me a greater work ethic," and "I learned what I can and can't do." In short, this category encompassed the ways in which athletes felt that their injury psychologically enhanced their approach to training and/or performing.

The final category, physical-technical developments was mentioned by 48% of the athletes. This third category of responses encompassed comments such as "I got more aggressive with my physical training," "I learned to ski technically better," and "I learned what my body can handle." Hence, this category of responses captured that idea that injured athletes felt they learned more about their bodies and how the body responds to training demands.

At this time the Udry et al. (1997) work is one of the few systematic explorations of the possible long-term positive consequences of athletic injuries. Therefore, numerous unanswered questions remain relative to understanding what psychological and/or contextual factors contribute to athletes' perceptions of the positive consequences of injuries. For example, it is not known whether certain *dispositional* variables (e.g., optimism, hardiness, locus of control) are likely to be associated with an increased likelihood that athletes will report positive consequences from their injuries. Oltjenbruns (1991), reporting on research with adolescents who experienced the death of family member or friend, found that individuals with an internal (versus external) locus of control were more likely to report having improved communication with others as a positive consequence of their grief experience. Thus, there has been some suggestion that dispositional factors influence how individuals interpret life's misfortunes. Alternatively, it may be that certain *situational* factors contribute to whether injured athletes perceive positive consequences from their injuries. Bulman and Wortman (1977) conducted interviews with individuals who had experienced severe accidents. They noted that people who were involved in freely chosen activities (e.g., diving) at the time of their accident tended to cope better with their loss of health than did those who were injured in other ways (e.g., paralyzed from a car accident whereby the other driver was at fault). Implication? It may be that athletes are more likely to derive meaning from their injuries because sport is typically an activity in which athletes make a decision on whether or not to participate. To summarize, although research in related areas has hinted at some of the factors that contribute to individuals' perceptions of the meaning and positive consequences of adversity, the extent to which these findings apply to injured athletes is not known. Thus, additional research is needed to identify more precisely the dispositional and situational factors that contribute to the extent to which athletes derive positive consequences from their injuries.

Recommendations for Facilitating Positive Consequences From Athletic Injuries

The previous sections have explored whether individuals in general and athletes in particular may grow from unfortunate circumstances such as injuries. However, it would be naive and unrealistic to simply assume that athletes will universally and effortlessly experience numerous benefits from their injuries. In fact, it would be argued that if these types of assumptions are made by individuals who come into contact with injured athletes, the stress associated with injuries may be exacerbated. Rather, the approach that is taken here is that it may be possible to facilitate the process by which athletes derive positive consequences from their injuries. It is in this light that the following recommendations are forwarded (and summarized in Table 1).

Table 1. Summary of Recommendations for Facilitating Positive Consequences From Athletic Injuries

• Recognize that deriving positive consequences takes effort.
• Recognize different problem-solving strategies can be used (e.g., reversals, extrications).
• Recognize that reframing may not occur immediately.
• Avoid secondary victimization.
• Acknowledge that positive consequences may extend beyond the individual athlete.

Recognize That Deriving Positive Consequences Takes Effort

Counseling therapists often use the term "grief work" to describe the process by which individuals learn to deal with the sudden loss of a loved one. This language implies that the process of coming to terms with loss is one that requires effort. It is suggested that this perspective is useful when thinking about the possible positive consequences of athletic injuries. That is, injured athletes must not passively assume positive consequences will occur; rather they must also do this "work." This notion is reinforced if one examines the language used by injured athletes in the Udry et al. (1997) study relative to the positive consequences of injuries. Specifically, athletes used terms such as "learned" or "recognized" to describe how they felt they grew from their injuries. These types of descriptions suggest these athletes were engaged in the process of counterbalancing their misfortune. As Thoits (1995) has noted when we try to understand how individuals respond to adversity we should not ignore the fact that individuals are often activists on their own behalf.

Recognize Different Problem-Solving Strategies Can Be Used

If deriving positive outcomes from injuries requires effort then the next question becomes "What types of problem-solving efforts can be used to counterbalance adversity?" Thoits (1994) highlights two types of problem-solving efforts that may have implications for injured athletes: *reversals* and *extrications*. Reversals occur when individuals act to "reverse" or convert a negative situation into a positive one, or at the very least, into a less negative situation. For instance, Leslie Visser, a well-known television sportscaster was severely injured when she fell while running in New York City's Central Park. Visser's injuries included shattered bones in her legs, a dislocated hip, torn hamstring and groin muscles, and facial lacerations. Fortunately for Visser, a passerby saw Visser lying on the ground and quickly called an ambulance. Visser's advocate ordered the ambulance to go to New York's Lenox Hill Hospital—a hospital renowned for its reputation for treating orthopedic injuries. Despite her serious injuries and lengthy rehabilitation, Visser optimistically commented:

> I suppose I've always looked at the glass as half full, but I really believe I was lucky. Of all the places I could have been injured, it was New York, with the best emergency care in the world. Of all the hospitals I could have ended up in, it was Lenox Hill, the very top for my type of injury. (quoted in Donaldson, 1994, p. 35)

In this instance, Visser reversed what many would have viewed as a negative situation (i.e., being severely injured) and chose to view her situation as positive because she was able to access highly competent medical care. Alternatively, individuals may extricate themselves from a negative situation by voluntarily relinquishing problematic roles (Thoits, 1994). For instance, an injured athlete who has been unable to make a successful return to sport following an injury may free him- or herself from the ongoing problems of being in this situation by leaving the sport. In this instance, the athlete is first extricated; then he or she must reverse the situation by finding a new and, it is hoped, better situation in which to be immersed.

Recognize That Reframing May Not Occur Immediately

Although Udry et al. (1997) found that the majority of injured athletes reported one or more positive outcomes from their injuries, it is important to note that it may not be possible for injured athletes to immediately derive any positive outcomes from their injuries. The work of Udry et al. was based on interviews with athletes who were interviewed, on average, 2.7 years after experiencing their injury. It is not yet known at what stage in the injury recovery process that athletes are likely to be able to perceive that they derived any long-term benefits from their injuries. In the general psychology literature, Miller and Porter (1980) have presented evidence that attributions for events change over time. Based on the above, it would be realistic to expect that a considerable amount of time may be needed before injured athletes are able to counterbalance the negative aspects of their injuries.

Avoid Secondary Victimization

Although it has been suggested that injured athletes at some point grow from their injury experiences, it is imperative for those who come in contact with injured athletes not to trivialize or minimize the experiences of injured athletes. Shumaker and Brownell (1984) discuss the notion of "secondary victimization" whereby victims are victimized once again by awkward or inadequate expressions of concern. Thus, statements to an injured athlete such as "You're lucky to be injured because now you'll have time to concentrate on school" or "It's not that bad—you'll grow from this" may serve to increase rather than diminish the stress athletes experience from being injured.

Acknowledge That Positive Consequences of Injuries May Extend Beyond the Individual Athlete

Although athletic injuries occur to individuals, they often have significant ramifications for those close to the injured athletes. As a result individuals whose lives are intertwined with the injured athletes must often also work to counterbalance the negative impact of injuries. Consider the case of Chamique Holdsclaw, a gifted player who went to play for the legendary University of Tennessee women's basketball team. In her freshman year, Holdsclaw partially tore a ligament in her right knee. Holdsclaw's injury clearly diminished her ability to perform up to the high expectations of this championship team. Interestingly, Holdsclaw's coach, Pat Summit noted, "When she (Chamique) went down, all the others realized they had to do more. It made us a better team . . . " (quoted in Gelin, 1996, p. 104). Thus, the growth processes associated with injuries are not necessarily limited to the athlete who is injured but may extend to those close to the injured athlete.

Conclusion

The emotional turmoil that is frequently associated with athletic injuries is not disputed. However, it is suggested that there may be important positive consequences associated with athletic injuries. Three conceptual models of stress and adversity have been examined: Selye's (1974) General Adaptation Syndrome (GAS), Erikson's normal personality development (1959), and Danish, Petitpas, and Hale's (1995) Life Development Model (LDM). A similarity of these models is that they all suggest that individuals' growth and development may be stimulated by some form of stress or crisis (e.g., injuries). Research with injured athletes has supported the idea that athletes may experience a variety of positive outcomes from injures (Udry et al., 1997). Recommendations for facilitating the development of positive consequences from injuries were discussed.

References

Brewer, B. W., Linder, D. E., & Phelps, C. M. (1995). Situational correlates of emotional adjustment to athletic injury. *Clinical Journal of Sports Medicine, 5,* 241–245.

Brewer, B. W., Petitpas, A. J., Van Raalte, J. L., Sklar, J. H., & Ditmar, T. D. (1995). Prevalence of psychological distress among patients at a physical therapy clinic specializing in sports medicine. *Sports Medicine Training and Rehabilitation, 6,* 139 145.

Bulman, R. J., & Wortman, C. B. (1977). Attributions of blame and coping in the "real world". Severe accidents victims react to their lot. *Journal of Personality and Social Psychology, 35,* 351–363.

Crossman, J., & Jamieson, J. (1985). Differences in perceptions of seriousness of disrupting effects of athletic injury as viewed by athletes and their trainer. *Perceptual and Motor Skills, 61,* 1131–1134.

Danish, S. J., Petitpas, A., & Hale, B. D. (1995). Psychological interventions: A life developmental model. In S. Murphy (Ed.), *Sport psychology interventions* (pp. 19–38). Champaign: Human Kinetics.

Donaldson, G. (1994, October). Adding insight to injury. *Women's Sports and Fitness,* 33–37.

Erikson, E. H. (1959). Identity and the life cycle. *Psychological Issues, 1*(1), 18–171.

Gelin, D. (1996, December 2). Bound for glory. *Sports Illustrated,* 100–104.

Gould, D., Udry, E., Bridges, D., & Beck, L. (1997). Stress sources encountered when rehabilitating from season-ending ski injuries. *The Sport Psychologist, 11,* 381–403.

Heil, J. (1993). *Psychology of sport injury.* Champaign: Human Kinetics.

Leddy, M. H., Lambert, M. J., & Ogles, B. M. (1994). Psychological consequences of athletic injury among high level competitors. *Research Quarterly for Exercise and Sport, 65,* 347–354.

Lieber, J. (1991, July 29). Deep scars. *Sports Illustrated,* 37–44.

Miller, D. T., & Porter, C. A. (1980). Effects of temporal perspective on the attribution process. *Journal of Personality and Social Psychology, 39,* 532–540.

Oltjenbruns, K.A. (1991). Positive outcomes of adolescents' experience with grief. *Journal of Adolescent Research, 6*(1), 43–53.

Petitpas, A., & Danish, S. (1994). Caring for injured athletes. In S. Murphy (Ed.), *Sport psychology interventions* (pp. 255–281). Champaign: Human Kinetics.

Reissman, C. K. (1990). *Divorce talk: Women and men make sense of personal relationships.* New Brunswick: Rutgers University Press.

Selye, H. (1974). *Stress without distress.* New York: Signet.

Shumaker, S. A., & Brownell, A. (1984). Toward a theory of social support: Closing conceptual gaps. *Journal of Social Issues, 40*(4), 11–36.

Silver, R. L., Boon, C., & Stones, M. H. (1983). Searching for meaning in misfortune: Making sense of incest. *Journal of Social Issues, 39*(2), 81–102.

Smith, A., Scott, S., O'Fallon, W., & Young, M. (1990). Emotional responses of athletes to injury. *Mayo Clinic Proceedings, 65,* 38–50.

Thoits, P. A. (1994). Stressors and problem-solving: The individual as psychologist. *Journal of Health and Social Behavior, 35,* 143–159.

Thoits, P. A. (1995). Stress, coping, and social support processes: Where are we? What next? *Journal of Health and Social Behavior*(extra issue), 53–79.

Turner, R. J., & Avison, W. R. (1992). Innovations in the measurement of life stress: Crisis theory and the significance of event resolution. *Journal of Health and Social Behavior, 33,* 36–50.

Udry, E., Gould, D., Bridges, D., & Beck, L. (1997). Down but not out: Athlete responses to season-ending injuries. *Journal of Sport and Exercise Psychology, 19,* 229–248.

Weisman, A. D., & Worden, J. W. (1976). The existential plight in cancer: Significance of the first 100 days. *International Journal of Psychiatry in Medicine, 7,* 1–15.

7

Personality Correlates of Psychological Processes During Injury Rehabilitation

J. Robert Grove
Theresa Bianco
The University of Western Australia

Psychological theory suggests a link between personality and the thoughts, feelings, and behaviors of athletes during rehabilitation. Research on the personality correlates of cognitions, mood states, and coping behaviors indicates that neuroticism, explanatory style, optimism, and hardiness might be particularly important dispositional factors in this regard. Knowledge about these traits may therefore help sports medicine personnel to anticipate, understand, and deal with undesirable rehabilitation responses. For that reason, formal and informal assessment approaches are examined, and behavior management strategies are discussed in relation to these personality traits.

Theoretical models of the rehabilitation process identify a variety of situational and personal factors that could influence an injured athlete's thoughts, feelings, actions, and rehabilitation outcomes (Brewer, 1994; Gordon, 1986; Grove, 1993; Wiese-Bjornstal & Smith, 1993). Situational factors include injury-related variables (e.g., type, severity, progress/status) as well as treatment-related variables (e.g., facilities, time demands, pain, medical personnel) and various "external influences" (e.g., life stress, social support, pressure to return). Personal factors include general demographic variables (e.g., age) as well as injury history, coping resources, psychological skills, and personality traits. In this chapter, we focus on personality factors as a correlate of cognitions, mood states, and coping strategies in injury rehabilitation. We review research findings that link selected personality traits to these psychological processes, and we outline the possible implications of these relationships for the rehabilitation behavior of injured athletes. We conclude by discussing ways that sports medicine personnel can obtain information about relevant personality traits, and we suggest potential uses for this information.

Personality and Health

Reviews of the connection between personality and health suggest that a number of traits are potential correlates of health status (Eysenck, 1988; Friedman, 1990; Friedman & Booth-Kewley, 1987; Rodin & Salovey, 1989; Scheier & Bridges, 1995; Taylor, 1990). Four of these personality factors (neuroticism, explanatory style, dispositional optimism, and hardiness) are examined here. These particular factors have been selected because their documented connection to thought processes, emotional reactions, and/or coping behaviors suggests that they are likely to influence the athlete's psychological and behavioral responses during injury rehabilitation.

Neuroticism

Neuroticism is a basic dimension of personality that reflects a general tendency toward emotional lability and negative affect (Eysenck & Eysenck, 1985; McCrae & John, 1992; Watson & Clark, 1984). This trait has logical and empirical links to recovery-relevant constructs such as stress reactivity, distress proneness, and symptom reports (Bolger & Schilling, 1991; Ormal & Wohlfarth, 1991; Watson & Pennebaker, 1989). For example, Bolger and Zuckerman (1995) reported that students high in neuroticism experienced more conflict in their daily lives than did those low in neuroticism. In addition, those high in neuroticism used more confrontive coping, which, in turn, contributed to more interpersonal problems. Thus, neuroticism contributed to both greater exposure and greater reactivity to stress.

Although there is limited evidence linking neuroticism with cognitive, emotional, or behavioral responses to sport injuries, there is abundant evidence that such injuries produce generalized negative affect, especially when they are severe (Daly, Brewer, Van Raalte, Petitpas, & Sklar, 1995; McDonald

& Hardy, 1990; Meyers, Sterling, Calvo, Marley, & Duhon, 1991; Pearson & Jones, 1992; Smith, Scott, O'Fallon, & Young, 1990). In a study of elite skiers who had sustained serious sport injuries, for example, Bianco (1996) reported that typical emotional responses included disappointment, frustration, confusion, and depression. One athlete who suffered a career-ending injury summarized it this way: "There was pain because I had the surgery; pain because I knew my career was over. It was probably the moment I suffered the most in my life, both mentally and physically. It was pain all over" (quoted in Bianco).

If high levels of neuroticism are associated with selective attention to (or an exaggeration of) these negative emotions in response to injury, then various types of maladaptive behavior and rehabilitation difficulties could ensue (cf. Sanderson, 1981). Inappropriate displays of anger could be one form of maladaptive behavior exhibited by individuals with strong neurotic tendencies. Impatience, irritability, and hostility are known to correlate positively with neuroticism (Costa & McCrae, 1992), and the stressful nature of the rehabilitation process increases the likelihood of these sorts of negative reactions. Hostile outbursts can also contribute to relationship strain between the patient and health professional and therefore result in withdrawal of support. Silver, Wortman, and Crofton (1990) have shown that communicating a need for social support by showing distress often led to rejection rather than eliciting support, and Ford and Gordon (1993) have also reported that injured athletes who exhibited distress were rated as least desirable to treat by sport physiotherapists. Unfortunately, the distress of injury can frequently cause athletes to direct negative emotional reactions toward health-care professionals: "I was not a nice person to be around. I just wasn't easy to get along with. I'd be moody and was just not happy a lot of the time. I was kind of frustrated, and I got into arguments with my doctor" (quoted in Bianco, 1996).

Another form of maladaptive behavior among highly neurotic athletes could be a tendency to rely on inefficient coping strategies. Neurotic tendencies have been reliably linked to the use of certain types of coping strategies, and these same strategies appear to be negatively related to coping effectiveness in the health domain. More specifically, various measures of neuroticism have exhibited positive correlations with avoidance-oriented and emotion-oriented coping strategies, such as denial, escapist fantasy, withdrawal, passivity, selfblame, wishful thinking, indecisiveness, emotional focus/venting, sedation, and mental/behavioral disengagement (Costa & McRae, 1989; Endler & Parker, 1990; Kardum & Hudek-Knezevic, 1996; McCrae & Costa, 1986; Scheier, Carver, & Bridges, 1994). At the same time, neuroticism has been shown to correlate negatively with problem-focused coping strategies involving direct action and active coping (Endler & Parker, 1990; Parkes, 1986; Rim, 1986; Scheier et al.,

1994). These relationships between neurotic tendencies and coping behaviors could have important consequences for injury rehabilitation because the medical literature shows that patients who use passive/avoidant, emotion-focused coping strategies often have more difficulty adjusting to health problems than do those who use more active, problem-focused strategies (Maes, Leventhal, & de Ridder, 1996; Zeidner & Saklofske, 1996).

Explanatory Style

Explanatory style is the way an individual typically accounts for significant events in his or her life. In other words, it is a relatively permanent tendency to explain things in a certain way. Individuals who exhibit a *pessimistic explanatory style* tend to explain negative events as personally caused (e.g., "It's my own fault I got injured"), stable over time (e.g., "I'm never going to get back all my mobility"), and global in nature (e.g., "It's going to affect my entire life"). At the same time, these individuals tend to explain positive events as externally caused (e.g., "Healing just takes time"), unstable over time (e.g., "My progress is likely to be up and down"), and specific in nature (e.g., "My recovery depends on this particular therapist and treatment").

A decade of research investigating the links between explanatory style and health has demonstrated a connection between pessimistic explanatory style and negative health consequences. Simply put, individuals who attribute bad events to internal, stable, and global causes experience poorer health than do their more optimistic counterparts who explain bad events with external, unstable, and specific causes (Peterson, 1995). Kamen and Seligman (1987) suggested that links between pessimism and immune system function might underlie this relationship, and in a study investigating this hypothesis, they found that older adults with a pessimistic explanatory style did indeed exhibit lowered immunocompetence (Kamen-Siegel, Rodin, Seligman, & Dwyer, 1991). Mundane passivity in the face of disease could be another possible mechanism contributing to the relationship between pessimistic explanatory style and poor health (Lin & Peterson, 1990). Kamen and Seligman noted that pessimists are passive with regard to self-help, self-care, and life challenges. Finally, it is also possible that pessimistic explanatory style increases the chances of social isolation, loneliness, and/or depression. Interestingly, all three of these factors have been noted as indicators of poor psychological adjustment among injured athletes (Gordon, Milios, & Grove, 1991a).

Dispositional Optimism

Scheier and Carver (1985, 1987, 1992) have discussed the health-related consequences of a personality variable that bears some resemblance to explanatory style. They call this variable *dispositional optimism* and define it simply as a general expectancy for good rather than bad outcomes to occur. It has been suggested that these positive expectancies might influence health via physiological or behavioral/interpersonal pathways, or both (Peterson & Bossio, 1991; Scheier & Carver, 1987). Investigations of the proposed physiological mechanisms have not obtained consistent results, but some studies have found differences in cardiovascular reactivity and immunological functioning to be associated with individual differences in optimism. Van Treuren and Hull (1986), for example, found that optimists were less reactive than pessimists when blood pressure and pulse rate responses were monitored during exposure to positive and negative events (Scheier & Carver, 1987). There is also some evidence that an optimistic orientation is positively related to natural killer-cell activity (Bachen et al., cited in Scheier & Carver, 1992; Levy & Wise, 1987), whereas a pessimistic orientation is associated with disease progression (Goodkin, Antoni, & Blaney, 1986).

Studies of the proposed behavioral mechanisms have been more consistent in their findings. Taylor and Aspinwall (1996) summarize these findings by suggesting that optimism may mitigate the stress-illness relationship by facilitating successful coping efforts, preventing stressful events from intruding into other aspects of life, and encouraging better health practices. Coping appears to be a particularly important behavioral mechanism, and it has been repeatedly shown that optimists tend to cope by accepting the reality of negative situations, seeking social support, engaging in positive reinterpretation, and using direct, problem-focused coping strategies (Scheier & Carver, 1987, 1992). At the same time, optimists tend *not* to deny the reality of negative situations, disengage from their coping efforts, and become preoccupied with their emotional distress:

> As soon as you can start moving your toes, you move your toes. As soon as you can start moving your leg, you move your leg. As soon as you can walk, you walk . . . I think you have highs and lows. But I always say to myself, no matter how bad it gets, it always gets better. So even if I was really down, I didn't worry about it. I just looked on ahead and knew that it would get better. (quoted in Bianco, 1996)

A compelling demonstration of the potential link between optimism and health was provided in a study of recovery from coronary artery bypass surgery (Scheier et al., 1989). In that investigation, optimists and pessimists were compared on mood states and coping strategies prior to surgery, physiological reactions during surgery, and recovery progress after surgery. The findings indicated that optimism had positive consequences at all three points in time. Specifically, optimists reported less hostility and depression than did pessimists immediately prior to surgery. Optimists also made plans and set goals for recovery prior to the operation to a greater extent than pessimists did, and optimists exhibited fewer adverse physiological reactions during surgery than did the pessimists. In addition, optimists tended to recover faster than pessimists, both in terms of objective recovery indices and in terms of subjective ratings of improvement by members of the rehabilitation team. Finally, there was a strong relationship ($r = .57$, $d = 1.39$) between presurgery optimism and self-reported quality of life 6 months after the operation.

The importance of an optimistic outlook has also been demonstrated in relation to sport injury rehabilitation. More specifically, Ievleva and Orlick (1991) found that such an outlook correlated negatively ($r = -.21$, $d = .44$) with the time needed for athletes to recover from Grade II ankle and knee injuries.[1] Bianco (1996) obtained additional evidence for the central role of an optimistic orientation during sport injury rehabilitation in her interview study of elite skiers confronted with long and difficult recovery periods:

> The more positive you keep, the more you can really believe that you can come back full strength to compete as good, or better, than you did before the injury. That's what really keeps you driving and working through the pain and the setbacks . . . I'm a pretty positive person. I see the good in everything. You've got to turn everything into good. Sometimes when bad things happen, I just remember that in a month or two, I'll look back at the situation and laugh—so that makes it a lot easier. (quoted)

Hardiness

Hardiness is another personality trait believed to moderate the effects of stress on physical and mental health. Hardiness represents a "constellation of personality characteristics that function as a resistance resource in the encounter with stressful life events" (Kobasa, Maddi, & Kahn, 1982, p. 169). It is composed of three interrelated elements: commitment, challenge, and control. *Commitment* refers to a strong belief in one's own value and self-worth as well as a sense of purpose and involvement in whatever one is doing. *Challenge* refers to a tendency to view difficulties and change as problems to be over-

---

1. We provide Cohen's d as an estimate of effect size rather than the more traditional p-value because of the disparate sample sizes in the studies cited. Unlike significance levels, this statistic is independent of sample size, with small, moderate, and large effect sizes indicated by ds of approximately .20, .50, and .80, respectively (Cohen, 1988).

come rather than threats to one's personal security. Individuals scoring high in challenge exhibit a high degree of cognitive flexibility that permits effective appraisal of potentially threatening events. *Control* involves a sense of personal power over the events in one's life. Individuals with a strong sense of control assume responsibility for their actions and are able to avert feelings of helplessness through the use of effective thinking, decision-making, and coping strategies. Simply put, hardy people are committed to what they are doing in their lives; they believe they have personal control over the solutions to life problems; and they view adaptation and change as opportunities for growth rather than as threats.

Research conducted by Kobasa and colleagues has linked hardiness to physical health both retrospectively and prospectively. Kobasa (1979), for example, measured various elements of the hardiness construct and self-reported illness among executives from a utility company. Groups of executives experiencing low rather than high levels of illness over the previous 3 years were characterized by a high level of commitment (vs. alienation), a perception of meaningfulness in their activities, and an internal locus of control. These findings were viewed as consistent with the three-dimensional model of hardiness outlined above. In another study, Kobasa et al. (1982) collected data on personality and previous illness from a group of middle-aged male executives. These individuals were then followed for 2 years, with illness data recorded at the end of each 12-month period. Results once again supported the importance of the hardiness construct within the health domain. Specifically, the executives who were low in hardiness experienced high levels of illness when exposed to stressful environments, but the executives who were high in hardiness had self-reported illness scores that were close to baseline under these conditions.

The mechanisms underlying the connection between hardiness and health have been debated (cf. Hull, Van Treuren, & Virnelli, 1987), but it has been suggested that both appraisal and coping processes contribute to this relationship (Florian, Mikulincer, & Taubman, 1995; Gentry & Kobasa, 1984). More specifically, individuals high in hardiness seem to evaluate and interpret potentially stressful experiences in a way that minimizes their negative impact (Allred & Smith, 1989; Wiebe, 1991). Even when stress is perceived, however, hardy individuals have a tendency to rely on adaptive rather than maladaptive coping strategies (Blaney & Ganellen, 1990; Nowack, 1989). This tendency is nicely illustrated by the findings of Williams, Wiebe, and Smith (1992), who examined relationships between hardiness and coping in a group of university undergraduates. Williams et al. observed significant negative correlations between avoidance-oriented coping and three hardiness variables (commitment, control, total hardiness score) as well as significant positive correlations between problem-focused coping, seeking of social support, and the commitment component of hardiness.

Studies of Injured Athletes

Although personality variables have not been extensively examined in connection with cognitions, emotions, and coping among injured athletes, there is some evidence that neuroticism, explanatory style, dispositional optimism, and hardiness are related to these psychological processes. Grove, Stewart, and Gordon (1990), for example, investigated emotional reactions among 21 sport performers who underwent knee reconstruction surgery because of anterior cruciate ligament (ACL) damage. The athletes completed questionnaire measures of hardiness and dispositional optimism, and they provided periodic explanations for their rehabilitation progress that were transformed into an index of explanatory style. The athletes also responded to a mood state inventory once a week for 3 months following surgery. The mood state inventory assessed seven moods (tension, depression, anger, fatigue, confusion, vigor, and esteem-related affect) that were then correlated with scores on the personality measures. The results are summarized in Table 1.

Several aspects of the data in Table 1 deserve comment. First, all three personality factors exhibited potentially meaningful relationships to mood during the first 3 months of recovery from knee reconstruction surgery. Second, the direction of these relationships was generally consistent with expectations based on a conceptual understanding of the hardiness, optimism, and explanatory-style constructs. More specifically, negative emotions, such as tension, depression, and anger, exhibited inverse relationships with hardiness and optimism but direct relationships with explanatory pessimism. Positive emotions, such as vigor and esteem-related affect, on the other hand, exhibit mostly direct relationships with hardiness and optimism but inverse relationships with explanatory pessimism. Third, depression, fatigue, confusion, and vigor were the most consistent correlates of the personality factors assessed in this study, with 8 of 9, 6 of 9, 6 of 9, and 5 of 9 relationships exhibiting effect sizes of .50 or more, respectively. Finally, although hardiness appeared to be the least influential of the three personality measures, this might have been due to the use of a composite hardiness index rather than separate indices of the three hardiness components. Hull et al. (1987) as well Carver (1989) have taken issue with Kobasa's (1979) claim that hardiness is a unitary, higher order personality factor, and they recommend separating the challenge, commitment, and control dimensions for purposes of analysis. Supplementary analyses of our data using separate hardiness dimensions indicated that the challenge component exhibited a larger number of substantial correlations in

Table 1. Personality and Mood State Relationships in the 3 Months Following Knee Reconstruction Surgery (Grove et al., 1990).

Time Period and Mood Variable	Hardiness Total	Optimism Total	Explanatory Pessimism
First month			
Tension	-.22*	-.30*	+.46**
Depression	-.24*	-.27*	+.37**
Anger	-.06	-.12	+.26*
Fatigue	-.38**	-.32*	+.47
Confusion	-.22*	-.32*	+.37**
Vigor	-.03	+.04	-.44**
Esteem	-.17	+.01	-.34*
Second Month			
Tension	-.08	-.04	+.44**
Depression	-.25*	-.28*	+.42**
Anger	-.04	-.13	+.36**
Fatigue	-.20	+.01	+.35*
Confusion	-.16	-.25*	+.50**
Vigor	-.03	+.26*	-.41**
Esteem	-.08	+.16	-.28*
Third Month			
Tension	-.15	+.04	+.30
Depression	-.24*	-.35	+.19
Anger	-.15	-.35*	+.13
Fatigue	-.31*	-.21	+.38**
Confusion	-.23*	-.33*	+.37**
Vigor	+.22*	+.48**	-.39**
Esteem	+.16	+.39**	-.20

* Moderate effect size ($d > .45$, but $d < .75$)[1]
** Large effect size ($d > .75$)

the expected direction than did the composite index, the commitment dimension, or the control dimension.

In a subsequent study of coping among injured athletes (Grove & Bahnsen, 1997), neuroticism was also investigated as a correlate of psychological processes during rehabilitation. In that study, 72 athletes who had received 4–6 weeks of treatment for a sport-related injury during the past 6 months completed a neuroticism scale and also supplied information about the strategies they had used to cope with the stress of the injury and its rehabilitation. Relationships were then examined among neuroticism, injury severity, coping strategies, and the amount of time needed for full physical recovery. Selected findings are summarized in Table 2. The data indicated that the use of certain coping strategies during rehabilitation was positively related to neuroticism but unrelated to injury severity. The types of coping strategies exhibiting the strongest relationships to neuroticism were primarily emotion focused or avoidant in nature, or both, and they included emotional focus/venting, denial, mental disengagement, and alcohol/drug use. Several of these same coping strategies also exhibited positive correlations with the length of the recovery period. That is, increased use of emotional focus/venting, denial, and mental disengagement was associated not only with higher levels of neuroticism but also with longer recovery periods. Although not noted in Table 2, it is worth mentioning that these relationships occurred in the absence of a direct association between neuroticism and recovery time ($r = -.02$, $d = .04$).

Table 2. Correlations of Neuroticism, Injury Severity, and Recovery Time With Self-Reported Use of Selected Coping Strategies by Injured Athletes (Grove & Bahnsen, 1997)

Coping Strategies	Neuroticism	Injury Severity	Recovery Time (Weeks)
Focus on Vent Emotions	-.42**	+.02	+.30*
Positive Reinterpretation	+.36**	+.17	+.32*
Denial	+.34*	-.04	+.27*
Mental Disengagement	+.33*	+.01	+.36**
Behavioral Disengagement	+.32*	-.01	+.14
Turning to Religion	+.28*	+.14	+.13
Alcohol & Drug Use	+.28*	+.01	+.08
Restraint Coping	+.20	-.02	-.01
Emotional Social Support	+.18	+.07	+.05
Active Coping	-.16	-.13	-.13
Instrumental Social Suport	-.14	-.14	-.32*
Suppress Competing Activities	+.11	+.03	-.02
Planning	-.10	-.03	-.01
Humor	+.02	+.12	-.03
Acceptance	-.01	+.11	-.11

* Moderate effect size ($d > .45$, but $d < .75$)[1]
** Large effect size ($d > .75$)

Overall, the findings from these two studies are consistent with the more general literature on the psychological correlates of neuroticism, explanatory style, optimism, and hardiness in the health domain. More important, however, they show that these dispositional constructs are related to the cognitive and behavioral responses of injured athletes during rehabilitation. Individuals who interact with injured athletes might therefore be in a better position to understand their reactions and offer assistance if they know how to obtain information about these personality traits.

Methods of Obtaining Personality Information

There are basically two ways that personality information can be collected by practitioners. These two procedures are best used in a complementary fashion, but they will be discussed separately here for ease of exposition. A "formal" approach to personality assessment involves the use of written scales. The advantage of this approach is that it is time-efficient and quantifiable. At the same time, however, it can sometimes be perceived as impersonal by the athlete. The alternative method, "informal" personality assessment, involves an analysis of statements or behaviors, or both, that arise spontaneously in face-to-face interactions. This approach is less directive and allows the therapist considerable latitude to pursue issues that he or she thinks are meaningful. It does tend to be less precise than the formal approach, however, and, for that reason, may require more experience on the part of the therapist.

Formal Assessment Procedures

The personality factors discussed in this chapter can be measured with relatively short pen-and-paper scales, and sports medicine personnel can obtain written information on these traits with very little inconvenience to the athlete. Relevant scales can be administered in the waiting area prior to treatment, during periods of passive treatment (e.g., icing), or as part of a posttreatment debriefing. If the athlete is presented with one scale per session, practitioners can obtain a reasonably comprehensive personality profile in just three or four treatment sessions.

Neuroticism. Because neuroticism is recognized as a basic dimension of personality in numerous theoretical models, many different scales are available to assess this trait. The classic measure, however, is the 23-item neuroticism subscale from the Eysenck Personality Questionnaire (EPQ-N; Eysenck & Eysenck, 1975). This subscale requires simple yes/no responses to questions like "Does your mood often go up and down?" and "Are your feelings easily hurt?" Scores range from 0 to 23 according to the number of "yes" responses. Similar items appear in form of statements on the 48-item neuroticism subscale of the Revised NEO Personality Inventory (NEOPIR-N; Costa & McCrae, 1992), but responses are made on a 5-point scale ranging from strongly disagree to strongly agree. Although longer than the EPQ-N scale, the NEOPIR neuroticism scale offers the advantage of providing separate scores for six different aspects of neuroticism rather than just a single neuroticism score. Information about these subcomponents (anxiety, angry hostility, depression, self-consciousness, impulsiveness, and vulnerability) could be useful to sports medicine personnel in some circumstances. A shortened, 12-item version of the NEOPIR neuroticism scale is also available, but it is less reliable than the 48-item scale and does not provide scores for the subcomponents (Costa & McCrae, 1992). Nevertheless, this brief scale could be useful if time constraints are a problem.

Explanatory style. Scales that measure explanatory style typically list a series of positive and/or negative events and ask the respondents to indicate what the most likely cause of each event would have been if it had happened to them. The causal statements are then categorized along several different dimensions, and conclusions are drawn about the person's typical ways of interpreting good and bad events. A number of general explanatory-style scales could be used to measure explanatory pessimism among injured athletes in this fashion. These general scales include several versions of the Attributional Style Questionnaire (ASQ; Peterson et al., 1982; Peterson & Villanova, 1988; Whitley, 1991), the Balanced Attributional Style Questionnaire (BASQ; Feather & Tiggemann, 1984), and the Attributional Style Assessment Test (ASAT; Anderson, Horowitz, & French, 1983; Anderson & Riger, 1991). The Revised Causal Dimension Scale (CDSII; McAuley, Duncan, & Russell, 1992) could also be used, but its standard format specifies a single event rather than multiple events. Two sport-specific instruments are also available: the Wingate Sport Achievement Responsibility Scale (WSARS; Tenenbaum, Furst, & Weingarten, 1984) and the Sport Attributional Style Scale (SASS; Hanrahan & Grove, 1990a; Hanrahan, Grove, & Hattie, 1989). The SASS allows the athlete to generate his or her own causal statements in an open-ended response format, whereas the WSARS uses forced-choice responses. A short form of the SASS has also been developed (Hanrahan & Grove, 1990b), and it, therefore, may be the instrument of choice in sport medicine settings.

Dispositional optimism. A variety of instruments are available to measure trait optimism. These instruments include the Expected Balance Scale (EBS; Staats, 1989), the Optimism and Pessimism Scale (OPS; Dember, Martin, Hummer, Howe, & Melton, 1989), and the Life Orientation Test (LOT; Scheier & Carver, 1985). The LOT offers the advantages of being brief, well researched, and readily accessible, so it is arguably the instrument of choice for assessing this construct in sport medicine settings. The most recent version of this instrument (Revised LOT; Scheier et al., 1994) contains just 10 items, with 3 of them worded in a positive direction and 3 of them worded in a negative direction. The remaining 4 statements are filler items and do not contribute to the score on the scale (Scheier et al., 1994). Respondents are simply asked to indicate the extent to which they agree or disagree with each of the statements. Response categories and their numerical equivalents are as follows: strongly agree (4); agree (3); neutral (2); disagree (1); strongly disagree (0). A total score for dispositional optimism is obtained by reverse-scoring the ratings for the negatively worded items and then totaling the numerical values for the 6 relevant items. Scores can range from 0 to 24, and higher scores indicate more optimism on the part of the athlete. Separate scores can also be calculated for optimism and pessimism if that is preferred.

Hardiness. Numerous hardiness scales have appeared in the psychological literature during the past two decades. The original Hardiness Scale (HS; Kobasa et al., 1982) contained 71 items drawn from pre-existing scales believed to measure constructs related to commitment, challenge, and control. An abbreviated, 36-item version of this original instrument, the Revised Hardiness Scale (RHS), subsequently became available. Two additional hardiness scales were also developed in an effort to overcome measurement problems associated with the HS and the RHS. These "third-generation" scales are the 50-item Personal Views Survey (PVS; Hardiness Institute, 1985) and the 45-item Dispositional Resilience Scale (DRS; Bartone, Ursano, Wright, & Ingraham, 1989). Despite the relatively large item pools in the third-generation scales, we recommend their use in sports medicine settings because they appear to possess better psychometric properties than those of the earlier scales (Funk, 1992).

Informal Assessment

Some sports medicine personnel may decide that informal assessment procedures are more appropriate than formal ones. This decision could arise because the desired personality scales are unavailable, because the practitioner is uncomfortable with written scales, or because the athlete indicates that he or she is uncomfortable with such scales. For purposes of this discussion, adopting an informal approach to personality assessment means (a) talking to the injured athlete on a one-to-one basis in an effort to gain insight into his or her character and (b) paying attention to comments made by the athlete either spontaneously or in response to others in the rehabilitation setting (including other injured athletes). Effective use of this approach requires a thorough understanding of the personality factors that may influence rehabilitation behavior as well as good communication skills. The practitioner must be able to establish trust and rapport with the athlete, ask appropriate questions at appropriate times, listen attentively to statements made by the athlete, and draw inferences about the athlete's character and likely behavior based on these statements.

A tendency to experience negative emotions such as fear, sadness, embarrassment, guilt, and anger is the core feature of neuroticism (Costa & McCrae, 1992). Although some degree of negative emotionality is to be expected during rehabilitation, practitioners should be alert for comments or behaviors that suggest inappropriate amounts of anxiety or hostility for a given injury. Persistent feelings of guilt, rapid discouragement, and/or obvious withdrawal and isolation from teammates could also indicate neurotic tendencies, as could hypersensitivity and strong feelings of inferiority. Neurotic individuals may also be prone to experience and/or express feelings of being overwhelmed with the demands of rehabilitation and being unable to cope. They may also exhibit very low frustration tolerance and engage in impulsive behaviors, such as experimenting with unconventional treatments or attempting to perform physical actions that they are clearly not well enough to perform.

Insight into the athlete's explanatory style will be obtained most directly by paying attention to "why" statements. These statements might refer to events that have actually occurred or to hypothetical events. For example, if actual recovery has been either slower than expected or faster than expected, the athlete could be asked why he or she believes this has occurred. Similarly, the athlete could be asked to generate a likely cause for a hypothetical setback during rehabilitation. If explanations for positive rehabilitation events tend to be external, unstable, and specific (e.g., "I had a different therapist for those 2 weeks where I did really well") and/or explanations for negative events tend to be internal, stable, and global (e.g., "I never have been able to handle pain and discomfort too well"), then a pessimistic explanatory style may be indicated. In order to confirm such an impression, it is essential that the practitioner obtain several explanations and carefully consider both their dimensional properties and their legitimacy. If, for example, one of the therapists really *is* much more competent than another, then such an attribution may reflect accurate perception more than pessimistic style.

Dispositional optimism could be assessed informally by asking specific questions at opportune times during treatment. An athlete who is handling a particular phase of treatment in a positive manner could be asked something like "Are you always so positive about things?" or "Do you approach everything with such a bright outlook?" Similarly, an athlete who has experienced a setback could be asked, "I tend to believe that every cloud has a silver lining; how do you feel about that?" If responses to several of these questions and/or other comments made by the athlete indicate a consistently positive or negative outlook, then the practitioner may be able to make an inference about the degree of general optimism possessed by the individual.

The defining characteristics of the hardy personality are a tendency to view obstacles as challenges rather than threats (challenge), a tendency to become absorbed in what one is doing rather than just "going through the motions" (commitment), and a tendency to believe that one's outcomes are self-determined rather than determined by external forces (control). Statements and behaviors that occur in response to setbacks during rehabilitation can provide valuable information about the athlete's perceptions of challenge versus threat. Similarly, comments or actions indicating a lack of enthusiasm for studies, sport, work, or life in general could indicate low levels of commitment and, if pronounced, could suggest the need for psychological intervention. The therapist should note such comments and discuss them with other members of the rehabilitation team. Statements or behaviors that reflect a denial of personal responsibility and control during rehabilitation are also noteworthy. Refusing to set recovery goals or blaming the therapist or rehabilitation program, or both, for lack of progress may reflect such an attitude. Placing responsibility for recovery primarily in the hands of an external spiritual entity could also indicate a low level of perceived control, although one must be cautious in this regard because of the central role of religion in some people's lives.

When evaluating information obtained through either formal or informal assessment procedures, it is very important to bear in mind that, regardless of their personality traits, athletes are likely to cycle among denial, distress, and determined coping throughout the recovery process (Heil, 1993). Denial refers to a sense of disbelief regarding injury severity; denial can range from mild to profound and may vary across time and circumstances. Distress can include shock, anger, bargaining, anxiety, depression, and helplessness. Finally, determined coping implies acceptance of the injury and is characterized by the purposeful use of coping resources in working through the process of recovery. Distress and denial will tend to be at their peak in the early stages of injury, whereas determined coping will usually prevail as rehabilitation proceeds. It is important to assess the magnitude of distress and how appropriate it is relative to the severity of the injury and the phase of recovery. Similarly, denial can sometimes be advantageous in that it allows athletes to maintain a positive outlook and cope with the situation at hand, but it can also become problematic if it allows the athlete to avoid the emotional work of recovery.

Implications for Practice

Effective provision of sports medicine services involves more than the facilitation of physical recovery. Indeed, if practitioners do not also take steps to help athletes cope with the psychological stress of injury and rehabilitation, then physical recovery may be delayed. Members of the sports medicine team are in an excellent position to help athletes cope with the stress of rehabilitation, and, as observed in Bianco's (1996) study of elite skiers, injured athletes often look to them for this type of support:

> The person that I wanted to talk to the most was the person that was going to help me get better, and that was my physiotherapist. We had the best relationship ever. He knew what I was thinking; he knew what I was going through. He was my moral supporter, a helper, a psychologist. He was pretty much everything for me. (quoted)

Personality information can help medical personnel to provide a more complete (and, therefore, more effective) service by enabling them to recognize interrelated patterns of thought, emotion, and behavior during rehabilitation. Although we know very little about the specific effects of neuroticism, explanatory style, dispositional optimism, or hardiness on the thoughts, emotions, and behaviors of *injured athletes,* the research literature does offer some clues about what we can generally expect from individuals who differ substantially on these traits. Because maladaptive rehabilitation responses are likely to concern sports medicine personnel more than adaptive ones are, a summary of probable responses from individuals at the negative extremes of these traits will be presented.

Highly neurotic athletes are prone to overreactions, negative emotions, quick frustration, and impulsive actions. They also have a tendency to exaggerate physical symptoms and to use denial, disengagement, and emotional venting as injury-related coping mechanisms (Costa & McCrae, 1992; Grove & Bahnsen, 1997). Practitioners may need to make a conscious effort to model rational behavior when dealing with this type of athlete. At the same time, they should be prepared for emotional reactions and questioning of what might seem like well-planned and thoughtful treatment regimes. Maintaining precise records of progress and making even the smallest gains known to the athlete may be beneficial. Within limits, a tolerance may also need to be exhibited for impatience with conventional treatment modalities. At the same time, the athlete should be encouraged to develop skills in stress management (e.g., Greenberg, 1990), thought management (e.g., Bunker, Williams, & Zinsser, 1993), and problem-focused coping strategies such as goal setting (e.g., Locke & Latham, 1990; Weinberg, 1996).

Injured athletes with a highly pessimistic attributional style may be predisposed to feelings of helplessness and depression. Therefore, they may tend to isolate themselves from coaches and teammates and/or feel overwhelmed by the adjustments necessary because of their incapacitation. These adjustments could include retaining a job during convalescence, scheduling time for treatments, depending on others for transportation, and handling unexpected medical expenses (Gordon, Milios, & Grove, 1991b). Athletes with pessimistic attributional styles may also fail to follow recommended treatment programs (especially the unsupervised aspects of their programs) and may exhibit a lack of persistence in the face of poor progress or setbacks (Laubach, Brewer, Van Raalte, & Petitpas, 1996; Shaffer & McAuley, 1993). Therapists should take steps to short-circuit such responses if they detect a highly pessimistic orientation on the part of the athlete. Encouraging continued attendance at training sessions and offering advice about how to cope with the extra demands of injury may prevent the athlete from feeling isolated and overwhelmed. In addition to providing such pragmatic advice, medical personnel may also need to provide emotional social support to these athletes (cf. Bianco, 1996).

Scheier and Carver (1987, 1992) have noted a number of similarities between the concepts of explanatory pessimism and dispositional optimism. They go on to say that pessimistic attributions may influence behavior primarily through their effect on generalized expectancies (i.e., optimism). Thus, therapists might expect to see many of the same reactions from athletes high in explanatory pessimism and those low in dispositional optimism. This similarity would seem especially relevant for depressive emotions, absence of self-initiated behavior change, and lack of persistence in times of difficulty. Because individuals low in dispositional optimism tend to use avoidance-oriented and/or emotion-oriented strategies to cope with stress (Grove & Heard, in press; Scheier et al., 1994), therapists might also expect these athletes to deny the seriousness of their injury and/or express anger during the course of rehabilitation. Denial tendencies might be diminished somewhat by providing the athlete with objective evidence about the extent of damage. In most cases, anger can be diffused by listening empathetically, confronting the athlete in a calm and rational manner if expressions of anger become disruptive, and/or providing information on thought management techniques (Novaco, 1995). In cases where anger persists, Faulkner, Maguire, and Regnard (1994) suggest that (a) the individual should first be invited to consider whether there are "hidden" reasons for their anger; (b) a situation-specific assessment should then be made of its causes, focus, and rationality; and (c) the athlete should be given "space" to recover before addressing further rehabilitation issues.

Individuals low in hardiness (particularly the commitment and control dimensions of hardiness) share several common tendencies. Specifically, these individuals tend to worry about their public image, overgeneralize negative aspects of their character, and experience depressive moods (Hull et al., 1987). They also tend to view potentially stressful events as threatening, suffer high levels of anxiety and apprehension about their ability to cope, and make infrequent use of social support resources (Florian et al., 1995; Maddi & Khoshaba, 1994). Thus, practitioners might expect injured athletes who are low in hardiness to ruminate about the way others view them and their injury, to become nervous and tense when faced with stressful treatment procedures, and, perhaps, to grow depressed about their incapacities. In addition, they might be inclined to isolate themselves from coaches and teammates and might fail to adhere to recommended treatment regimes. Therapists should take care to communicate clearly with these athletes about the severity of the injury and should consider the need for supplying information on stress management (e.g., Greenberg, 1990). Contacts with coaches, teammates, and other recovering athletes should be actively encouraged, and steps should be taken to reinforce personal initiative/effort in relation to rehabilitation. Active involvement in the determination of rehabilitation goals and self-monitoring of rehabilitation progress via charts or graphs may also be desirable for these athletes in order to enhance feelings of personal commitment and control.

Conclusion

Personality is one of several factors that influence the thoughts, feelings, and behaviors of athletes during rehabilitation. Research indicates that explanatory pessimism, dispositional optimism, and hardiness have health-related consequences, and it was suggested that these traits might also affect psychophysiological processes during recovery from injury. Preliminary data collected from athletes in the 3 months following knee surgery suggest that mood states are, indeed, influenced by these personality factors. Knowledge of an athlete's personality may help sports medicine personnel to anticipate, understand, and deal with undesirable rehabilitation responses. For that reason, formal and informal approaches to personality assessment were examined, and potential problems were discussed with reference to specific personality characteristics. Effective resolution of these problematic responses will require knowledge, awareness, compassion, and creativity on the part of the practitioner.

References

Allred, K.D., & Smith, T.W. (1989). The hardy personality: Cognitive and physiological responses to evaluative threat. *Journal of Personality and Social Psychology, 56,* 257–266.

Anderson, C.A., Horowitz, L.M., & French, R. (1983). Attributional style of lonely and depressed people. *Journal of Personality and Social Psychology, 45,* 127–136.

Anderson, C. A., & Riger, A. L. (1991). A controllability attributional model of problems in living: Dimensional and situational interactions in the prediction of depression and loneliness. *Social Cognition, 9,* 149–181.

Bartone, P. T., Ursano, R., Wright, K., & Ingraham, L. (1989). The impact of military air disaster on the health of assistance workers. *Journal of Nervous and Mental Disease, 177,* 317–328.

Bianco, T. (1996). *Social support influences on recovery from sport injury.* Unpublished master's thesis, University of Ottawa, Ottawa, Ontario, Canada.

Blaney, P. H., & Ganellen, R. J. (1990). Hardiness and social support. In I. G. Sarason, B. Sarason, & G. Pierce (Eds.), *Social support: An international view* (pp. 297–318). New York: Wiley.

Bolger, N., & Schilling, E. A. (1991). Personality and the problems of everyday life: The role of neuroticism in exposure and reactivity daily stressors. *Journal of Personality, 59,* 355–386.

Bolger, N., & Zuckerman, A. (1995). A framework for studying personality in the stress process. *Journal of Personality and Social Psychology, 69,* 890–902.

Brewer, B. W. (1994). Review and critique of models of psychological adjustment to athletic injury. *Journal of Applied Sport Psychology, 6,* 87–100.

Bunker, L., Williams, J. M., & Zinsser, N. (1993). Cognitive techniques for improving performance and building confidence. In J. M. Williams (Ed.), *Applied sport psychology: Personal growth to peak performance* (pp. 225–242). Mountain View, CA: Mayfield.

Carver, C. S. (1989). How should multifaceted personality constructs be tested? Issues related to self-monitoring, attributional style, and hardiness. *Journal of Personality and Social Psychology, 56,* 577–585.

Cohen, J. (1988). *Statistical power analysis for the behavioral sciences* (2nd ed.). Hillsdale, NJ: Erlbaum.

Costa, P. T., & McCrae, R. R. (1989). Personality, stress, and coping: Some lessons from a decade of research. In K. S. Markides & C. L. Cooper (Eds.), *Aging, stress, and health* (pp. 269–285). New York: Wiley.

Costa, P. T., & McCrae, R. R. (1992). *Professional manual: Revised NEO Personality Inventory and NEO Five-Factor Inventory.* Odessa, FL: Psychological Assessment Resources.

Daly, J. M., Brewer, B. W., Van Raalte, J. L., Petitpas, A. J., & Sklar, J. H. (1995). Cognitive appraisal, emotional adjustment, and adherence to rehabilitation following knee surgery. *Journal of Sport Rehabilitation, 4,* 23–30.

Dember, W. N., Martin, S., Hummer, M. K., Howe, S., & Melton, R. (1989). The measurement of optimism and pessimism. *Current Psychology: Research & Reviews, 8,* 102–119.

Endler, N. S., & Parker, J. D. A. (1990). Multidimensional assessment of coping: A critical evaluation. *Journal of Personality and Social Psychology, 58,* 844–854.

Eysenck, H. J. (1988). Personality, stress and cancer: Prediction and prophylaxis. *British Journal of Medical Psychology, 61,* 57–75.

Eysenck, H. J., & Eysenck, M. W. (1985). *Personality and individual differences.* New York: Plenum.

Eysenck, H. J., & Eysenck, S. B. G. (1975). *Manual of the Eysenck Personality Questionnaire.* London: Hodder & Stoughton.

Faulkner, A., Maguire, P., & Regnard, C. (1994). Dealing with anger in a patient or relative: A flow diagram. *Palliative Medicine, 8,* 51–57.

Feather, N.T., & Tiggemann, M. (1984). A balanced measure of attributional style. *Australian Journal of Psychology, 36,* 267–283.

Florian, V., Mikulincer, M., & Taubman, O. (1995). Does hardiness contribute to mental health during a stressful real-life situation? The roles of appraisal and coping. *Journal of Personality and Social Psychology, 68,* 687–695.

Ford, I., & Gordon, S. (1993). Social support and athletic injury: The perspective of sport physiotherapists. *The Australian Journal of Science and Medicine in Sport, 25,* 17–25.

Friedman, H. S. (Ed.). (1990). *Personality and disease.* New York: Wiley.

Friedman, H. S., & Booth-Kewley, S. (1987). The "disease-prone personality": A meta-analytic view of the construct. *American Psychologist, 42,* 539–555.

Funk, S. C. (1992). Hardiness: A review of theory and research. *Health Psychology, 11,* 335–345.

Gentry, W. D., & Kobasa, S. C. (1984). Social and psychological resources mediating stress-illness relationships in humans. In W. D. Gentry (Ed.), *Handbook of behavioral medicine* (pp. 87–116). New York: Guilford Press.

Goodkin, K., Antoni, M. H., & Blaney, P .H. (1986). Stress and helplessness in the promotion of cervical intraepithelial neoplasia to invasive squamous cell carcinoma of the cervix. *Journal of Psychosomatic Research, 50,* 67–76.

Gordon, S. (1986, March). Sport psychology and the injured athlete: A cognitive behavioral approach to injury response and injury rehabilitation. *Science Periodical on Research and Technology in Sport, 1*–10.

Gordon, S., Milios, D., & Grove, J. R. (1991a). Psychological aspects of the recovery process from sport injury: The perspective of sport physiotherapists. *Australian Journal of Science and Medicine in Sport, 23,* 53–60.

Gordon, S., Milios, D., & Grove, J. R. (1991b). Psychological adjustment to sports injuries: Implications for athletes, coaches, and family members. *Sports Coach, 14* (2), 40–44.

Greenberg, J. S. (1990). *Comprehensive stress management* (3rd ed.). Dubuque, IA: Wm. C. Brown.

Grove, J. R. (1993). Personality and injury rehabilitation among sport performers. In D. Pargman (Ed.), *Psychological bases of sport injuries* (pp. 99–120). Morgantown, WV: Fitness Information Technology.

Grove, J. R., & Bahnsen, A. (1997). *Neuroticism, injury severity, and coping with rehabilitation.* Manuscript submitted for publication.

Grove, J. R., & Heard, N. P. (in press). Optimism and sport-confidence as correlates of slump-related coping among athletes. *The Sport Psychologist.*

Grove, J. R., Stewart, R. M. L., & Gordon, S. (1990, October). *Emotional reactions of athletes to knee rehabilitation.* Paper presented at the annual meeting of the Australian Sports Medicine Federation, Alice Springs.

Hanrahan, S. J., & Grove, J. R. (1990a). Further examination of the psychometric properties of the Sport Attributional Style Scale. *Journal of Sport Behavior, 13,* 183–193.

Hanrahan, S. J., & Grove, J. R. (1990b). A short form of the Sport Attributional Style Scale. *Australian Journal of Science and Medicine in Sport, 22,* 97–101.

Hanrahan, S. J., Grove, J. R., & Hattie, J. A. (1989). Development of a questionnaire measure of sport-related attributional style. *International Journal of Sport Psychology, 20,* 114–134.

Hardiness Institute. (1985). *Personal Views Survey.* Arlington Heights, IL: Author.

Heil, J. (1993). A psychologist's view of the personal challenge of injury. In J. Heil (Ed.), *Psychology of sport injury* (pp. 34–46). Champaign, IL: Human Kinetics.

Hull, J. G., Van Treuren, R. R., & Virnelli, S. (1987). Hardiness and health: A critique and alternative approach. *Journal of Personality and Social Psychology, 53,* 518–530.

Ievleva, L., & Orlick, T. (1991). Mental links to enhanced healing: An exploratory study. *The Sport Psychologist, 5,* 25–40.

Kamen, L., & Seligman, M. E. (1987). Explanatory style and health. *Current Psychology: Research & Reviews, 6,* 207–218.

Kamen-Siegel, L., Rodin, J., Seligman, M. E., & Dwyer, J. (1991). Explanatory style and cell-mediated immunity in older men and women. *Health Psychology, 10,* 229–235.

Kardum, I., & Hudek-Knezevic, J. (1996). The relationship between Eysenck's personality traits, coping styles and moods. *Personality and Individual Differences, 20,* 341–350.

Kobasa, S. C. (1979). Stressful life events, personality, and health: An inquiry into hardiness. *Journal of Personality and Social Psychology, 37,* 1–11.

Kobasa, S. C., Maddi, S. R., & Kahn, S. (1982). Hardiness and health: A prospective study. *Journal of Personality and Social Psychology, 42,* 168–177.

Laubach, W. J., Brewer, B. W., Van Raalte, J. L., & Petitpas, A. J. (1996). Attributions for recovery and adherence to sport injury rehabilitation. *Australian Journal of Science and Medicine in Sport, 28,* 30–34.

Levy, S. M., & Wise, B. D. (1987). Psychosocial risk factors, natural immunity, and cancer progression: Implications for intervention. *Current Psychology: Research & Reviews, 6,* 229–243.

Lin, E. H., & Peterson, C. (1990). Pessimistic explanatory style and response to illness. *Behavior Research and Therapy, 28,* 243–248.

Locke, E. A., & Latham, G. P. (1990). *A theory of goal-setting and task performance.* Englewood Cliffs, NJ: Prentice-Hall.

Maddi, S. R., & Khoshaba, D. M. (1994). Hardiness and mental health. *Journal of Personality Assessment, 63,* 265–274.

Maes, S., Leventhal, H., & de Ridder, D. T. (1996). Coping with chronic diseases. In M. Zeidner & N. S. Endler (Eds.), *Handbook of coping: Theory, research, applications* (pp. 221–251). New York: Wiley.

McAuley, E., Duncan, T. E., & Russell, D. W. (1992). Measuring causal attributions: The Revised Causal Attribution Scale (CDSII). *Personality and Social Psychology Bulletin, 18,* 566–573.

McCrae, R. R., & Costa, P. T. (1986). Personality, coping, and coping effectiveness in an adult sample. *Journal of Personality, 54,* 385–405.

McCrae, R. R., & John, O. P. (1992). An introduction to the five-factor model and its applications. *Journal of Personality, 60,* 175–215.

McDonald, S. A., & Hardy, C. J. (1990). Affective response patterns of the injured athlete: An exploratory analysis. *The Sport Psychologist, 4,* 261–274.

Meyers, M. C., Sterling, J. C., Calvo, R. D., Marley, R., & Duhon, T. K. (1991). Mood state of athletes undergoing orthopaedic surgery and rehabilitation: A preliminary report [Abstract]. *Medicine and Science in Sports and Exercise, 23*(Supplement), S138.

Novaco, R. W. (1995). Clinical problems of anger and its assessment and regulation through a stress coping skills approach. In W. O'Donohue & L. Krasner (Eds.), *Handbook of psychological skills training: Clinical techniques and applications* (pp. 320–338). Boston: Allyn & Bacon.

Nowack, K. M. (1989). Coping style, cognitive hardiness, and health status. *Journal of Behavioral Medicine, 12,* 145–158.

Ormal, J., & Wohlfarth, T. (1991). How neuroticism, long-term difficulties, and life situation change influence psychological distress: A longitudinal model. *Journal of Personality and Social Psychology, 60,* 744–755.

Parkes, K. R. (1986). Coping in stressful episodes: The role of individual differences, environmental factors, and situational characteristics. *Journal of Personality and Social Psychology, 51,* 1277–1292.

Pearson, L., & Jones, G. (1992). Emotional effects of sports injuries: Implications for physiotherapists. *Physiotherapy, 78,* 762–770.

Peterson, C. (1995). Explanatory style and health. In G. M. Buchanan & M. P. Seligman (Eds.), *Explanatory style* (pp.233–246). Hillsdale, NJ: Erlbaum.

Peterson, C., & Bossio, L. M. (1991). *Health and optimism.* New York: Free Press.

Peterson, C., Semmel, A., Von Baeyer, C., Abramson, L.Y., Metalsky, G.I., & Seligman, M. E. P. (1982). The Attributional Style Questionnaire. *Cognitive Therapy and Research, 6,* 287–299.

Peterson, C., & Villanova, P. (1988). An Expanded Attributional Style Questionnaire. *Journal of Abnormal Psychology, 97,* 87–89.

Rim, Y. (1986). Ways of coping, personality, age, sex and family structure variables. *Personality and Individual Differences, 7,* 113–116.

Rodin, J., & Salovey, P. (1989). Health psychology. *Annual Review of Psychology, 40,* 533–579.

Sanderson, F. H. (1981). The psychological implications of injury. In T.P. Reilly (Ed.), *Sports fitness and sports injuries* (pp. 37–41). London: Faber & Faber.

Scheier, M. F., & Bridges, M. W. (1995). Person variables and health: Personality predispositions and acute psychological states as shared determinants for disease. *Psychosomatic Medicine, 57,* 255–268.

Scheier, M. F., & Carver, C. S. (1985). Optimism, coping, and health: Assessment and implications of generalized outcome expectancies. *Health Psychology, 4,* 219–248.

Scheier, M. F., & Carver, C. S. (1987). Dispositional optimism and physical well-being: The influence of generalized outcome expectancies on health. *Journal of Personality, 55,* 169–210.

Scheier, M. F., & Carver, C. S. (1992). Effects of optimism on psychological and physical well-being: Theoretical overview and empirical update. *Cognitive Therapy and Research, 16,* 201–228.

Scheier, M. F., Carver, C. S., & Bridges, M. W. (1994). Distinguishing optimism from neuroticism (and trait anxiety, self-mastery, and self-esteem): A reevaluation of the Life Orientation Test. *Journal of Personality and Social Psychology, 67,* 1063–1078.

Scheier, M. F., Matthews, K. A., Owens, J. F., Magovern, G. J., Lefebvre, R. C., Abbott, R. A., & Carver, C. S. (1989). Dispositional optimism and recovery from coronary artery bypass surgery: The beneficial effects on physical and psychological well-being. *Journal of Personality and Social Psychology, 57,* 1024–1040.

Shaffer, S., & McAuley, E. (1993). Attributions and self-efficacy as predictors of rehabilitative success [Abstract]. *Journal of Sport and Exercise Psychology, 15* (Supplement), S71.

Silver, R. C., Wortman, C. B., & Crofton, C. (1990). The role of coping in support provision: The self-representational dilemma of victims of life crisis. In B. R. Sarason, I. G. Sarason, & G. R. Pierce (Eds.), *Social support: An interactional view* (pp. 397–426). New York: Wiley.

Smith, A. M., Scott, S. G., O'Fallon, W. M., & Young, M. L. (1990). Emotional responses of athletes to injury. *Mayo Clinic Proceedings, 65,* 38–50.

Staats, S. (1989). Hope: A comparison of two self-report measures for adults. *Journal of Personality Assessment, 53,* 366–375.

Taylor, S. E. (1990). Health psychology: The science and the field. *American Psychologist, 45,* 40–50.

Taylor, S. E., & Aspinwall, L. G. (1996). Mediating and moderating processes in psychosocial stress: Appraisal, coping, resistance, and vulnerability. In H. B. Kaplan (Ed.), *Psychosocial stress: Perspectives on structure, theory, life-course, and methods* (pp. 71–110). San Diego, CA: Academic Press.

Tenenbaum, G., Furst, D., & Weingarten, G. (1984). Attribution of causality in sport events: Validation of the Wingate Sport Achievement Responsibility Scale. *Journal of Sport Psychology, 6,* 430–439.

Van Treuren, R. R., & Hull, J. G. (1986, October). *Health and stress: Dispositional optimism and psychophysiological responses.* Paper presented at the annual meeting of the Society for Psychophysiological Research, Montreal, Canada.

Watson, D., & Clark, L. A. (1984). Negative affectivity: The disposition to experience aversive emotional states. *Psychological Bulletin, 96,* 465–490.

Watson, D., & Pennebaker, J. W. (1989). Health complaints, stress, and distress: Exploring the central role of negative affectivity. *Psychological Review, 96,* 234–254.

Weinberg, R. S. (1996). Goal setting in sport and exercise: Research to practice. In J. L. Van Raalte & B. W. Brewer (Eds.), *Exploring sport and exercise psychology* (pp. 3–24). Washington, DC: American Psychological Association.

Whitley, B. E. (1991). A short form of the Expanded Attributional Style Questionnaire. *Journal of Personality Assessment, 56,* 365–369.

Wiebe, D. J. (1991). Hardiness and stress moderation: A test of proposed mechanisms. *Journal of Personality and Social Psychology, 60,* 89–99.

Wiese-Bjornstal, D. M., & Smith, A. M. (1993). Counseling strategies for enhanced recovery of injured athletes within a team approach. In D. Pargman (Ed.), *Psychological bases of sport injuries* (pp. 149–182). Morgantown, WV: Fitness Information Technology.

Williams, P. G., Wiebe, D. J., & Smith, T. W. (1992). Coping processes as mediators of the relationship between hardiness and health. *Journal of Behavioral Medicine, 15,* 237–255.

Zeidner, M., & Saklofske, D. (1996). Adaptive and maladaptive coping. In M. Zeidner & N. S. Endler (Eds.), *Handbook of coping: Theory, research, applications* (pp. 505–531). New York: Wiley.

8

The Malingering Athlete: Psychological Considerations

Robert J. Rotella
University of Virginia

Bruce C. Ogilvie
Professor Emeritus
San Jose State University

David H. Perrin
University of Virginia

The malingering athlete presents one of the greatest challenges for the sport psychologist, athletic trainer, and coach. This chapter describes malingering in general terms and discusses the causes or origins of malingering in athletics. Although it is impossible to know with complete certainty that an athlete is a malingerer, several persistent characteristics and/or causal factors related to the malingering athlete are presented. Several strategies for changing the behavior of the malingerer are presented that should be useful for the athletic trainer, coach, and sport psychologist. It is recommended that these strategies be considered with respect to the individual athlete and that the entire rehabilitation team be involved in the development of an effective plan of treatment.

Introduction

Attempting to understand and help the malingerer in sport has been a frequent topic of interest to coaches, athletic trainers, and sport psychologists. It is argued that teams have underachieved and that careers have been wasted as a result of malingering. Coaches and athletic trainers have been frustrated and have had their patience and love for their work challenged by athletes whom they felt to be malingering. The necessity of athletic trainers functioning as counselors to prevent such difficulties and referring athletes to better trained specialists when appropriate has been emphasized for several years (Kane, 1984; Nack, 1980).

Although malingering has been discussed in the sport psychology literature since at least 1966, it is still not completely understood (Rogers, 1990). In fact, it is presently impossible to know with absolute certainty that an individual is a malingerer. This is one aspect that makes the topic so intriguing, confusing, and controversial. This chapter, combining the perspectives of specialists in clinical sport psychology, sport psychology, and sport medicine-athletic training, is intended to provide a more clear understanding of the malingerer, the background of the malingerer, and the motivation of the malinger; and to provide experientially tested strategies for helping malingerers (Ogilvie & Tutko, 1966; Rotella, 1988; Shank, 1989). Yet, it must be understood from the onset that years of empirical research are needed before the malingering athlete is completely understood.

Prior to discussing the "whys" of malingering, it is crucial that all members of the rehabilitation team be patient and trust that athletes are telling the truth about how their bodies feel. It is a serious mistake to make a snap judgment about an athlete that leads to the malingerer label (Kane, 1984; Nack, 1980). Caution should be exercised before an athlete is considered to be a malingerer, and the athlete should receive benefit of doubt about his or her alleged inability to perform optimally due to injury. The entire rehabilitation team must believe in the athlete's claim and not be influenced by past experiences with the same athlete or with other athletes. Mental health practitioners can never be certain of the accuracy and reliability of their diagnosis of malingering. No completely definite way of identifying this behavior is available. However, through careful observation of behavior patterns, insightful professionals may find support for such a diagnosis.

Understanding Malingering

Some reasons for malingering may be logical and justifiable, at least in the mind of a particular athlete; and some reasons may lead to a short-term problem that will surface only in certain predictable situations. In some cases, underlying motives may lead to continued and repeated malingering if effective intervention is not provided. The primary focus for the remainder of this chapter will be on athletes who have a serious, recurring problem with malingering.

Table 1 provides some common reasons for malingering in sport that derive from the experiences of this chapter's authors.

Table 1. Common Reasons for Malingering in Sport

- An ex-star player is demoted to a less prized position and decides to use an insignificant injury as an excuse or justifiable explanation as to why he is no longer starting, starring, playing well.

- Use of disability or injury to prevent the loss of an athletic scholarship.

- Exaggeration of an injury to prevent the loss of an athletic scholarship.

- An excuse for loss of motivation during a losing season, a slump in personal performance, or an absence of opportunity to play.

- Use of an injury or a disability to protect the athlete's ego upon realizing or believing he or she has insufficient talent to compete.

- Use of an injury to escape from activity when competing needs become more important.

- Use of symptoms to gain attention and interest that cannot be fulfilled by opportunities outside sport.

- Seeking special recognition by playing "hurt" as a demonstration of "courage" or "guts."

- Hiding behind an injury as a protection against the expectation of coach, parents, or teammates.

- For some athletes, when their physical threshold is breached, they feign injury as an acceptable escape.

- There will be those malingerers who hide behind injury or disability in order to get even or punish those they think have been unfair or uncaring. The withholding of their talent is an expression of hostility or anger.

- A highly talented athlete may malinger because he or she sees the coach as a hypocrite. Coach always tells the team that those who practice the hardest will start or play the most and the player knows it is a lie and wishes to throw the lie in the coach's face. This athlete usually has no respect for the coach but fakes it in front of the coach.

- The athlete malingers in order to prepare in advance an acceptable excuse in case of failure to perform well in an upcoming important contest or in one against a skilled team or individual.

- A talented athlete hates his or her sport and feels forced to play it because he or she is talented. This athlete is often willing to compete but not to practice, and thus is willing to test the coach.

- A talented athlete always did well in competition from a very early age, never practiced, and does not see any reason to change.

- The athlete malingers in order to save his or her body for the next level of competition, such as college or the professional level, where the payoff for skills is greater.

- The athlete has heard stories of athletes who always practiced hard, wasted their bodies in practice, and destroyed their careers. He or she does not wish to do the same.

- The athlete does not feel the athletic trainer and/or coach is looking out for his or her best interests, so he or she assumes responsibility.

- The athlete has a lack of self-discipline and has always tried to get out of anything he or she did not really enjoy doing.

Malingering is not restricted to the world of sport. For instance, in industrial medicine, it has proven to be an extremely costly psychological and behavioral problem (Brink, 1989; Labbate & Miller, 1990; Lees-Haley, 1986a). The difficulties range from the assessment and identification of malingerers to the provision of effective treatments for modifying behavior patterns to the making of legal decisions regarding workers' compensation (Brink, 1989).

Malingerers, casually labeled by coaches and athletes as those who intentionally lie about an injury in order to avoid practice or competition, have been studied closely for many years (Kane, 1989; Ogilvie & Tutko, 1966). "One major cue to malingering is the potential for gain or loss as a consequence of having problems" (Lees-Haley, 1986b, p. 68). The presence of a clearly definable goal differentiates malingerers from persons with other forms of fictitious illness (Swanson, 1984). Assessment, although plagued with uncertainty even today, has included the Minnesota Multiphase Personality Inventory (MMPI), the Bender-Gestalt Test, the Wechsler Adult Intelligence Scale (WAIS) (Lees-Haley, 1986a), the Rorschach, and the Structural Interview of Reported Symptoms (SIRS) (Rogers, Gillis, & Bagby, 1990). Beal (1989) has argued that other scales are more appropriate and sensitive depending upon the specific kind of malingering in question.

Recent models of malingering attempt to explain malingering as the result of an adaptive response to adverse circumstances. It has been suggested that malingering may be understood by examining the underlying psychopathology or criminal backgrounds of malingerers (Rogers, 1990). However, within the context of sport it seems more helpful to consider this behavior as an adaptive response to adverse circumstances requiring the presence of an external incentive for being injured (Labbate & Miller, 1990). Travin and Proffer (1984) attempted to reconceptualize malingering along a continuum ranging from other-deceptive to self-deceptive depending upon the degree of one's self-awareness.

Historically, attempts have been made to distinguish between malingering and other forms of pathological avoidance behavior. Much clinical insight derives from the comparisons with mentally aberrant avoidance reactions such as those found in conversion hysteria. Such a comparison can contribute greatly to our understanding of malingering. Malingerers may present a considerable challenge to the clinical psychologist because there is no foolproof way to confirm that a person is consciously faking symptoms of discomfort or physical distress. This is especially true when such individuals seem to cling to their symptoms or disability in the absence of physiological support for such behavior. When the various categories of the hysterical disorders are examined, it is found that it is possible to mimic almost every known disease and physical disorder. Malingerers may mimic disorders of entire systems such as hysterical blindness or aphonia, a loss of speech, and a wide range of other motor systems. The range of visceral symptoms also covers the entire range of possible somatic disorders (Overholser, 1990).

In view of the manifold opportunities for deception, it is indeed a challenge for a rehabilitation team to determine if malingering is present. Critical to such a determination is the unique way in which the individual communicates the nature of the disability and how such is expressed in terms of pain or state of recovery. Extremely subtle forms of communication are necessary in order for a rehabilitation team to find support for a malingering diagnosis. As has been outlined, experience suggests that identifiable behavior patterns may indicate malingering. What becomes apparent in the face of an unsuccessful treatment program is the issue of intentionality. The athlete who fails to respond to treatment or to a physician's assurance as to the athlete's state of physical recovery may be driven by unconscious as well as conscious motives. Some athletes are content to continue expressing their symptoms and receive consequential attention. They tend to be highly verbal, and their descriptions of their physical limitations are considerably detailed. They appear to be emotionally detached from even the most disabling symptoms.

Malingerers will be characterized by their guile and deceit as they seek to manipulate others with their verbal skills. To avoid expectations that require them to behave maturely and confront their personal responsibility to team, teammates, treatment staff, and coaches, these athletes (or malingerers) engage in various forms of deception (Ogilvie & Tutko, 1966).

Treatment for malingering is always confounded by the issue of secondary gain. In the workplace, when workers fake disability, the secondary gain becomes a financial settlement or material support for life. Athletes who fabricate or maintain symptoms are provided with an escape route from any appropriate demand that may be placed upon them. Experience in a military rehabilitation center causes Ogilvie to argue "that you have to outcon the conman" in order to force such individuals to expose their own preferred form of deceit. In World War II, it seemed that the number one symptom for the malingerer was low back pain. This remains one of the most difficult differential diagnoses for the physician to make.

Based on the present knowledge of the available literature and experience in the athletic environment, most athletes who have a repeated habit of malingering do so primarily as a result of (a) a need for attention or (b) fears. The need for *attention* is typically at the top of the list of causes for malingering (Ogilvie & Tutko, 1966). For a variety of reasons the need for attention becomes a more important priority than does the need to perform (practice or compete).

The malingerer is an immediate problem. The team suffers; the individual athlete suffers; and the coach and athletic trainer feel frustrated, helpless, and discouraged by their inability to help. The malingerer's response is extreme. This athlete's response is almost in direct opposition to the highly dedicated athlete who feels guilty because he or she is injured and is not able to help the team that is struggling. This type of athlete usually attends every practice and game if allowed to do so and gets treatment for an hour before and after every practice. The goal is to return as soon as possible to practicing and competing. In contrast, the malingerer is completely free of guilt related to responsibility to the team and goes for treatment with the goal of getting out of practice and/or competition while still receiving attention, perhaps in the form of sympathy.

The true malingerer is plainly and simply a fraud, a fake, and often a great actor. When attempting to fool coaches, athletic trainers, and teammates, the malingerer's performance may be deserving of an Oscar Award. The malingerer can show pain and suffering upon a moment's notice. Often the giveaway for the malingerer is *the degree to which the drama is overdone*. Instead of wanting to melt into the background until healthy again, the malingerer, while demonstrating a lack of commitment to rehabilitation, wants everyone to know he or she is hurt in order to obtain the desired attention. If such an athlete in any way becomes concerned about getting caught in the lie, expression of the severity of the injury and the anguish being felt will be further exaggerated. *For the typical malingering athlete the greatest need is attention, and the greatest fear is getting caught.* Honesty and naturalness are never the malingerers' calling card. It is the exaggerated response that often allows the malingering athlete to be identified and differentiated from athletes who have low pain threshold or low pain tolerance, or both. Again, it must be emphasized that even experienced experts are unable to know for sure if an athlete is faking or truly experiencing pain.

Background

What factors explain the causes or origins of malingering behavior? This section attempts to provide some answers to this question by way of exemplifying childhood experiences that may have contributed to the tendency to malinger. A key to understanding is the realization that an athlete *learns* to be a malingerer. It may be learned from personal experiences; it may be learned indirectly from observing someone viewed as a model, such as a parent, coach, or older athlete; or it may have been taught to the athlete directly by an older athlete. However it occurs, malingering is a behavior that has been *learned, adopted as acceptable, rewarded,* and is now done *willfully* and *intentionally* or *habitually* (Ogilvie & Tutko, 1966).

It is believed that typical malingering athletes were often spoiled in their early years. Regardless of the reasons for being spoiled, lying and deception were allowed. Quite commonly as a child (or in one's early sport experiences), the malingerer perceived that lying was acceptable and justifiable in order to get his or her way. This devious behavior was either directly reinforced or learned indirectly by observing parents, teachers, coaches, or older athletes being reinforced for dishonest behavior. The athlete may have simply observed others behaving in ways that belie what they expressed as a personal philosophy. Such hypocrisy in others whom the athlete considered to be models may have contributed to the malingering tendencies he or she now demonstrates.

Typically, malingerers learn at an early age that family members would always intervene and rescue them from trouble. Moreover, they learn that if caught, the result would be a simple reprimand or lecture. Thus, behaving improperly and yet avoiding due punishment became a frivolous and almost pleasant game-like experience. Talented athletes from such backgrounds tend to enjoy knowing the team's success depends on them. Such athletes typically enjoy the potential for exercising control the attention received and the disturbances they may cause to their team.

Some gifted athletes do not become malingerers because of home- or family-related conditioning. For instance, when their athletic talents were first recognized in middle school or junior high school, they discovered that many adults held their abilities in very high esteem. Soon the young, elite athletes learn that unacceptable behaviors such as skipping class, cheating, or stealing would be overlooked. They revel in their immunity from punishment and enjoy very special attention. Later, they are likely to acknowledge their dishonesty, but assert that it was in part fueled by adult hypocrisy.

Before we continue to discuss some of the more persistent characteristics and causal factors related to malingerers, three factors should be emphasized. As stated previously, the condition we label malingering is typically a *manifestation of complex motives*. Social and family influences that undermine the maturity of malingerers vary considerably; however, they seem to produce individuals with a *shallow conscience*. This, in turn, tends to result in the shirking of responsibility to others. Avoidance reactions then become the standard response when such persons are confronted with the demands of reality. Malingering is a consequence of faking, deceit, or selfish manipulation that is related in some way to underlying forms of *inadequacy*.

A malingerer is usually fearful of being exposed as such and is, therefore, always on guard. However, self-confrontation of the inclination to be deceitful is unlikely because admission of such behavior is frightening. A malingerer, therefore, tends to cling to the strategy of dishonesty at all cost, making it very difficult to provide help. It must be emphasized that the authors, in describing malingerers, have listed a variety of causes of this kind of behavior. These may be defined as character disorders. Should such observations represent individuals who demonstrate sociopathic tendencies, the treatment team is faced with an unusual challenge. Such individuals will be extremely skilled at rationalization, denial, and projection of responsibility. They will tend to have a history of manipulating and exploiting others. Having been in confrontations with authority figures most of their lives, they have become skilled in the avoidance of responsibility.

Helping Malingerers

It should be stated that becoming involved in a battle of wills in order to salvage an athlete who exhibits the foregoing traits may place too many demands upon the treatment team. Knowledge may be most effectively utilized by preventing the treatment team from being exploited by such athletes. At some point, cost-effectiveness must be evaluated and a decision made as to whether or not the time and energy required for changing a particular athlete is worth it. It is appropriate at some point to accept that some athletes are too immature to be helped at the present time, but this should be a last alternative, rather than a first choice decision.

The following generalizations about the malingerer may provide members of the treatment team with insight that enables them to feel empowered to be a positive service provider. During interviews, verbal communication, and treatment sessions, it will be helpful to observe the following (Lees-Haley, 1986b; Ogilvie & Tutko, 1966; Overholser, 1990; Swanson, 1984):

1. The extent to which the athlete exhibits narcissistic behavior patterns, that is, the athlete is self-centered, shows low interest in pain or nature of other's disabilities, is demanding, complains that he or she never receives the same care as others, or tends to rationalize away his or her responsibility for following the treatment program.
2. The tendency to want to avoid talking about the real or imagined disability. Watch eye contact, avoidance of personnel, failure to keep appointments, criticisms of treatment program.
3. The extent to which the athlete senses any responsibility with regard to supporting the team or coach and the effect the athlete's absence might be having on the team.
4. Unguarded moments, checking for consistency/inconsistency in behavior.
5. Lack of true emotional involvement in the injury. Athletes who are genuinely injured tend to grieve and deny loss.
6. A lack of cooperation with diagnostic and/or therapeutic regimes.

7. The presence of external incentives that are greater for being injured than for being healthy.

Because athletes malinger for a variety of reasons, there are many different strategies for changing their behavior (Kane, 1984; Ogilvie & Tutko, 1966; Olmstead, 1976; Shank, 1989). Athletic trainers, coaches and sport psychologists may find one or all of the following to be useful. It is recommended that each suggestion be considered in terms of individual athletes and that the entire rehabilitation team be involved in developing an effective strategy.

1. As a first step, attempt to understand the individual athlete's problems and the underlying reason for malingering. This will require taking the time to develop a trusting relationship with an athlete whom it may initially be difficult to like, respect, and admire. *Listening* to the athlete is a necessary second step, but the coach, sport psychologist, or athletic trainer must go beyond listening. It is important to show care, concern, and interest in the athlete. Yet, it is crucial not to let such athletes use the discussion or counseling session as another opportunity to lie and manipulate. Expect that a malingering athlete will likely try to do this, but attempt not to take such ploys personally. These are simply well-learned habits. Listening must be combined with frank, honest, straightforward feedback to the athlete.

2. If, after in-depth observation and thoughtful evaluation, it is difficult to ascertain that the athlete is faking, it is important to sit with the athlete and confront the issue honestly and directly. Do not attack or accuse the athlete of lying, and be sure to display empathy for the possibility of an undetected injury. Make it clear that the best interests of the athlete and the team are the only concerns. Allow the athlete to express his or her thoughts and concerns. Encourage honesty and openness, and question the athlete on statements perceived as inconsistent with behavior.

3. Remember that empathy and understanding of the athlete's situation promotes growth and positive development, whereas sympathy breeds weakness, stagnation, and self-pity.

4. Malingering is done only if it produces gain for the athlete. It will not occur in the absence of perceived gain.

5. Attempt to determine if the athlete malingers due to fear of playing, need of help in managing stress or fear, need to reduce internally or externally imposed pressure, or need of attention.

6. Honestly explain to the malingering athlete that both the athletic trainer and coach are very frustrated and are either lost or still searching for answers. Ask the athlete for suggestions and admit that your patience is running thin. Tell the athlete that you feel he or she seems to defy get-

ting well and you are wondering if the athlete really wants to get well or *if you as an athletic trainer or sport psychologist are failing to do something that might help.* Make it clear that you do not care whose fault it is. You simply want to solve the problem and help the athlete because that is your job and responsibility and you care about the athlete.

7. At some point, a malingering athlete must be given strictly defined boundaries for behavior and detailed consequences of stepping outside those boundaries. Make it clear that these steps are being taken in the best interest of the athlete and the team. Be certain to establish and maintain that you are in charge of the team and that you will make and enforce the rules for the team members. It is ideal to establish team rules in the preseason that make expectations and consequences perfectly clear. A simple rule stating that athletes who cannot practice for 2 days prior to a game will not play in the game regardless of the athlete's talent often works wonders in eliminating malingering in a sport such as football. Doing this makes a definite statement—that the team will not rely on any one athlete for its success and that no athlete will be permitted to manipulate the coach, sport psychologist, or athletic trainer. Thus malingerers will not receive the attention they desire: If they cannot practice, they cannot play. Nothing personal is implied by this strategy. It is simply a team rule. (Table 2 lists several other techniques important to the prevention of malingering.)

8. Establish and record with the athlete's agreement specific rehabilitation goals. Agree upon times for treatment, length of program, and exact responsibilities for athlete, counselor, and athletic trainer. Be sure to determine the date and time for the next appointment.

9. Assign the athlete to talk with other athletes who have successfully recovered from a similar injury and who have returned to a preinjury level of performance.

10. Develop a treatment team including a sport psychologist.

11. Provide rewards for the desired behavior (going to practice) or retract a reward (playing in game, starting) for malingering. Initially it is useful to give malingerers rewards for desired behaviors and withdraw rewards for unwanted behaviors. In the early stages give continuous reinforcement or praise and attention every time the desired behavior occurs, but as behavior shaping continues, provide feedback on a variable schedule (e.g., every fourth, seventh time the desired behavior occurs). Finally, be sure that what you offer as a reward is indeed viewed as such by the athlete.

12. In most cases, it is best to avoid using a word like "malingerer" when speaking to the athlete, as it will most likely only serve to raise defenses

and further hinder honest communication. On the other hand, the term may be applied strategically when the athletic trainer's, coach's, or sport psychologist's patience, care, and concern have been provided to no avail.

Table 2. Coaching Techniques Important for Prevention of Malingering

- Keep practice challenging and demanding but keep it stimulating and strive to keep it fun.
- Privately and publicly reward athletes who practice and play despite being sore and in some pain but who are not at risk of further damage to their bodies.
- Do everything possible to give starters and nonstarters equal amounts of attention.
- Keep eyes open for signs of overtired athletes and be willing to give the team a day off when necessary or to give particularly overtired players an easy day of practice.
- Be sure to take the time to teach star players the special responsibilities of being gifted and emphasize such players' impact on other team players.
- Regularly check to make sure that coaches and athletic trainers are sticking to guidelines set in the preseason.
- Emphasize that rules established are to benefit athletes rather than to hurt athletes.
- Particularly in the first 2 years in a program, be sure that developing the right attitude is more important than winning a particular game.
- As soon as possible after an athlete is injured, set short-term and long-term goals and be certain to show athletes that they are making forward progress.
- Be open-minded toward normally dedicated athletes who may malinger for a day or two because they are tired, in a lousy mood, having personal or family problems.
- Be committed to being particularly enthusiastic and encouraging following losses or any time the team is in a losing streak. This is not a time when athletes need to be criticized and/or emotionally beat up. Failure to follow this advice is likely to lead to an increase in malingering.

Summary

Although data depicting the actual incidence of malingering in sport are not available, it is likely that although real and prevalent, the problem is not overwhelming. Nonetheless, for obvious reasons pertaining to the athlete, the team, and its management, malingering should be eradicated whenever possible. To this end, this chapter attempts to clarify reasons for such behavior in sport as well as to recommend strategies for its elimination or reduction. Also important is the establishment of a trusting and respectful relationship with the malingering athlete. The athletic trainer, coach, and counselor may demonstrate caring by setting and enforcing rules for their athlete's practice and on-the-field behaviors. Helping malingerers requires tremendous patience, but the long-term benefits of doing so are enormous. Finally, athletic trainers and coaches must remember that some injuries may have unusual or subtle signs and symptoms. Thus, although malingering may be suspected, the potential always exists that the athlete is in fact injured.

References

Beal, D. C. (1989). Assessment of malingering in personal injury cases. *American Journal of Forensic Psychology, 7,* 59–65.

Brink, N. E. (1989). The power struggle of Workers Compensation: Strategies for intervention. *Journal of Applied Rehabilitation Counseling, 20,* 25–28.

Kane, B. (1989). Trainer counseling to avoid three face-saving maneuvers. *Athletic Training, 19,* 171–174.

Labbate, L. A., & Miller, R. W. (1990). A case of malingering. *American Journal of Psychiatry, 47,* 257–258.

Lees-Haley, P. R. (1986a). How to detect malingerers in the workplace. *Personnel Journal, 65,* 106–110.

Lees-Haley, P. R. (1986b). Psychological malingerers. *Trial, 21,* 68–69.

Nack, W. (1980). Now everyone believes him. *Sports Illustrated, 53,* 12–17.

Ogilvie, B., & Tutko, T. (1966). *Problem athletes and how to handle them.* London: Pelham Books.

Olmstead, A. E. (1976). Malingering and stroking. *Transactional Analyses Journal, 6,* 268–269.

Overholser, J. C. (1990). Differential diagnoses of malingering and fictitious disorders with physical symptoms. Special issue: Malingering and deception: An update. *Behavioral Sciences and the Law, 8,* 55–65.

Rogers, R. (1990). Development of a new classification model of malingering. *Bulletin of the American Academy of Psychiatry and the Law, 18,* 323–333.

Rogers, R., Gillis, J., & Bagby, R. (1990). The SIRS as a measure of malingering. *Behavioral Sciences and the Law, 8,* 85–92.

Rotella, R. (1988). Psychological care of the injured athlete. In D. N. Kuland (Ed.), *The injured athlete* (pp. 213–224). Philadelphia: J. P. Lippincott.

Shank, R. H. (1989). Academic and athletic factors related to predicting compliance by athletes to treatments. *Athletic Training, 24,* 125.

Swanson, D. A. (1984). Malingering and associated syndromes. *Psychiatric Medicine, 2,* 287–293.

Travin, S., & Proffer, B. (1984). Malingering and malingering-like behavior: Some denial and conceptual issues. *Psychiatry Quarterly, 56,* 189–197.

SECTION 3

COUNSELING ATHLETES WHO ARE INJURED

Chapter 9
Counseling Strategies for Enhanced Recovery
of Injured Athletes Within a Team Approach
Diane M. Wiese-Bjornstal
Aynsley M. Smith

Chapter 10
Patient-Practitioner Interactions in Sport Injury Rehabilitation
Britton W. Brewer
Judy L. Van Raalte
Albert J. Petitpas

Chapter 11
Social Support and Injury:
A Framework for Social Support-Based Interventions With Injured Athletes
Charles J. Hardy
R. Kelly Crace
Kevin L. Burke

Chapter 12
Mental Paths to Enhanced Recovery From a Sports Injury
Lydia Ievleva
Terry Orlick

Chapter 13
Seeing Helps Believing: Modeling in Injury Rehabilitation
Frances A. Flint

Chapter 14
The Use of Imagery in the Rehabilitation of Injured Athletes
Lance B. Green

The direction taken by this section is counseling. Here, the authors dwell upon specific methods and techniques recommended for use with rehabilitating athletes.

Diane M. Wiese-Bjornstal and **Aynsley M. Smith** bring attention to the appropriateness of a team effort in rehabilitating athletes. In the first chapter of Section 3 (chapter 9), they describe the efforts of peer athletes, physicians, athletic trainers, and sport psychology consultants in assisting the rehabilitating injured athlete. Examples of how the influence of these persons contributes to the rehabilitation effort are provided.

In the section's second chapter (chapter 10), **Britton W. Brewer**, **Judy L. Van Raalte**, and **Albert J. Petitpas** address interactions/communications between the rehabilitating athlete and various health professionals. In addition, patient as well as practitioner perceptions about the injury and rehabilitation process are discussed.

In chapter 11, **Charles J. Hardy**, **R. Kelly Crace**, and **Kevin L. Burke** elaborate upon the role of social support interventions in rehabilitation programs.

In chapter 12, **Lydia Ievleva** and **Terry Orlick** discuss findings from a study they conducted that examined the comparative effectiveness of various mental activities used by slow- and fast-healing injured athletes. Examples are given of athletes who were led to important understanding and acceptance of their injuries that enabled them to rehabilitate successfully.

Two of the most unusual contributions in this book, **Frances A. Flint's** chapter and that of **Lance B. Green** (chapters 13 and 14, respectively) provide creative approaches for the rehabilitation of injured athletes. Modeling is described as an effective method by **Flint** and mental imagery by **Green**.

9

Counseling Strategies for Enhanced Recovery of Injured Athletes Within a Team Approach

Diane M. Wiese-Bjornstal
University of Minnesota

Aynsley M. Smith
Mayo Clinic Sports Medicine Center

Athletes experience a variety of cognitive, emotional, and behavioral responses following athletic injury occurrence, ranging on a continuum from no change in the athlete's psychological state to extreme distress, such as attempted suicide. During the time span from immediate postinjury to full recovery, there are a variety of sports medicine team members with whom the athlete comes in contact, all of whom have important psychological roles to play in the recovery process. It is the purpose of this chapter to identify counseling and other psychological and social strategies to be employed by these various members of the sports medicine team, with the ultimate goal being the enhancement of the physical and psychological recovery of the athlete.

Introduction

Both sport-related and health care professionals have expressed concerns about the psychosocial impact of incurring athletic injury. Eldridge (1983) stated that health care professionals must understand the psychosocial dynamics accompanying sports injuries to appreciate the significance of the injury to the athlete. For example, among other possible psychological consequences, it has been noted by Scott (1984) that clinical depression, often present in injured athletes, must be identified early if optimal rehabilitation is to occur.

Limited empirical evidence exists, however, to document systematically the emotional responses of athletes to injury. In general, the preliminary research that we do have suggests that some, but not all, injured athletes manifest a variety of negative emotional reactions. For example, some very recent studies have provided preliminary data on postinjury emotional responses. Significant mood disturbances, such as elevations in depression, tension, and anger, have been found in more seriously injured athletes (Grove, Stewart, & Gordon, 1990; A. M. Smith, Scott, O'Fallon, & Young, 1990), in injured collegiate athletes (McDonald & Hardy, 1990), and in injured runners who were forced to remain out of running for two weeks (Chan & Grossman, 1988). In the A. M. Smith, Scott, O'Fallon, and Young study, it was found that mood disturbance paralleled the rating of perceived recovery, that severity of injury was the major determinant of the emotional response, and that athletes with minor injuries actually had less mood disturbance than college norms. Connelly (1991) found that physical self-efficacy was affected by injury, but that self-esteem and physical acceptance were not. These initial findings illustrate the importance of avoiding the assumptions that all injured athletes will experience psychological trauma and that they will experience the same cognitive and emotional responses. Many, it appears, may handle the injury experience quite well.

Among those athletes who do experience psychological disturbance, it is clear that negative mood states, such as depression, tension, and anger, may occur almost immediately postinjury. These negative mood states may continue in the absence of intervention until the athlete returns to sport or adapts to alternative interests. In our clinical experience, athletic injury has combined with serious preinjury stress to prompt at least five suicide attempts (A. M. Smith & Milliner, 1991). The work of Gordon, Milios, and Grove (1991) suggested that physiotherapists working with injured athletes noted many postinjury behavioral reactions resembling stages of the grief response previously identified by Kübler-Ross (1969) in her work with terminal patients. Clearly, counseling interventions are often appropriate as soon as the injury is diagnosed, the prognosis established, appropriate medical interventions arranged, and cognitive and emotional responses assessed.

However, the clinical utility of using "loss of health" models (e.g., Cassem & Hackett, 1971; Kübler-Ross, 1969) for understanding athlete reactions to injury has yet to be established. Existing loss of health models were developed from responses of patient populations very different from injured athletes. For example, Kübler-Ross based her model on the consolidation of numerous interviews with elderly terminally ill patients and with children having leukemia who were coping with pending death, during an era when treatment was ineffective for this form of cancer. Her stages of anger, denial, bargaining, depression, and acceptance represented the nonsequential coping stages of the terminally ill and may not be the same as those experienced by injured athletes. The Cassem and Hackett model, on the other hand, describes the emotional experiences of patients who sustained heart attacks and were admitted as "critical" to an intensive care unit. Referrals of these patients to psychiatric services were primarily for anxiety, denial, and depression—responses that differ somewhat from the Kübler-Ross model.

In addition to the possibility of emotional response differences between athletes and nonathletes, there is evidence to suggest the existence of behavioral differences. Carmen, Zerman, and Blaine (1968), for example, found that athletes used a psychiatric counseling service at Harvard less than nonathletes did. Furthermore, when they finally were seen, the athletes had more severe problems than nonathletes did. The reluctance of athletes to seek help was attributed to a determination not to "give in" to weakness. Pierce (1969) found that athletes held more negative attitudes toward emotional illness and were less intellectual in their interests than were nonathletes. Furthermore, Linder, Pillow, and Reno (1989) reported that athletes who seek help or counseling from a sport psychologist may well experience discrimination. This study found that in a "mock-up" of the draft selection process, athletes were rated lower if they sought assistance from a sports psychologist than if they obtained assistance for stress management from a coach.

Although the previously cited studies suggest that athletes may be reluctant to seek assistance or counseling for their problems, the work of Little (1969) underscores the importance of having counseling services available to injured athletes. In a study of males who were experiencing depression and anxiety, approximately 75% of the middle-aged athletic group had sustained injury or illness that precipitated their symptoms, compared to 11% of the nonathletes. Furthermore, the athletic group took longer in treatment and had a less favorable prognosis than did the nonathletes. Little believed that the athletic persons experienced a deprivation crisis secondary to the injury or illness that required cessation of physical activity.

In summary, differences have been noted among the following: (a) individual differences in the emotional responses of athletes to injury, (b) the ages and situation severity of psychological response models designed around terminally ill and heart attack populations, and the psychological responses of injured athletes, and (c) the reported differences between athlete and nonathlete help-seeking behaviors.

Theoretical Model of Postinjury Response

Taken together, the results just cited suggest a need to consider athletic injury as a unique phenomenon. To better appreciate the specific psychosocial impact of athletic injury, a preliminary model of response is proposed in Figure 1. The preinjury psychosocial model outlined by Andersen and Williams (1988) has been extended in this illustration to include the postinjury phase, incorporating the stress model of injury response proposed by Wiese and Weiss (1987). Some of the predicted precursors to athletic injury, such as coping resources, social support availability, history of stressors, and personality certainly impact on the postinjury responses as well. For example, injured athletes who experience high life stress and who lack coping skills (R. E. Smith, Smoll, & Ptacek, 1990) will likely not have these preinjury issues resolved by the time they are seen for postinjury counseling. In fact the presence of preinjury stress and impaired coping will likely amplify the postinjury mood disturbance. An attempt is made in this model to identify some of the psychosocial factors influencing the postinjury cognitive and emotional responses and, subsequently, psychological and physical recovery from injury. The key aspects of this extended model relate to the mediating role of severity of injury; sport-specific situational factors; interactions with the sports medicine team; individual differences; and the resultant emotional, cognitive, and behavioral responses of the athlete. In addition to providing a preliminary theoretical model for much needed research in this area, this model may also prove to have clinical utility in assessing the postinjury cognitive and emotional responses for planning appropriate interventions. The specific predictions of this model will be discussed in a future article.

Inherent within this model are the various persons with whom the athlete comes into contact during rehabilitation. Each person in the sports medicine network encountered by the athlete plays an important role in his or her recovery, both physically and psychologically. Thus, the adoption of a comprehensive sports medicine team approach to assist the athlete in dealing psychologically with the injury is strongly advocated. Figure 2 identifies some of the sports medicine team members with whom injured athletes at different levels

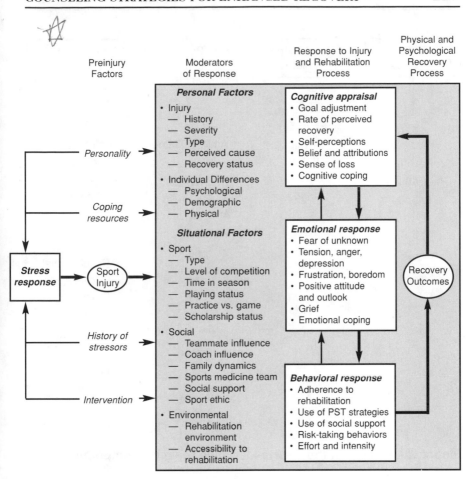

Figure 1. An Operational Model of Psychologic Response to Athletic Injury and Rehabilitation

Adapted and reprinted with permission from Wiese-Bjornstal, D. M., Smith, A. M., & LaMott, E. E. (1995). A model of psychologic response to athletic injury and rehabilitation. *Athletic Training: Sports Health Care Perspectives, 1*(1), 17–30.

of sport participation may interact. Each member of the sports medicine team can contribute unique and complementary psychosocial support services to the rehabilitation program to enhance full recovery. However, the key is that the athlete is the captain of the team, and it is ultimately those factors that the athlete takes ownership of and has commitment to that best determine rehabilitation and recovery.

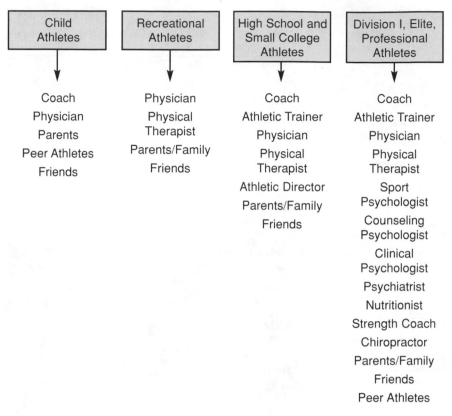

Figure 2. Members of the Sports Medicine Team by Competitive Level

Purpose of the Chapter

The primary goal of this chapter to identify strategies for enhancing the coping resources and social support networks of athletes, as well as to suggest psychological counseling and intervention strategies. To accomplish our purpose, this chapter is organized around the framework of the various roles and responsibilities of sports medicine team members, viewed from an educational and a counseling approach. It is of primary importance to involve both the sport personnel and the medical and clinical personnel in the rehabilitation process. Clear communication among the various members of the team is integral to the effectiveness of this approach.

The contents of the chapter reflect the authors' perspectives derived from our professional experiences as a sport psychology educator and researcher in a university setting and as a nurse-counselor in sport psychology at a sports medicine center. A number of case studies are presented with the intent of illustrating the authors' recommendations. These use a first-person style in an effort to stress that reported interactions and practices on behalf of one or both of the authors actually occurred. Although these case studies are based on our actual experiences with injured athletes, some aspects have been altered to protect the identity of those involved.

Social Support and Educational Strategies for Sport-Related Practitioners

The involvement of sport-related practitioners in the rehabilitation of the athlete will depend to some extent on the competitive level and sponsor (e.g., school-based, national team, youth sport) as identified in Figure 2. The work of Duda, Smart, and Tappe (1989) suggested that adherence to rehabilitation programs is related to athlete perceptions about the effectiveness of the rehabilitation protocol, social support for injury rehabilitation, degree of self-motivation, and involvement in sport for primarily task-related motives. Clearly the first two factors can be influenced by various sport-related members of the sports medicine team. Some suggested strategies follow.

Athletic Trainers

The recent establishment of the Nuprin Comeback Award at the U.S. Olympic Festival 1990 in Minneapolis/St. Paul pays tribute to the important role athletic trainers play in the rehabilitation of athletes from injury. The award, presented again at the 1991 festival in Los Angeles, recognizes not only athletes who make an exceptional recovery from sport-related injuries to distinguish themselves in elite level competition, but also their athletic trainers, who enhanced their rehabilitation.

In understanding the role of trainers, it is important to examine their psychosocial contributions, as well as their more familiar physical responsibilities in the rehabilitation process. Clear, controlled communication is a primary responsibility of athletic trainers during the initial management of injury (Wiese & Weiss, 1987). Often athletic trainers are the first responders when athletic injury occurs. What they say, and perhaps even more important *how* they say it, immediately following injury is extremely critical. All interactions should be calm and professional when injury occurs, as many athletes will turn to the trainer for reassurance and information about the nature of the injury. Trainers should be empathic and reassuring. It is sometimes helpful to encourage athletes to talk, thereby distracting them from overreaction to injury. Diagnoses and hasty impressions must be avoided, as they might precipitate unnecessary emotional reactions.

Later in the chronological progression, at least in high school and university team settings, the athletic trainers are the ones to plan, monitor, and evaluate rehabilitation programs. Thus the training staff has the most frequent contact with injured athletes, usually even more than do coaches and teammates. Rehabilitation must be viewed as an educational process, and the psychosocial role that the trainer plays at this time is crucial to the recovery process. Athletes experience many different emotional and cognitive states during the course of an extended rehabilitation. Usually, depending on the nature and severity of the injury and the rehabilitation protocol, performance plateaus occur when the athlete does not seem to make further progress. Support, encouragement, and reassurance that this is a normal part of the rehabilitation is helpful from the trainer during these times. Positive rather than negative communication skills are essential, including good listening skills on the part of the trainer. The focus should be on aspects of the rehabilitation program that have been performed correctly, and emphasis should be placed on the use of praise and rewards as a means of further encouraging desired recovery behaviors. Corrective feedback may be inserted between positively reinforcing comments, adopting the "sandwich approach" described in another chapter of this book.

Trainers should also ensure that athletes have realistic goals and expectations for their recovery. Some athletes apply their same high levels of self-motivation enjoyed in sport to their rehabilitation programs; for these athletes the biggest challenge will be helping them to be realistic and not overdo, consequently risking reinjury. Other athletes may have a tendency to give up in the face of a difficult rehabilitation. In this case the challenge to the trainer is to find appropriate motivational strategies. In both of these situations, realistic, short-term goals (i.e., daily goals) should be employed to allow plenty of room for goal adjustment based on the current progress. The provision of specific performance-based feedback regarding attainment of goals should be central to trainer's job.

The athletic training staff can provide social support to the athlete in the form of encouragement, as just described. However, the athlete must not rely solely on the trainer for social support. The trainer may have to remind the athletes to also rely on others, such as their coaches, teammates, parents, and significant others. One tool that might be helpful in assessing both the available social support networks and the desires of the athlete with respect to involvement by these persons is provided in Figure 3. This simple questionnaire allows the athlete to express his or her preferences. However, it may not be best administered by the athletic trainer if other options are available.

1. Name: _____ Date: _____

2. Injury: _____ Sport: _____

3. What would you like from your coaches during rehabilitation? (e.g., encouragement, keeping you involved with the team, leaving you alone, monitoring your progress, etc.)

   Types of support desired: _____

   Strategies for requesting this support: _____

   Time frame: _____

4. What would you like from your athletic trainer or physical therapist? (e.g., explaining more about the injury to you, taking an interest in you outside your sport background, helping you set goals, etc.)

   Types of support desired: _____

   Strategies for requesting this support: _____

   Time frame: _____

5. What would you like from your teammates? (e.g., telling you about practice, checking up on how you are doing, asking you to help them with their technique, not talking about the team in front of you, etc.)

   Types of support desired: _____

   Strategies for requesting this support: _____

   Time frame: _____

6. What would you like from your family? (e.g., taking time to talk to you, not fussing over you, still attending games, transportation, etc.)

   Types of support desired: _____

   Strategies for requesting this support: _____

   Time frame: _____

7. What would you like from your friends? (e.g., spending more time with you, encouragement, an ear to bend, transportation, etc.)

   Types of support desired: _____

   Strategies for requesting this support: _____

   Time frame: _____

8. What are some ways in which you can provide support to others during the time of your injury and rehabilitation? (e.g., attending practices and games, encouraging teammates, peer coaching, etc.)

   Types of support you can provide: _____

   Strategies for providing this support: _____

   Time frame: _____

Figure 3. Social Support Survey

Because the effect of social desirability is potentially high, it may be more beneficial to have a sport psychology consultant, when available, administer and read the questionnaires and convey the information to the appropriate persons, or, better yet, to have the injured athletes express their own thoughts honestly and directly to the persons involved if the athletes are assertive enough to do so. In either case, the survey encourages injured athletes to think through what behaviors they desire from various individuals.

Other specific psychosocial strategies that can be employed by athletic trainers are highly dependent upon their personal training and education. Results of studies that have tapped an important source of psychological data based on the interactions of athletic trainers and physiotherapists with injured athletes (e.g., Gordon et al., 1991; Wiese, Weiss, & Yukelson, 1991) have demonstrated that these practitioners have experiential knowledge about responses to injury, but often lack systematic and specific educational preparation that might provide a context or framework for understanding and interpreting these emotional, cognitive, and behavioral responses. It is of the utmost importance that future preparation programs for athletic trainers mandate formal educational consideration of involved psychosocial factors (Wiese et al., 1991). If trainers have such an educational preparation, they may well be able to assist the athlete with such strategies as more systematic goal setting, relaxation training, and imagery as methods of enhancing recovery. We are attempting to work toward this end at the University of Minnesota, where students preparing to become athletic trainers are strongly encouraged to take at least one course in applied sport psychology. In this course they receive at least basic education regarding psychosocial factors related to athletics and experience in employing Psychological Skills Training (PST; Martens, 1987) techniques. These may prove to be beneficial to athletes in enhancing their recovery, and it is hoped that in the future such education will be central to the preparation of all athletic trainers.

Coaches

In some cases, unfortunately, coaches pay little attention to injured athletes because they are no longer useful to the team or perhaps because coaches feel awkward around injured athletes and do not know what to say or do. When this occurs, it may be because the coach knows little about the athlete's life outside of the sport context, his or her responses to stress, the injury and rehabilitation protocol, or even whether or when the athlete can return to sport. Unfortunately, many coaches expect athletes to "tough it out" and feel that they should not need support from the coach or others during rehabilitation.

▲

Case 1: A collegiate athlete playing for a national caliber hockey program sustained several serious knee injuries during the course of his career. After his collegiate career ended, he retrospectively expressed to me several concerns about the rehabilitation process that he experienced. One concern was that injured athletes were virtually ignored by the coaching staff, indicative in his opinion of the coaches' general attitude toward "treating athletes as pieces of meat." His feeling lends support to the suggestion stated earlier that some coaches lose interest in athletes when they are no longer of immediate usefulness to the team and, more importantly, in winning games. On the other hand, this athlete expressed a preference, perhaps learned during the course of several rehabilitation experiences, not to be too extensively involved with the team during his recovery. He felt that he wanted to prove to the coaches and his teammates that he could come back from the injury on his own and return to play. This may possibly be reflective of high self-motivation and determination. More likely, however, his behavior was in response to his perception that if the coaches did not care about him, he would not care about the team. This athlete took great pride in recovering faster than the time line initially determined for him, perhaps in part due to the use of short- and long-term goal setting. It was almost as though his pride was based primarily on his recovery in spite of being ignored by the coaches, sort of an "in your face" response. In either case, this athlete recovered successfully and has gone on to become a high school coach.

▼

Coaches should strive to provide evidence that they care about their injured athletes. This may be done by recognizing and supporting the athletes' rehabilitative progress, whether or not their return to team activities is anticipated during the current season or in the future. Coaches are educators, and it therefore behooves them to be concerned with the psychosocial and physical aspects of their athletes' growth and development.

Moreover, it is important to keep injured athletes integrated with the team in order that they retain a sense of self-worth and importance to the team. For example, injured athletes may continue to attend practice and participate as drill leaders or peer coaches. They may be able to help referee or officiate a scrimmage, thereby freeing the coach to evaluate the performance of others. They can keep scores, times, or statistics during contests. Some young athletes might wish to serve as an extra team manager as a means of retaining involvement with the team. Injured athletes can provide support and encouragement to teammates during practice and competition, although this may be difficult for those who are used to receiving high and frequent praise for their past competitive performance. In fact, this may be a good lesson for some elite injured athletes to learn.

In addition, the coach may also suggest activities to injured athletes in order to keep their sport knowledge and insights current. Mental rehearsal of individual skills or team strategies might prove helpful to athletes. Athletes may also be referred to books about their sport, be encouraged to take coaching or officiating classes, or attend a clinic to learn more about various aspects of their sport. Injured athletes who are interested could even obtain officiating certification. The coach might make the injured athlete feel involved in the team effort by asking her or him to view game films and provide notes, comments, or feedback. The goal of these strategies is to further the injured athlete's skills, knowledge, and understanding about competitive sport during a time of reduced physical involvement, given that the athlete expresses an interest in learning about other aspects of the sport. However, the coach must be sensitive to maintaining realistic time demands for injured athletes, as they will have the added time commitment of their rehabilitation regimens. Certainly athletes should not be expected to accomplish all of the above, but rather should be allowed some choice from among involvement alternatives.

Peer Athletes

Peer athletes play an important role in the rehabilitation process. Both healthy and injured peers can offer social support to the injured athlete. For example, healthy teammates and other peer athletes can simply serve as friends who take an interest in both the recovery of the athlete and in the life of the athlete outside sport, as appropriate. These peers may also keep the athlete informed and involved in the activities of the team, so that the injured athlete still feels an integral part of the group. Teammates should make sure to include the injured athlete in social gatherings and other functions.

Another more structured way in which peer athletes might become involved is via establishment of injury support groups (Weiss & Troxel, 1986). This involves meeting with a facilitator and other injured athletes to discuss thoughts, emotions, and challenges associated with injury and rehabilitation. Injured athletes may share common concerns; this provides an opportunity to find out that they are not alone in their recovery triumphs and struggles.

This strategy has been tried in a limited fashion at the University of Minnesota, with injured athletes attending group meetings led by a licensed clinical psychologist who is also knowledgeable about sport. Many of the recommendations for future efforts that arose from this initial attempt related to the frequency of meeting and attendance requirements. For example, some athletes recommended meeting with limited frequency, such as once every month, due to the other time constraints that they faced in rehabilitation and practice. Others suggested that attendance not be made mandatory by coaches or athletic trainers, but that each injured athlete make a personal decision about attending. Some athletes indicated that they found the groups very useful and that meeting gave them a chance primarily to share the emotions associated with injury, whereas others did not feel that they needed to attend because they were coping with the injury quite well on their own.

An example of the important role played by peer athletes, particularly those who have sustained the same injury, was provided following the recent permanent paralysis sustained by football guard Mike Utley of the Detroit Lions. Former New England Patriots wide receiver Darryl Stingley was quoted as saying,

> It doesn't mean that life is over. It means you have to make a few more adjustments. My advice is to be strong. If he survives, the sky is the limit as to what he can do, depending on his competitive nature and spirit. Just never get down. (quoted in "NFL Notebook," 1991).

His public support and encouragement to Utley was likely gratefully received.

Other Sport Professionals and Nonsport Individuals

Examples of other professionals who are often involved with the injured athlete are the athletic director, strength coach, and sport nutritionist, whereas non-sport-related persons involved in the process might be teachers, friends, peers, and family members. It is important for these individuals to share in the rehabilitative process and show concern for athletes' recovery efforts. Because injured athletes frequently maintain keen interests in their sport, efforts should be made by nonsport as well as sport-related peers, friends, and acquaintances to discuss sport issues, results of current competitions, and other pertinent events. It is also important to discuss other aspects of the athlete's life, such as school, work, or church activities. Parents, family, and friends are perhaps the most important source of social support for injured athletes, depending on the level of competitive involvement and age of the athlete. For example, in the youth sport setting, parents and family members provide the primary social network for the young athlete and thus must be extremely sensitive to their cognitive and emotional responses during recovery. Just "being there" for the injured athlete to talk to is very important during the recovery process. However, injured athletes will need to feel a sense of trust in the relationship before they will reveal their innermost fears and concerns. It is also important to be sensitive to the motives, desires, and values of the athlete, rather than to impose those of the parents or friends. In many cases, what the athlete wants and is willing to risk in order to return to sport may be quite different from that which the parent desires. Sometimes injured athletes feel the stakes and demands are too high, and they are not prepared to take further risk. In other situations, the athletes are insistent on a return to sport even though it means persevering in spite of recommendations.

In summary, the sport-related professionals and personal relatives and friends are very important in helping athletes recover from injury and return to sport. Should the return to sport not be possible or desired, the same persons play an important role in helping injured athletes recover and adapt to normal life without their sports.

Counseling Strategies for Psychological and Medical Practitioners

The extent to which psychological and medical practitioners will be involved in an athlete's rehabilitation will depend on such factors as the severity of the injury, the athlete's competitive level, and sport sponsor (e.g., school, national

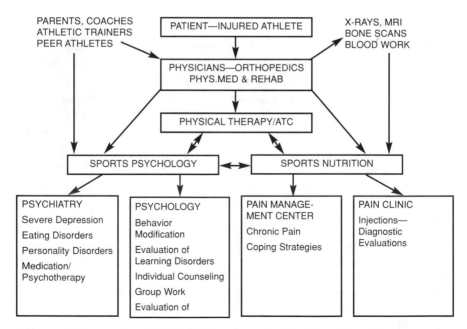

Figure 4. Example of Patient Flow in a Sports Medicine Center

team, youth sport league) as previously identified in Figure 2. Figure 4 illustrates a specific example of a sports medicine team approach flowchart. Injured athletes who seek treatment at the Mayo Clinic Sports Medicine Center may interact with these and other sports medicine team members, depending on the nature of the presenting problem.

Coping and the Counseling Approach

Coping has been defined by Folkman and Lazarus (1986) as transient behavioral efforts to change specific external and internal demands that are appraised as taxing or exceeding a person's resources. As described by Tunks and Bellissimo (1988), some individuals seem able to transform calamities into opportunities for growth whereas others transform everyday hassles into overwhelming adversities. Coping skills vary in appropriateness, may be adaptive or maladaptive, and can be taught and used as a situation requires. Coping skills are organized primarily into three domains: (a) The appraisal aspect of coping attempts to understand and find meaning in a crisis, evaluating what the demands are of a situation (primary appraisal) and the coping resources available (secondary appraisal); (b) problem-focused coping confronts the reality of the crisis and deals with tangible consequences by constructing a more satisfying situation; and (c) emotion-focused coping aims to manage the feelings provoked by the situation (stressor) and to obtain effective equilibrium. It is believed that most stressful situations are responded to with both problem-focused and emotion-focused coping.

Extensive research on the effectiveness of counseling interventions with injured athletes is not yet available, but based on what is known of athlete and nonathlete differences, it seems likely that athletes in general would prefer a rehabilitation program that "stresses concrete, behavioral goal setting and accurate data feedback on their progress in preference to a program of abstract planning and detailed scientific explanation" (Rohe & Athelstan, 1982, p. 290). These recommendations are consistent with suggestions by other health care researchers who suggest problem-focused coping strategies for their heart attack (Christman,1988), adolescent (Yarcheski & Mahon,1986) and spinal cord-injured patients (Rohe & Athelstan, 1982). This approach seems ideal for injured athletes, as it is congruent with goal-setting and performance-enhancement programs common to exercise and sport training.

Sport Psychology Counselor

Medical History and Intervention Plan

Sport psychology counselors, particularly those in hospital or medical clinic settings, are often asked to see injured athletes within a few days of their injury.

Prior to meeting the athlete, the first task is to conduct a thorough assessment of the athlete's situation, which begins with a review of the patient's medical history, relevant physician and physical therapy notes, as well as X-ray, bone scan, and M.R.I reports. Associated illnesses or conditions, such as insulin-dependent diabetes, exercise-induced asthma, scores on standardized psychological tests, and the presence of a psychiatric history should be noted. The medical plan for the patient (e.g., surgical or nonsurgical rehabilitation) should be identified and the patient and physician expectations recorded. Review of these records and any additional necessary communication with the physician or physical therapist should take place before the patient is directed to the counselor.

Assessment Meeting with Injured Athlete

Ideal counseling atmosphere. Counseling offices in a sports medicine center can be designed specifically to decrease athlete discomfort and enhance a sense of trust and intimacy. Ideally, the injured athlete and counselor are seated in chairs of the same size so that both parties occupy the same space. A round table allows for a sense of togetherness and mutuality as the guided interview progresses and necessary forms are completed. Colors in the office should be attractive and coordinated, with the decor reflecting an interest in sport (e.g., sport photos or pictures on the wall). These physical details reflect a desire on the part of the interviewer for mutual respect and understanding, a necessary prerequisite to a meaningful interaction.

Interviewing alone. By interviewing the athlete alone, in the absence of coaches, parents, athletic trainers, teammates, or other members of the sports medicine team, the athlete has the opportunity to convey honest concerns and not simply say what others want to hear. When interviewed alone, athletes are often inclined to acknowledge the pressures they experience, their readiness to quit a sport, the degree of physical and emotional pain they experience, or on the other hand, their sincere desire and intent to continue, despite injury and the need to persevere with their extensive rehabilitation therapy. For example:

▲

Case 2: A few years ago, an injured college athlete, captain of his varsity football team, was seen in the sports medicine center. The athlete was on a scholarship and had experienced 2 years of severe, chronic back pain. The athletic trainer had accompanied the athlete to all of his previous appointments. I gently stopped the athletic trainer from entering the counseling room, and later, the athlete expressed appreciation. "This is the first time I've seen a member of the sports medicine team alone. Frankly, I've had 2 years of pain. I've worked hard for my scholarship, and I've produced well. I don't plan to continue my sport beyond college, and I'd rather stop now, rehabilitate, and know I won't be risking permanent disability. I'm O.K. with not playing any more, focusing on my academic career and on life beyond sport." As a nurse-counselor, my role is to serve as the patient's advocate. With the athlete's permission, I shared his concerns and other pertinent findings from our interview with the sports medicine physician who was directing the evaluation and treatment. The physician has the difficult task of considering and coordinating all professional input and then, together with the injured athlete, determining the best course of action.

▼

Interview format. When the counselor meets initially with the injured athlete, it is important that a thorough explanation of the counselor's role and qualifications be provided. The guided interview then follows the Emotional Responses of Athletes to Injury Questionnaire (ERAIQ), adapted slightly from the version previously published (A. M. Smith, Scott, & Wiese, 1990). The clinical version of this questionnaire was developed over a period of several years and is based on interviews with hundreds of injured athletes (see Figure 5).

The instrument's first question offers an opportunity for the interviewer to gain insight into the athlete's values and priorities. The athlete can share dreams of music, academics, and nonsport career goals. The athlete who is tired, burned out, or, conversely, burning with desire can often be identified through question number one. The second question helps the interviewer determine the athlete's perception of whether the injury has occurred at a more or less critical time in the year or season relative to the athlete's priority sports. This information allows a better understanding of the psychosocial impact of injury. The third question permits the interviewer a glimpse into the athlete's motivation for sport or exercise and heightens the interviewer's appreciation of what is lost to the athlete when injury occurs. Postinjury intervention strategies often incorporate information from this question. The questions on perceived athleticism, goals, nature of the injury (patient's perception), pressures to be in sport and perform up to the expectations of others, stress, and social support are self-explanatory. The last two factors are integrated into the view taken of the injured athlete, illustrated in our earlier model of postinjury response.

The question that asks the athlete to rank emotional responses is central to the ERAIQ. This question is deliberately placed well into the interview, so that ideally a trusting relationship has already been established. More seriously injured athletes have rated frustration, depression, and anger highest on

Name ....   Date ....

Address ....   Age ....   DOB ....

City .... State .... Zip ....   Clinic # ....

Phone (H) ....   (W) ....   Ht.............................   Wt.........................

If you could be anything you wanted in life, what would your dream be? ....

List in order of preference the sports and activities that you participate in: ....

1 ....   2 ....

3 ....   4 ....

Why do you participate in sports? (please rank order, 10=high, 0=low)

...... Self-discipline   ...... Stress management
...... Competition   ...... Personal improvement
...... Socialization   ...... Outlet of aggression
...... Fitness   ...... Weight management
...... Fun   ...... Other, i.e., well-being

Would you describe yourself as an athlete?

1   2   3   4   5
(absolutely not)   (absolutely yes)

When did your injury occur? .... / .... / ....
Before season, mid-season, or end-season?

What is the nature of your injury? ....

What sport were you injured in? ....
How did it happen? ....

What specific goals do you have in sports? ....

Have they changed since the injury? ....
Yes   No   If yes, how? ....

Are you encouraged in sports by your significant others? Yes   No ....
Is this support: pressure or just right?
Who exerts the most pressure? (circle)
Self   Mother   Father   Coach   Other ....

What are the major sources of stress in your life right now?

1 ....   2 ....

3 ....   4 ....

Were you under any recent stress (life changes) before the injury?(circle)
Yes   No   If yes, please describe ....

Do you have a strong family support system or close friends who know about your injury? (circle)
Yes   No
If yes, who are they? (i.e., coach, friend, Parents, teammates, other) ....

How have you been feeling emotionally since the injury? ....

Please rank how these emotions describe how you are feeling because of the injury (12=high, 0=low):

...... Helpless   ...... Tense
...... Bored   ...... Depressed
...... Angry   ...... Frustrated
...... Shocked   ...... Discouraged
...... Frightened   ...... Optimistic
...... In pain   ...... Relieved
...... Other

If 0% is no recovery, what % recovery have you made to your preinjury status (circle):

0%   10%   20%   30%   40%   50%   60%
70%   80%   90%   100%

When is your estimated date of return to sports?

Do you have fears about returning to sport? (circle) Yes   No   If yes, what are they? ....

Are you a motivated person for exercise?

1   2   3   4   5   6   7   8   9   10
(not at all)   (extremely)

How well do you generally handle pain?

1   2   3   4   5
(not at all)   (somewhat)   (very)

What do you think is the most important thing necessary for a successful recovery? ....

Is the most important thing something you have power over? (circle)

1   2   3   4   5
(not at all)   (somewhat)   (very)

How optimistic are you about fully recovering from your injury/surgery? (circle)

1   2   3   4   5
(not at all)   (somewhat)   (very)

What is your current rehab program?
Exercises ....
Times per week ....

Are you able to work out on exercise equipment or modalities? (circle) Yes   No
If yes, please describe.......................................

Figure 5. Emotional Reponses of Athletes to Injury Questionnaire (ERAIQ)

From "Psychological Impact of Athletic Injuries," by A. M. Smith, 1996, *Sports Medicine*, 22(6), 391–405. Reprinted with permission.

the ERAIQ, which correspond with the depression, tension, and anger scales of the Profile of Mood Scales (POMS; McNair, Lorr, & Droppleman, 1971) a popularly used standardized instrument used to assess mood. This information tells the interviewer which emotions are the most bothersome to the injured athlete and thus need to be addressed with appropriate intervention so they do not adversely impede rehabilitation. When interviewing athletes who have a chronic injury or who are being seen preoperatively, pain may be ranked near the top of the athlete's concerns. The interviewer has an obligation to ensure that the injured athlete is physically comfortable during the interview.

The injured athlete's understanding of the injury and the planned surgical procedure or the goals of the nonoperative rehabilitation program should also be assessed. If the athlete does not understand the problem or procedure, the counselor can provide the correct information. If this is not within the counselor's expertise, assistance should be sought. Usually the physicians and therapists have instructed the patient carefully, and the athlete's understandings are accurate.

Information of a subjective nature obtained during the interview (e.g., tendency towards making eye contact with the counselor, energy level, and posture) is considered in addition to the athlete's answers to the interview questions. Sometimes information omitted from the athlete's responses is very important. For example, an athlete suffering from an exercise addiction or an eating disorder will frequently rank weight management and stress management lowest on the list of motivators, perhaps in a conscious or unconscious effort to draw the interviewer's attention away from some major concerns and areas of discomfort.

The POMS or other psychological tests may be used when appropriate, if the counselor is trained in their use. The POMS measures several aspects of mood state and had been used in other sport and medical research and practice. The results from this test provide objective quantitative data to support the emotional response findings on the ERAIQ. On occasion, high depression, tension, and anger scores have been seen in injured athletes, prompting a referral—with the patient's permission—to a clinical psychologist or psychiatrist for therapeutic intervention. Most often, mood disturbance, measured objectively on the POMS, is moderate and simply supports the mood state identified on the ERAIQ. However, more elevated depression, tension, and anger scores, reinforced by the ranking of emotional responses on the ERAIQ, provide a blueprint for counseling intervention.

Again, assessment of the injured athlete is based on a review of the medical findings, the treatment plan (contingent upon severity of injury), the interview (ERAIQ), subjective findings, and any appropriate psychometric testing. Emphasis is also placed on how the athlete's personality, history of stressors, and coping resources might influence the postinjury emotional response. Personality vulnerabilities, frequent and intense life stressors, and poor coping skills do not disappear when injury occurs; rather, they may become exacerbated, and injury may be the last link in a culmination of events.

The most significant factor that determines the magnitude of emotional response related to sport injury appears to be the athlete's perception about the severity of the injury and its consequences (A. M. Smith, Scott, O'Fallon, et al., 1990). Typically, the most seriously injured athletes will demonstrate the most significant emotional response. An example of this is seen in the following case, which also serves to illustrate how the assessment criteria discussed above may be incorporated by the counselor.

▲

Case 3: This athlete was a high school senior from the southwestern United States. He excelled in baseball, football, and basketball. His older brother had received numerous college scholarship offers in several sports, but was seriously injured during his senior year and regretted being unable to accept one. During the athlete's sophomore year, he sustained a foot injury that was diagnosed as a ligament sprain. He played on the foot all season, despite pain. Later it was discovered that his foot had been fractured. Despite the necessity of surgery due to the trauma of having played all season on an undiagnosed fracture, the pain and swelling lingered. Some months later, he was injured again, this time by a jealous teammate, and seriously damaged his shoulder. In spite of his doctor's and therapist's rigorous efforts, he failed to respond to therapy and was referred to our sports medicine center. On clinical examination, the physicians found the shoulder sore and range of motion impaired. Consultation was made with the sports counselor to assess the psychosocial impact of injury. It was apparent from the onset of consultation that the injury had tremendous psychosocial impact on this young athlete. He was the second son and, according to his coaches, a "gifted athlete." He often scored nearly 75% of his team's total points per game in basketball and gained at least half of the total team yardage in football. In baseball, his defensive play at third base and his offensive production kept the team together. His dream was to be a professional athlete, and he wanted a college scholarship. The shoulder injury "robbed" him of his junior season, which was very crucial as he felt this was "when scouts notice ballplayers." He was very depressed and angry. He described himself as "straight" (i.e., someone who did not attend parties involving alcohol or drugs), and he felt totally left out of any peer group when he could not play and help the team. During our interview, his affect was flat, and he sat slouched in the chair, unable to make eye contact. It became increasingly apparent that he was very depressed and was unable to assure me that he would not harm himself before our next visit. I suggested he see our sport psychiatrist. He resisted, stating he was tired of doctors. I asked him to complete the POMS to obtain objective data to support our interview findings (which followed the ERAIQ) and my subjective observations. His resulting mood scores were depression = 49, tension = 37, and anger = 35. These negative mood state scores were significantly higher than college norms and than those observed in our study (A. M. Smith, Scott, O'Fallon, et al., 1990) for seriously injured athletes (in which the mean scores were depression = 23.1, tension = 19.1, and anger = 19.1). When these findings were integrated with his highly self-motivated personality, the stress of physical and emotional violation, pressure from parents and coaches, a lost season in his preferred sport, pain and reduced range of motion, and the lack of a supportive peer group, it was apparent that profound mood disturbance existed. Somewhat reluctantly, he granted me permission to discuss the situation with his parents. They agreed that a consultation with our sport psychiatrist was appropriate. I wondered if the physicians might feel that he was a candidate for short-term intensive psychotherapy and possibly a course of antidepressant drugs. However, he failed to keep his appointment with the psychiatrist. His reluctance may have been related to his determination not to give in to weakness (Carmen et al., 1968), a negative view of emotional illness (Pierce, 1969), or a fear of discrimination (Linder et al., 1989). It may also be that he had simply lost hope. Fortunately, he returned one week later to see me, and we worked through several other major issues. He was provided with support, coping skill interventions, homework, some inspirational reading, and hope. When he returned for his final visit one month later, his affect, shoulder, and POMS scores all showed marked improvement. Although professional licensed psychotherapy was offered, the patient declined and fortunately seemed to work through this situational depression with the support of both family and the nurse-counselor.

▼

Counseling interventions. Referrals to the sports counselor may involve preoperative, postoperative, or nonoperative counseling, each requiring different emphases. Overall, the pre- and postoperative counseling sessions are ordered by the physician, and counseling interventions are based on the athlete's injury and concerns that are identified from the medical history and guided interview (ERAIQ). Most sports medicine surgical and nonsurgical rehabilitation programs require a great willingness on the part of the patient to commit a large amount of time and energy to regaining pre-injury status. The flexibility and strengthening exercises are often demanding and force athletes to push through pain and swelling, whereas adhering to rigorous appointment schedules or, equally difficult, maintaining the motivation to exercise on their own. The goals of each individual athlete are integrated with the reality of the injury, the potential for rehabilitation, and any short- or long-term limitations. The counselor must decide which strategies will help athletes cope psychologically with present and future events.

Preoperative consultation. In preoperative counseling the primary focus should be on helping the athlete to understand the goals of the forthcoming surgical procedure and on developing or strengthening the commitment to rehabilitation. Athletes are asked to make decisions about anesthetic choices, pain management, and certain aspects of the rehabilitation regimen that will follow. Aspects of attribution theory (Weiner, 1974), which explain differential tendencies to account for behavior outcomes, may be described to athletes in order to emphasize the need for intrinsic motivation for rehabilitation. Athletes should be made aware that much of the potential for successful rehabilitation is under their control. Specifically, athletes are encouraged to become involved in their own stress management, pain control, and motivation and to assist the sports medicine team in setting and revising daily rehabilitation goals.

This attributional approach appeals to the problem-focused athlete as it increases the athlete's sense of control. However, in spite of helping the athlete exercise control over some aspects of the postinjury experience, it is also important to discuss prospective issues of dependency, helplessness, and potential lapses in motivation that occur during the long rehabilitation process (Dishman, 1985; Duda et al., 1989; Fisher, Domm, & Wuest, 1988). Practical issues, such as dealing with 6 weeks on crutches or in casts, transportation to rehabilitation sessions, and boredom resulting from repetitive performance of exercise routines, are also addressed.

A goal-setting model used for rehabilitation can be applied (A. M. Smith, 1991). Following an interview, it is helpful for the counselor to draw a target model and insert the individual athlete's dream goal and rehabilitation program. The target model (see Figure 6) has appeal to injured athletes and integrates long-, intermediate-, and short-term or daily goals. In the outer ring the "dream goal" is inserted, which serves to stimulate motivation. Nested inside

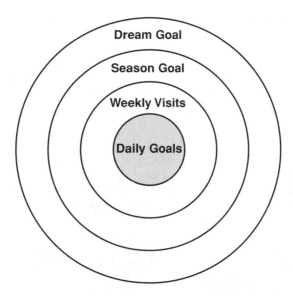

Figure 6. Target Approach for Goal Setting

can be any number of rings. The center is always anchored with the bull's-eye, which is darkened to attract the eye. The model is bidirectional in the sense that having a dream provides the inspiration to meet daily goals but only by doing the daily exercises will athletes return to sport and fulfill their dreams.

For example, the counselor can explain that during the postsurgical rehabilitation of an anterior cruciate ligament reconstruction, the postoperative course to recovery might resemble a "rum line in sailing." Just as a sailor tacks back and forth across the wind in order to progress to the destination, so will the injured athlete experience physical and psychosocial ups and downs during the rehabilitation period. Overall, the athlete must always mentally go back to the starting point to see how far he or she has come or how much progress has been made.

Relaxation and imagery are used preoperatively to reduce anxiety. The counselor suggests that relaxation and imagery may also be used prior to rehabilitation exercises when it may be appropriate to decrease muscle tension. A sample relaxation exercise that has been used with some success is provided in Figure 7. This technique combines elements of cognitive and physical relaxation, with an emphasis on clearing the mind of distracting thoughts and progressively tensing and relaxing various muscle groups of the body. In addition to the interventions discussed, sources of social support, recent stresses, and any maladaptive coping methods are identified. Issues of school and college

---

1. Find a quiet, comfortably warm room where distractions are minimal.
2. Attention must be focused on something such as your breathing.
3. It is essential to have a passive attitude and to let thoughts and images move through your mind in a passive manner. Gently bring your attention back to the object of focus when your mind wanders.
4. A comfortable position is essential, but you should not be so comfortable that you fall asleep.
5. Instructions:
   a. Sit in a comfortable position and close your eyes.
   b. Contract your muscles as hard as possible, harder yet, for count of 10.
   c. Start by pulling your toes up toward your nose (tightening calves) for a count of 10; tighten quadriceps (thighs); then abdominals; hand grip; biceps and triceps (make a muscle); and then pull your shoulders up toward your ears (muscles are contracted one group at a time starting with the toes).
   d. Feel the relaxation that follows, the warm feet, warm hands.
   e. Allow the muscles to remain deeply relaxed.
   f. Now settle in to the deep breathing phase. The breaths are slow, deep. On the way out say the word "calm."
   g. Allow all the air to escape so that you feel like a deflated balloon. Continue this practice for about 10 minutes. Keep your mind on the movement of air in and out of your lungs, gently bringing your attention back if your mind wanders.
6. Practice this at least once daily. Gradually use it as a form of emotional and arousal control for sport or stressful life situations. Learn how to use it to help you maintain an optimal flow zone for sport.

Figure 7. A Relaxation Method for Sports Medicine Patients

grades, drug and alcohol use and abuse, sexuality, and other concerns should be discussed and assistance provided as appropriate. Should factors such as single organs, infectious disease, or drug use, be identified as risks that might endanger the health of the patient or surgical team, they are discussed with both the patient and physician or that of the surgical team.

Relaxation and imagery are used preoperatively (a) to reduce anxiety, (b) to augment the effectiveness of pain medications, and (c) to prepare prior to range of motion or other stretching exercise. Care is taken to not use the operative limb in the relaxation method postoperatively until permission has been granted by the physician or physical therapist.

Postoperative consultation. During the first postoperative meeting the counselor may use the ERAIQ and a sport preference inventory to assess the athlete's psychosocial status in relation to the injury. Sometimes this is the first time the counselor and injured athlete have met, whereas at other times it is the postoperative follow-up to the preoperative interview. The interview is, therefore, conducted accordingly. It is also important at this time to evaluate the athlete's compliance with the actual rehabilitation protocol. The counselor must determine whether progress, or the lack thereof, relates to the injured athlete's attitude (i.e., motivation, ability, and effort) or to complicating factors, such as lack of insurance coverage for rehabilitation services; inadequate access to exercise or rehabilitation equipment; or medical complications, such as infections, thrombosis, or adhesions.

The counselor should assess stress, social support, and coping skills, as well as age-group, sex, team, and individual sport differences. It is preferable to assess the athlete's mood states and real and perceived progress on a monthly basis. The counselor must also discuss sleep deprivation and pain management issues. For example, pain and activity restriction due to large braces and immobilizers often interferes with sleep patterns. Other factors associated with athletic injury that have psychosocial ramifications for recovery include interactions with significant others, teammates, coaches, or parents as discussed earlier. These persons may be sources of stress or worry or, conversely, towers of strength and support. Additional factors that seem to affect athletes at this stage may relate to loss of social recognition (e.g., no rewards or positive feedback) and loss of financial and/or physical independence.

Strategies for intervention must be appropriate to the etiology of the problem. It may be necessary to see injured athletes every few days for a few weeks if they are very depressed. These injured athletes are also referred to a licensed clinical psychologist or a psychiatrist. The physician and physical therapist usually can best determine whether or not a lack of progress is related to factors under the athlete's control. Exercise logs or diaries are often helpful to increase compliance and permit evaluation of the effort exerted.

Nonoperative consultation. Nonoperative referrals to the sport counselor can be from athletes, physicians, patients, physical therapists, coaches, athletic trainers, athletic directors, or parents. Consultations that are not from physicians should be cleared by the medical directors for appropriateness before the appointment is made with the counselor. These athletes are usually referred for one of the following reasons:

1. To assess the impact of the injury on the athlete for whom surgery is not an appropriate solution. These injured athletes, for example, may have back pain, rotator cuff injuries, patellar-femoral pain, Osgood-Schlatter's disease, or stress fractures.
2. To assess performance decrements or assist with performance-enhancement strategies.

3. To determine the athlete's goals, motivation for rehabilitation, and existing pressures.
4. To explore concerns about eating disorders, exercise or substance abuse, fear of failure, or fear of success.
5. To interview injured athletes where pain is chronic and the injury has not resolved.

Some injured athletes have been seen at numerous institutions, have had several surgical procedures, and have pain that remains refractory to treatment, yet psychological or psychiatric intervention is glaringly absent in their medical history. Such patients are often frightened of, and therefore resistant to, psychological intervention. Occasionally they may be less inhibited by an interview with a nurse-counselor, but unfortunately, when a more in-depth evaluation by a psychologist or psychiatrist is warranted, these patients often leave the sports medicine center in search of yet another scalpel or surgical cure. Often chronic unresolved pain causes psychosocial issues that become associated with the physical pain. In such cases, breaking the cycle of pain should take priority over resolving issues of a psychological nature. Resolution or adaptation to chronic postinjury pain is a very different problem, one that usually requires a multidisciplinary or holistic approach. Professionals in the pain clinic or pain management center are often consulted to assist in the management of these patients.

As briefly discussed earlier, when appropriate to the situation, the counselor may introduce a variety of strategies, such as relaxation, guided imagery, cognitive restructuring (e.g., "channel-clicking," or cognitively switching from the negative talk channel to the positive talk channel), aerobic exercise (e.g, maintaining exercise logs with an emphasis on adherence to a training regimen for general, overall conditioning), and various performance-enhancement strategies (e.g., goal setting, mastery mental rehearsal of sport skills). Strategies to maintain reaction time, such as juggling and acu-vision, mental training programs, and biomechanical analysis of taped videos featuring the athletes in their sport, can be motivating, informational tools (A. M. Smith, Scott, & Wiese, 1990). Selected reading that is inspirational and appropriate to the athlete's sport may also be helpful (Wiese & Weiss, 1987).

Because injured athletes often respond to problem-focused coping, they may be engaged in sport-related experiences that interest them, such as participating in self-study programs to obtain coaching certification in the American Coaching Effectiveness Program (ACEP), acting as coordinator of marketing efforts for their teams, providing assistance in coaching younger athletes, reviewing available sport psychology tapes, or reading materials appropriate to their sport and level of participation. In addition, every attempt is made to maintain the athlete's strength and conditioning during the rehabilitation period to ensure readiness to return to sport. The following case study illustrates this strategy.

▲

Case 4: A 17-year-old female high school senior was referred to the sport psychology counselor by the high school athletic director. The injured athlete, whose aspiration was to play college tennis, had developed avascular necrosis of the hip. Our counseling strategy employed gradual attempts to change her dream from one of playing sport into one of a career in sport management. The athlete ultimately remained involved with sports by organizing a philanthropic marketing effort for a community sports team, giving a radio interview presenting an athlete's perspective on dealing with injury, and becoming affiliated with a high school athletic director in a clerkship role. After probing her interests further, it was discovered that she also wanted to learn more about coaching. We were able to provide her with the means to become leader-level certified through ACEP. At the time of this writing, she is coaching a youth tennis team and has been accepted to a fine college. We continue to emphasize her sense of self-control over her destiny, and she has responded well to this challenge. Consequently, we hope to minimize depressive tendencies that might otherwise occur. Communication of her progress, with her permission, is ongoing between the high school athletic director and sports medicine team.

▼

Physicians in Sports Medicine

As indicated earlier in Figure 4, physicians are often at the center of the injury treatment team. Consequently, it is of the utmost importance for them to keep abreast of both the physical *and* psychological progress of athletes during recovery. Physicians who treat sport injuries are usually trained in orthopedic surgery, physical medicine and rehabilitation, family practice, or community medicine. The practice of sports medicine, although primarily concerned with sport-related injuries, also encompasses prevention of injury, conditioning, performance enhancement, and other activity-related situations.

Most sports medicine centers try to accommodate injured athletes promptly to ensure accurate, immediate diagnosis and appropriate treatment. Many are equipped to serve as small emergency rooms with diagnostic, suturing, cast application, and cast removal capabilities. Frequently, the injured athlete meets the physician "on the field." The physician will diagnose the injury, explain the treatment options, perform whatever procedures are required, order pain and other medications as appropriate, and consult other members of the sports medicine team as indicated. If the athlete needs physical therapy, has nutritional concerns, or requires psychosocial assessment or counseling, the physician most often writes the orders. In some medical practices, physical therapists or athletic trainers are the first to evaluate the injured athlete, and they consult the physician as appropriate.

In either case, the key for these team members is to acknowledge the psychological reactions and progress of the athlete and to refer to sport psychology consultants, clinical psychologists, and psychiatrists as needed. A recent survey of sports medicine physicians conducted by Brewer, Van Raalte, and Linder (1991) found that behavioral and psychological problems were perceived by the physicians to occur with some frequency in conjunction with athletic injuries, thus suggesting the importance of having a referral network in place. Physicians were also found to have a moderately positive attitude toward the involvement of sport psychologists in the recovery process as appropriate. As these authors indicated, it is important to continue to build on this perceived value as physicians become more aware of the potential role of sport psychology practitioners as members of the medical team.

Physical Therapists in Sports Medicine

Physical therapists conduct a thorough evaluation of the injured area, determine the exercises or modalities that will be helpful, explain the therapy regimen, and set up goals for rehabilitation. The therapist instructs the injured athlete about when evaluations will be scheduled and accordingly provides appropriate feedback emanating from such evaluation. For example, on postsurgery status the athlete must satisfy prescribed and agreed-upon rehabilitation goals relative to regaining range of motion and strength. Such anticipated progress may be delineated and clarified by the physical therapist, who, in concert with the physician, decides upon treatment modification. Should the athlete not progress as expected, further diagnostic procedures may be indicated. Occasionally, if an aggressive nonoperative therapy program is unsuccessful, a surgical procedure may be indicated. Physical therapists use handouts, anatomical models, and actual demonstrations to instruct their patients. Physical therapists also initiate consultations with other members of the sports medicine team when additional input is in the best interests of the patient.

Psychiatrists and Psychologists in Sports Medicine

Psychiatrists and clinical psychologists may be consulted directly by physicians, although in the Mayo Clinic program many of these consultations are made on the recommendation of the sport psychology counselor. A telephone call is usually made to the sport psychiatrist regarding the appropriateness of a prospective referral. If the psychiatrist agrees that such intervention is indicated, an appointment is arranged. After the psychiatrist sees the injured athlete, we usually receive a call with a summary of the psychiatric interview and the goals of the recommended treatment regimen. A more detailed copy of the content from the interview is then placed in the confidential file. In this way, members of the sports medicine team who may continue to work with the injured athlete are informed of the basic treatment objectives, thus ensuring a consistent, integrated approach. Feedback from psychologists and dietitians seeing injured athletes occurs in a similar way.

Summary

Many team members from both the sport and medical communities are involved in the recovery process for injured athletes. Each has unique and, it is hoped, complementary offerings to enhance the injured athlete's physical *and* psychological rehabilitation. It must be emphasized that paramount in the process of rehabilitating the injured athlete is the delicate balance between confidentiality and the need for a holistic integrated sports medicine team approach to the client's care. Respect and empathy for injured athletes dictate the manner in which sports medicine is practiced.

It is also important to review information on academic progress, career goals, and alternative interests in the event that injury severity precludes return to sport in athletes. Athletes will benefit from working with a sports medicine team that communicates not only among themselves but also with the coach, family, and trainer to ensure a safe, productive return to sport.

References

Andersen, M. B., & Williams, J. M. (1988). A model of stress and athletic injury: Prediction and prevention. *Journal of Sport and Exercise Psychology,10,* 294–306.

Brewer, B. W., Van Raalte, J. L., & Linder, D. E. (1991). Role of the sport psychologist in treating injured athletes: A survey of sports medicine providers. *Journal of Applied Sport Psychology, 3,* 183–190.

Carmen, L., Zerman, J. L., & Blaine, G. B. (1968). The use of the Harvard psychiatric service by athletes and non-athletes. *Mental Hygiene, 52,* 134–137.

Cassem, M. H., & Hackett, T .P. (1971). Psychiatric consultations in a coronary care unit. *Annals of Internal Medicine, 75,* 9–14.

Chan, C. S., & Grossman, H. Y. (1988). Psychological effects of running loss on consistent runners. *Perceptual and Motor Skills, 66,* 875–883.

Christman, N. J. (1988). Uncertainty, coping and distress. *Research in Nursing and Health, 11,* 71–82.

Connelly, S. L. (1991). *Injury and self-esteem: A test of Sonstroem and Morgan's model.* Unpublished masters thesis, South Dakota State University, Vermillion.

Dishman, R. K. (1985). Medical psychology in exercise and sport. *Medical Clinics in North America, 69,* 123–142.

Duda, J. L., Smart, A. E., & Tappe, M. K. (1989). Predictors of adherence in the rehabilitation of athletic injuries: An application of personal investment theory. *Journal of Sport and Exercise Psychology, 11,* 367–381.

Eldridge, W. E. (1983). The importance of psychotherapy for athletic-related orthopedic injuries among adults. *International Journal of Sports Psychology, 14,* 203–211.

Fisher, A. C., Domm., M. A., & Wuest, D. A. (1988). Adherence to sports-injury rehabilitation programs. *The Physician and Sportsmedicine, 16,* 47–52.

Folkman, S., & Lazarus, R. S. (1986). Stress responses and depressive symptomatology. *Journal of Abnormal Psychology, 95,* 107–113.

Gordon, S., Milios, D., & Grove, J. R. (1991). Psychological aspects of the recovery process from sport injury: The perspective of sport physiotherapists. *Australian Journal of Science and Medicine in Sport, 23,* 53–60.

Grove, J. R., Stewart, R., & Gordon, S. (1990, October). *Emotional reactions of athletes to knee rehabilitation.* Paper presented at the Annual Meeting of the Australian Sports Medicine Federation, Alice Springs.

Kübler-Ross, E. (1969). *On death and dying.* New York: Macmillan.

Linder, D. E., Pillow, D. R., & Reno, R. R. (1989). Shrinking jocks: Derogation of athletes who consult a sports psychologist. *Journal of Sport and Exercise Psychology, 11,* 270–280.

Little, J. C. (1969). The athletes' neurosis: A deprivation crisis. *Acta Psychiatrica Scandinavia, 45,* 187–197.

Martens, R. M. (1987). *Coaches' guide to sport psychology.* Champaign, IL: Human Kinetics.

McDonald, S. A., & Hardy, C. J. (1990). Affective response patterns of the injured athlete. *The Sport Psychologist, 4*(3), 261–274.

McNair, D. M., Lorr, M., & Droppleman, L. F. (1971). *Manual: Profile of mood states.* San Diego, CA: Educational and Industrial Testing Service.

NFL notebook. (1991, November). *St. Paul Pioneer Press,* p. 3C.

Pierce, R. A. (1969). Athletes in psychotherapy: How many, how come? *Journal of the American College Health Association, 17,* 244–249.

Rohe, D. E., & Athelstan, G. T. (1982). Vocational interests of persons with spinal cord injury. *Journal of Counseling Psychology, 29,* 283–291.

Scott, S. G. (1984). Current concepts in the rehabilitation of the injured athlete. *Mayo Clinic Proceedings, 59,* 85–90.

Smith, A. M. (1991). *Power play: Mental toughness for hockey and beyond.* Unpublished paper, Mayo Clinic Sports Medicine Center, Rochester, MN 55905. (Available from Aynsley M. Smith, Mayo Clinic Sports Medicine Center, Rochester, MN 55905).

Smith A. M., & Milliner E. K. (1991). *Suicide risk in injured athletes.* Manuscript submitted for publication.

Smith, A. M., Scott, S. G., O'Fallon, W., & Young, M. L. (1990). The emotional responses of athletes to injury. *Mayo Clinic Proceedings, 65,* 38–50.

Smith, A. M., Scott, S. G., & Wiese, D. M. (1990). The psychological effects of sports injuries: Coping. *Sports Medicine, 9,* 352–369.

Smith, R. E., Smoll, F. L., & Ptacek, J. T. (1990). Conjunctive moderator variables in vulnerability and resiliency research: Life stress, social support and coping skills, and adolescent sport injuries. *Journal of Personality and Social Psychology, 58,* 360–370.

Tunks, T., & Bellissimo, A. (1988). Coping with the coping concept: A brief comment. *Pain, 34,* 171–174.

Weiner, B. (1974). *Achievement motivation and attribution theory.* Morristown, NJ: General Learning Press.

Weiss, M. R., & Troxel, R. K. (1986). Psychology of the injured athlete. *Athletic Training, 21,* 104–109, 154.

Wiese, D. M., & Weiss, M. R. (1987). Psychological rehabilitation and physical injury: Implications for the sportsmedicine team. *The Sport Psychologist, 1,* 318–330.

Wiese, D. M., Weiss, M. R., & Yukelson, D. P. (1991). Sport psychology in the training room: A survey of athletic trainers. *The Sport Psychologist, 5,* 15–24.

Wiese-Bjornstal, D. M. (in press, 1997). Psychosocial factors in sport injury. In M. K. Anderson & M. Martin (Eds.), *Field manual in athletic training.* Baltimore, MD: Williams & Wilkins.

Wiese-Bjornstal, D. M., Smith, A. M., & LaMott, E. E. (1995). A model of psychologic response to athletic injury and rehabilitation. *Athletic Training: Sports Health Care Perspectives, 1*(1), 17–30.

Yarcheski, A., & Mahon, M. E. (1986). Perceived stress and symptom patterns in early adolescents: The role of mediating variables. *Research in Nursing and Health, 9,* 289–297.

10

Patient-Practitioner Interactions in Sport Injury Rehabilitation

Britton W. Brewer
Judy L. Van Raalte
Albert J. Petitpas
Springfield College

Interactions between athletes with injuries and their sports medicine providers can exert an important influence on the athletes' psychological state, treatment adherence, and rehabilitation outcome. In this chapter, research on patient-practitioner interactions in the context of sport injury rehabilitation is reviewed. Topics such as patient-practitioner communication, patient and practitioner perceptions, and adherence to sport injury rehabilitation programs are addressed. Guidelines for referring patients for psychological services and recommendations for enhancing patient-practitioner interactions are presented.

Enhancement of physical well-being is the primary focus in sports medicine settings. It is abundantly clear, however, that sport injury rehabilitation occurs within a broader social context comprising patient interactions with orthopedic surgeons, physical therapists, athletic trainers, support staff, other patients, family members, and friends. The nature and quality of these interactions may have a profound impact on both processes (e.g., emotional adjustment, adherence) and outcomes (e.g., satisfaction, recovery of physical function) in sport injury rehabilitation.

Arguably the most important interactions in sport injury rehabilitation are those between patients and the sports medicine practitioners (i.e., physical therapists and athletic trainers) who direct their rehabilitation efforts on a day-to-day basis. In addition to facilitating physical recovery following injury, sport injury rehabilitation professionals can be an important source of social support for athletes with injuries (Ford & Gordon, 1993; Hardy & Crace, this volume; Udry, 1996). In a recent study of competitive and recreational athletes undergoing rehabilitation following knee surgery, physical therapists/athletic trainers were identified as second only to parents as providers of social support (Izzo, 1994). Social support has implications for the psychological distress (Brewer, Linder, & Phelps, 1995; Brewer, Petitpas, Van Raalte, Sklar, & Ditmar, 1995), rehabilitation adherence (Byerly, Worrell, Gahimer, & Domholdt, 1994; Duda, Smart, & Tappe, 1989; Fisher, Domm, & Wuest, 1988), and treatment outcome (Bianco & Orlick, 1996; Gordon & Lindgren, 1990) of patients with sport injuries.

Given the central importance ascribed to physical therapists and athletic trainers in sport injury rehabilitation, this chapter focuses on the interactions that these practitioners have with their patients. After presenting an overview of patient-practitioner communication in sport injury rehabilitation settings, empirical research exploring patient and practitioner perceptions in sport injury rehabilitation is examined, issues in patient adherence to rehabilitation regimens prescribed by sports medicine practitioners are discussed, and guidelines for referral of patients with sport injuries for counseling or psychotherapy are provided. The chapter concludes with recommendations for enhancing patient-practitioner interactions in sport injury rehabilitation.

Patient-Practitioner Communication

By definition, interactions between patients with sport injuries and the professionals supervising their rehabilitation involve communication. Although the importance of effective patient-practitioner communication in sport injury rehabilitation has been acknowledged by athletes (DeFrancesco, Miller, Larson, & Robinson, 1994; Fisher & Hoisington, 1993), sport rehabilitation professionals (Fisher, Mullins, & Frye, 1993; Gordon, Milios, & Grove, 1991; Larson, Starkey, & Zaichowsky, 1996; Wiese, Weiss, & Yukelson, 1991), and sport psychologists (e.g., Danish, 1986; Nideffer, 1983), it has received little empirical attention. The topic has, however, been examined extensively in the general medical literature, where a number of barriers to effective patient-practitioner communication have been identified. Patient characteristics that may interfere with communication include anxiety, inexperience with the medical disorder, and a lack of intelligence. Practitioner behaviors that may contribute to poor communication include not listening, using jargon and technical language, providing simplistic explanations, depersonalizing the patient, displaying worry, and holding perjorative stereotypes of patients (S. E. Taylor, 1995). Poor patient-practitioner communication can discourage the future use of medical services (S. E. Taylor, 1995) and hamper adherence to medical regimens (Meichenbaum & Turk, 1987; S. E. Taylor, 1995). For example, it has been found that patients are less likely to adhere to treatment recommendations when their physicians fail to give clear explanations, provide positive verbal communications, and answer questions (DiMatteo et al., 1993; Hall, Roter, & Katz, 1988).

In one of the few studies to examine patient-practitioner communication in the context of sport injury rehabilitation, Kahanov and Fairchild (1994) found that intercollegiate athletes with injuries and their athletic trainers had discrepancies in their perceptions of several aspects of communication during the initial evaluation. For example, more than one-third of the athletes indicated that they had summarized their athletic trainers' injury explanations when their athletic trainers indicated that they had not.

In a related investigation, Hokanson (1994) asked a sample of competitive and recreational athletes undergoing rehabilitation following knee surgery to describe the nature of their communication with the physical therapist or athletic trainer who was directing their rehabilitation efforts. Analyses of qualitative data revealed that patient-practitioner communication was predominantly informational, characterized by discussion of rehabilitation-related topics. To a lesser extent, there was empathic (or socioemotional) communication between patients and practitioners, in which common interests and patients' lives in general were discussed. Quantitative analyses in which patients' satisfaction with their communication with the rehabilitation professionals was assessed with the Sports Injury Clinic Athlete Satisfaction Scale (SICASS; A. H. Taylor & May, 1995b) indicated a nonsignificant relationship between satisfaction and adherence to the rehabilitation program.

Clearly, despite its importance, little is known about patient-practitioner communication in sport injury rehabilitation. Descriptive and inferential investigations are needed to provide a thorough understanding of the nature and implications of communication between athletes with injuries and the professionals attending to their rehabilitation.

Patient and Practitioner Perceptions

During the course of injury rehabilitation, patients and practitioners are likely to form impressions of rehabilitation-related processes and outcomes. These perceptions are important because they may both reflect and influence inter-actions between patients and practitioners. In this section of the chapter, re-search on patient and practitioner perceptions associated with sport injury re-habilitation is examined.

Rehabilitation Regimen

Several studies have investigated the congruence between patients and practi-tioners with regard to the content of sport injury rehabilitation regimens. Ka-hanov and Fairchild (1994) found that athletes with injuries and athletic train-ers had significant disagreement in terms of whether the athlete understood the rehabilitation program and whether a written protocol was given to the athlete. May and Taylor (1994) found that patients at a university-based sport injury clinic gave estimates of the amount of time required to complete their home rehabilitation exercises that were an average of 42% lower than their physiotherapists' estimates. A study by Webborn, Carbon, and Miller (1997) bolstered the findings of Kahanov and Fairchild and May and Taylor, demon-strating that 77% of sport injury clinic patients who were prescribed home re-habilitation exercises misunderstood at least some aspect of their rehabilita-tion program. Thus, it appears that patient and practitioner perceptions of something so vital and seemingly objective as the rehabilitation program itself may differ dramatically.

Recovery Progress

There is probably no aspect of the rehabilitation process more on the minds of patients and practitioners than the extent to which patients are progressing to-ward recovery. Perceptions of poor rehabilitation progress have been linked to negative emotional responses in athletes with injuries (McDonald & Hardy, 1990; Smith, Young, & Scott, 1988). Given the centrality and potential ad-verse impact of perceptions of recovery progress in sport injury rehabilitation, patient and practitioner perceptions of injury status have been assessed in a number of studies.

Crossman and Jamieson (1985) found that athletic trainer ratings of injury seriousness and injury disruptiveness were significantly correlated with those made by athletes with injuries ($r = .56$ and $r = .39$, respectively), indicating a degree of agreement between patients and practitioners on patients' current in-jury status. In contrast to their athletic trainers, however, the athletes with in-juries in this study tended to overestimate the seriousness and underestimate the disruptiveness of their injuries. Athletes who overestimated the seriousness or disruptiveness of their injuries tended to experience greater pain and mood disturbance than did athletes who did not overestimate the seriousness or disruptiveness of their injuries. In a follow-up study, Crossman, Jamieson, and Hume (1990) again found that athletes underestimated the disruptive impact of their injuries relative to the estimates of medical professionals.

Subsequent research has substantiated the findings of Crossman and her colleagues (Crossman & Jamieson, 1985; Crossman et al., 1990). Van Raalte, Brewer, and Petitpas (1992) documented significant correlations between patient and practitioner estimates of the number of days that the athletes would be prevented from participating in sport ($r = .92$) and ratings of the extent to which the athletes were fully rehabilitated ($r = .35$). Athletes in the Van Raalte et al. study viewed themselves as significantly more recovered than did their athletic trainers. Significant correlations between injury appraisals made by sports medicine clinic patients and their physicians were also obtained in investigations by Brewer, Linder, and Phelps (1995) and Brewer, Van Raalte, Petitpas, Sklar, and Ditmar (1995).

Thus, it appears that although patient and practitioner perceptions of recovery progress are often congruent, discrepancies sometimes occur and may influence the emotional state of patients. It should also be recognized that under certain circumstances, athletes may conceal symptoms and downplay the significance of their injuries to return to sport sooner than medically advisable (Nixon, 1994). In such situations, it may be difficult for patients and practitioners to see "eye to eye" with regard to patients' injury status. Fortunately, there is evidence that sport injury rehabilitation professionals are less susceptible than coaches to situational influences in judging the appropriateness of a given athlete's returning to sport following injury (Flint & Weiss, 1992).

Attributions for Recovery

One goal of sport injury rehabilitation practitioners is to instill a sense of responsibility for rehabilitation in their patients (Gordon et al., 1991). By encouraging their patients to take ownership of their rehabilitation, practitioners presume that patients will become more invested in completing therapeutic activities and will achieve a more rapid and complete recovery. Research indicates that the extent to which patients accept responsibility for their rehabilitation progress may depend upon the rate of recovery, with athletes who recover slowly being less likely to claim responsibility for their rehabilitation progress than are athletes who recover rapidly (Grove, Hanrahan, & Stewart, 1990; Laubach, Brewer, Van Raalte, & Petitpas, 1996). Because attributions for recovery have been associated with rehabilitation self-efficacy beliefs

92) and adherence to sport injury rehabilitation (Laubach et al., 1996), they merit further empirical attention.

Psychological Distress

Due in part to the psychological significance of sport participation to many athletes (Brewer, 1993; Kleiber & Brock, 1992), injury may be a major source of stress (Brewer & Petrie, 1995; Wiese-Bjornstal, Smith, & LaMott, 1995) and emotional disturbance (Brewer & Petrie, 1995; Chan & Grossman, 1988; Leddy, Lambert, & Ogles, 1994; Pearson & Jones, 1992; Smith et al., 1993). Because emotional disturbance is inversely related to rehabilitation adherence (Daly, Brewer, Van Raalte, Petitpas, & Sklar, 1995) and rehabilitation outcome (Wise, Jackson, & Rocchio, 1979), it is important for sport injury rehabilitation practitioners to recognize psychological distress in their patients to facilitate appropriate referral. Unfortunately, research indicates that rehabilitation personnel may have difficulty in identifying psychological distress in their patients. Brewer, Petitpas, et al. (1995) found that sports medicine clinic patients' self-reported psychological distress was uncorrelated with their physical therapists' or athletic trainers' ratings of patient behaviors indicative of psychological disturbance. This finding signals a potential need for additional emphasis on the psychological realm in the training of physical therapists and athletic trainers.

Adherence to Rehabilitation

Adherence to a sport injury rehabilitation program is a tangible outcome of patient-practitioner interactions. Encouraging patients to adopt treatment recommendations is an essential task of rehabilitation practitioners. Depending on the nature of the particular sport injury rehabilitation regimen, adherence may involve such behaviors as complying with practitioner instructions to restrict physical activity, completing home rehabilitation exercises, completing home cryotherapy (icing), complying with medication prescriptions, and participating in clinic-based rehabilitation exercises and therapy (Brewer, in press). A recent review of the literature indicated that, depending on how adherence to sport injury rehabilitation is assessed, adherence rates ranging from 40 to 91% have been documented (Brewer, in press).

Characteristics of both the patient and the rehabilitation context have been linked to adherence to sport injury rehabilitation. Patient characteristics positively associated with adherence include self-motivation (Brewer, Daly, Van Raalte, Petitpas, & Sklar, 1994; Culpepper, Masters, & Wittig, 1996; Duda et al., 1989; Fields, Murphey, Horodyski, & Stopka, 1995; Fisher et al., 1988; Noyes, Matthews, Mooar, & Grood, 1983), pain tolerance (Byerly et al., 1994;

Fields et al., 1995; Fisher et al., 1988), task involvement (Duda et al., 1989), and tough-mindedness (Wittig & Schurr, 1994). Ego involvement (Lampton, Lambert, & Yost, 1993) and trait anxiety (Eichenhofer, Wittig, Balogh, & Pisano, 1986) are patient characteristics that have been negatively correlated with adherence to sport injury rehabilitation programs. Thus, it appears that patients who are stoic, strong-willed, and self-motivated are more likely than other patients to stick with their rehabilitation.

A number of contextual variables have been linked to sport injury rehabilitation adherence. Factors related to greater adherence include belief in the efficacy of the treatment (Duda et al., 1989; Noyes et al., 1983; A. H. Taylor & May, 1996), comfort of the rehabilitation setting (Brewer, Daly, et al., 1994; Fields et al., 1995; Fisher et al., 1988), convenience of rehabilitation scheduling (Fields et al., 1995; Fisher et al., 1988), perceived exertion during rehabilitation exercises (Brewer, Daly, et al., 1994; Fisher et al., 1988), and rehabilitation practitioner expectancy of patient adherence (A. H. Taylor & May, 1995a). These factors highlight the importance of patients' interactions with the providers attending to their care and the sport injury rehabilitation environment as a whole. Adherence may be compromised when athletes with injuries are not confident in and comfortable with their rehabilitation regimens.

Fisher and his colleagues investigated the adherence-enhancing strategies and behaviors identified by previously injured athletes (Fisher & Hoisington, 1993) and athletic trainers (Fisher et al., 1993). The former patients noted that having practitioners who were caring, honest, and encouraging helped them through the rehabilitation process (Fisher & Hoisington, 1993). The practitioners indicated that providing patients with education about their injuries and rehabilitation programs, assisting patients with goal setting, offering encouragement to patients, and monitoring the progress of their patients were successful strategies for procuring patient adherence to rehabilitation (Fisher et al., 1993). Patients and practitioners both expressed disdain for athletic trainer threats and scare tactics in gaining adherence (Fisher & Hoisington, 1993; Fisher et al., 1993).

Although the strategies suggested by patients and practitioners may be effective in achieving increased adherence to sport injury rehabilitation programs, it is important to target the strategies appropriately. In particular, the adherence-enhancing interventions should be applied only to rehabilitation regimens for which there is substantial support for their efficacy. Poor adherence may hamper physical recovery for some rehabilitation regimens (Derscheid & Feiring, 1987; Meani, Migliorini, & Tinti, 1986; Satterfield, Dowden, & Yasamura, 1990), but not others (Noyes et al., 1983; Shelbourne & Wilckens, 1990), especially those that are "experimental" or lacking in formal documentation. Along these lines, practitioners are cautioned not to infer that patients are not adhering to the treatment program when their recovery is slower than expected. Healing rate is inappropriate for use as an index of adherence because it is not behaviorally based and therefore does not provide information on how well patients are complying with their rehabilitation programs (Johnson, 1993). In other words, athletes with slow-healing injuries may truly be doing all that has been asked of them, and to assume otherwise may damage the patient-practitioner relationship.

Referral for Psychological Services

Athletes, in general, exhibit a smaller range and frequency of mental disorders than are found in the population at large (Andersen, Denson, Brewer, & Van Raalte, 1994). Nevertheless, an estimated 5–13% of athletes report clinically meaningful levels of psychological distress, at least in the short term (i.e., one to two months), following injury (Brewer, Linder, & Phelps, 1995; Brewer, Petitpas, et al., 1995; Leddy et al., 1994; McDonald & Hardy, 1990; Smith, Scott, O'Fallon, & Young, 1990). Even for athletes with injuries who are not having difficulties in relationships, school, or work, referral to mental health professionals can improve their quality of life and enhance their sport involvement (Brewer, Petitpas, & Van Raalte, in press).

Referral is delicate process. The structure of the referral can set the stage for the quality and efficacy of the therapeutic relationship that follows (Bobele & Conran, 1988). When working with athletes, referrals can be complicated by the stigma associated with mental problems and the derogation of those who seek help from mental health practitioners (Linder, Brewer, Van Raalte, & DeLange, 1991). Although some athletes with injuries may be skeptical about the utility of psychological interventions in sport injury rehabilitation and express reluctance about receiving a psychological referral, research indicates that athletes have generally positive perceptions of psychological interventions in the context of injury rehabilitation (Brewer, Jeffers, Petitpas, & Van Raalte, 1994; DeFrancesco et al., 1994; Durso-Cupal, 1996; Pearson & Jones, 1992; Potter, 1995).

Referral Networks

Having gathered information about psychological problems that may require referral (e.g., anxiety/stress, depression, eating disorders, adjustment reaction to athletic injury, substance abuse), sports medicine practitioners should develop an appropriate referral network. A referral network is a group of people with expertise in a variety of areas to whom patients can be referred. Ideally, the mental health professionals in the referral network have knowledge of sport and experience working with athletes. At the least, they should be interested in learning about sport and exercise and open to working with an athletic population (Van Raalte & Andersen, 1996).

Establishing a referral network takes time and motivation. First, appropriate mental health professionals in the local area should be identified (Heyman, 1993). These might include psychologists, psychiatrists, and social workers. Selecting both male and female mental health professionals of various theoretical orientations and professional backgrounds can be useful. Second, an effort should be made to develop a relationship with these professionals. The referral process is often smoother and more comfortable if practitioners know the professionals to whom they are referring their patients and have asked the referral sources how they would like athletes to be referred (Bobele & Conran, 1988). Athletes seem to find this "team approach" in which various sport professionals work together to be appealing (Andersen, 1992). Third, the referral network should be evaluated and modified on an ongoing basis to provide the best service for athletes. Having a broad group of professionals available for referral allows sports medicine practitioners to have some flexibility in the referral process.

When developing a referral network, it is important to keep in mind some of the specific concerns that athletes may have. Athletes generally have limited time due to the demands of training and work or school, and many athletes have limited funds. Thus, it is useful to select local practitioners, at least some of whom provide services on a sliding scale basis. For student-athletes attending colleges or universities, there are usually "free" on-campus services available. Developing a relationship with these providers increases the likelihood that athletes will follow through on referrals made.

The Referral Process

Each athlete's needs and situation are different. Therefore, each referral is different. The likelihood of making successful referrals can be increased by carefully assessing the psychological needs of athletes who are injured, paying attention to the timing of referrals, and following up on referrals.

Sports medicine providers often observe athletes' psychological responses to injury as a normal part of treatment. For example, practitioners may ask their patients how they are feeling and how their recovery is progressing. Athletes who report that they are having difficulties may be good candidates for referral.

Before referring athletes, it is useful for sports medicine practitioners to consult with mental health professionals in their referral network to discuss the case. Consultation can help clarify the situation and, if referral is necessary, facilitate the referral process.

Sports medicine practitioners who have good relationships with their patients will probably have the easiest time making referrals. Nevertheless, the referral process is tricky, and there is no "perfect time" to make a referral. As a general rule, the more severe the psychological symptoms athletes are experiencing, the sooner athletes should be referred (Heil, 1993).

Sports medicine practitioners who decide to refer athletes should explain to athletes the reason for the referral and should describe what is involved in working with the mental health professionals to whom they have been referred (Bobele & Conran, 1988; Heil, 1993). Noting the important connection between mind and body and reassuring athletes that they are not "head cases" can also be useful (Heil, 1993).

After a referral has been made, sports medicine practitioners should follow up with the athletes. They might ask, "How is it going with Dr. Smith?" With the athlete's consent, it can also be helpful for the sports medicine and mental health practitioners to consult regarding the athlete's progress. The mental health professional should not reveal confidential details of the patient's discussions, but limited information about the patient's status can be shared.

In some cases, athletes may decide not to follow through on referrals. In these situations, the sports medicine practitioner and the patient might discuss alternate strategies for dealing with the problem. If appropriate, reintroduce the idea of referral at a later date (Heil, 1993).

Recommendations for Enhancing Patient-Practitioner Interactions

Although the importance of building effective patient-practitioner relationships has been recognized by both injured athletes and sport injury rehabilitation professionals (e.g., DeFrancesco et al., 1994; Gordon et al., 1991), there is little empirical evidence to suggest the best means for enhancing these interactions. However, extensive research from counseling psychology on the nature of the counselor-client relationship may provide a helpful framework for examining patient-practitioner interactions in the sports medicine setting.

The Working Alliance

It has long been believed that the quality of the counseling relationship is a critical variable in predicting successful therapeutic outcomes (Orlinsky & Howard, 1986). However, this relationship is quite complex, may change at different stages in the counseling process, and can be viewed quite differently by counselors and clients (Sexton & Whiston, 1994). Therefore, any recommendations for enhancing patient-practitioner interactions in the sport injury rehabilitation setting should also allow for individual differences, account for the time phase of the injury rehabilitation process, and consider the perceptions of both patients and practitioners.

Bordin (1979) suggested that the counselor-client relationship was a working alliance composed of three main components: agreement on goals, agreement on tasks, and development of an emotional bond between client and therapist. Clearly, agreement on goals and tasks would seem to be a critical component of most patient-practitioner interactions. However, as described earlier, it is not unusual to find discrepancies between patients' and practitioners' perceptions of patients' recovery progress, rehabilitation regimen, or level of psychological distress. In addition, even though athletic therapists may not perceive themselves as establishing emotional bonds with their patients, they have been identified as second only to parents as sources of social support for athletes with injuries (Izzo, 1994). Therefore, a closer examination of how to develop an effective working alliance may enhance sport injury rehabilitation practitioners' ability to facilitate treatment adherence and to positively influence rehabilitation outcomes.

In order to be effective in building working alliances, practitioners should consider their role within the context of the injury rehabilitation process. For the most part, initial interactions between patients and practitioners are marked by interpersonal complementarity. That is, the two participants in the interaction assume unequal status roles, with the practitioner being in the one-up position (Kiesler & Watkins, 1989). As such, athletes with injuries are likely to be dependent on athletic therapists for informational support and to wait for the therapist to take the lead and to establish norms for the interaction.

Ironically, premature attempts to explore feelings or to offer support and encouragement during initial interactions may have a negative impact on the working alliance by putting the patient in a passive role (Kivlighan & Schmitz, 1992). Instead, it may be better to initiate the interaction by providing clear information about the nature of the injury, treatment goals, possible side effects, and coping strategies for adjusting to the rehabilitation process (Petitpas & Danish, 1995). This type of information is often particularly helpful for athletes who experience anxiety over their injuries because it may provide them with a sense of control and predictability that could reduce the levels of stress they experience (Meichenbaum, 1985). However, practitioners must realize that how they present the information is critical in ensuring patient understanding (Henderson & Carroll, 1993), adherence to treatment regimens, and patient-practitioner collaboration (Petitpas & Danish, 1995).

Although practitioners may be in a one-up position in the working alliance, they need to take sufficient time to understand problems from the perspectives of the athletes with injuries and to ensure that the athletes understand clearly and accept the information that is provided to them. In addition, the anxiety or power differential that may be inherent in the initial patient-practitioner relationship may interfere with patients' abilities to listen attentively or to be willing to ask for further clarification. Even though practitioners may ask their patients if they have any questions or if everything is understood, many athletes with injuries may still be reluctant to respond. By adopting a working alliance perspective, patients would be required to demonstrate their understanding of the information provided through activities such as summarizing what they have heard, keeping notes, or explaining what the information meant to them. The main objectives at this point in the relationship are to reach agreement on goals and rehabilitation tasks. However, it is doubtful that these objectives will be accomplished unless patients are treated with respect and sensitivity to their unique situations (S. E. Taylor, 1995).

To develop an effective working alliance, practitioners must treat their patients with respect and dignity. All patients bring their own set of beliefs or fears about the injury rehabilitaion process, and practitioners should always focus first on the patients and not just their injuries (Danish, 1986). The counseling psychology literature suggests that respect, concreteness, genuineness, immediacy, and positive regard are counselor characteristics that are instrumental to the development of empathy and successful therapeutic relationships (Sexton & Whiston, 1994). Inherent in these characteristics is a belief in the dignity and worth of each individual. Therefore, a person sitting in the waiting room should not be treated as just another patient waiting for rehabilitation, but as a unique individual with beliefs, values, strengths, and fears.

Sport injury rehabilitation practitioners who demonstrate an empathic attitude and are able to understand patients' concerns and beliefs about their injuries are likely to create an emotional bond between themselves and their patients. However, care must be taken to understand the nature of this bond in order to avoid dependency or other issues that could negatively affect adherence or motivation. Used appropriately, a working alliance can empower patients to take responsibility for their own rehabilitation.

In addition, the nature of the working alliance may change as a result of the time frame of the rehabilitation process or the situational variables that may be present (e.g., severity of injury, time in athletic career, level of performance). For example, during the time period immediately following an injury, athletes may need a considerable amount of informational support and encouragement from their athletic therapists. However, once exercise regimens have been established and the athletes believe that they are making progress in their workouts, they may have less need for support. Nonetheless, this need could change markedly for athletes who are approaching their recovery target dates and are uncertain about their abilities to trust in their bodies to perform at preinjury levels (Petitpas & Danish, 1995).

Five Practical Suggestions for Enhancing the Working Alliance

1. *Check perceptions.* Do not assume that patients understand treatment goals, tasks, or exercise prescriptions. You can model the importance of gaining clarity by using paraphasing and summarization to ensure that you have accurately heard the communications of patients. Then, you can have patients demonstrate their understanding by having them explain what actions they are going to take.

2. *Get specifics.* One of the critical elements in building a working alliance is the use of concreteness. That is, you need to move from vague descriptions about what is happening during rehabilitation to specific, concrete examples. Remember the initial objectives of the working alliance are to reach agreement on goals and tasks. Specificity can provide a strong base for patient and practitioner problem solving (Ivey, Ivey, & Simek-Morgan, 1993).

3. *Listen before you fix.* Try to understand patients' problems from their perspectives before you offer suggestions for solving them. Do not make the mistake of assuming that you know what patients need. Instead, listen carefully to what they say about their circumstances, particularly their concerns and situational variables. Use active listening skills, such as paraphrasing and reflecting feelings, to allow patients to feel understood and accepted.

4. *Listen for the "but."* Because of the power differential inherent in the patient-practitioner dyad, many patients may be hesitant to assert their views or express their noninjury-related needs and concerns. Instead, they may simply go along with your lead and reluctantly allow you to set the agenda for your ongoing interactions. By listening carefully for "yes-but" patient responses, you may be able to identify their most pressing fears or concerns. For example, consider the following statement made by a female basketball player: "I can feel my knee getting stronger, but I hope I'm ready for the tournament." In this situation, the use of the "but" discounts the first part of the sentence and places most importance on her doubts about her ability to get back to playing strength in time to play in the league championships. If these doubts are not addressed, she may push herself too hard, which may cause a setback or an injury to another body part. It is also important to recognize that the "but" can be communicated nonverbally. If you have a sense that patients are simply agreeing with you and not fully expressing their doubts or concerns, you might ask them, "What's the but?"

5. *Value patient input.* One proven method for enhancing patient-practitioner interactions is to actively seek out input from patients in a manner that communicates respect (Meichenbaum & Turk, 1987). For example, it is better to ask patients a question like "What kinds of things are you doing to cope with your injury?" than to ask them a series of "Have you done this?" questions. In addition, allowing patients to complete their sentences, speaking at the appropriate technical level, and using collaborative problem solving have been shown to increase adherence to medical directives (Meichenbaum & Turk, 1987).

Summary

Social interaction between athletes with injuries and their sports medicine providers is a critical aspect of sport injury rehabilitation, influencing athlete adjustment, treatment adherence, and rehabilitation outcome. Sport injury rehabilitation personnel are in a key position to provide social support for athletes with injuries. However, the ability of practitioners to provide such support for their patients can be compromised by poor communication and discrepant perceptions of rehabilitation processes and outcomes.

Although personal factors undoubtedly contribute to patient adherence to sport injury rehabilitation regimens, adherence may also be affected by the social context in which rehabilitation occurs. Practitioner behavior can help facilitate adherence to prescribed rehabilitation programs.

In some cases, such as when patients are nonadherent or psychologically distressed, referral for psychological services may be warranted. Careful preparation and follow-through are needed to ensure the success of this most delicate and challenging of patient-practitioner interactions.

Sport injury rehabilitation practitioners can enhance their interactions with patients by adopting an approach to building effective therapeutic relationships derived from the counseling psychology literature. By forging an emotional bond with their patients and fostering patient-practitioner agreement on rehabilitation goals and tasks, sports medicine personnel can develop a working alliance that may contribute to positive physical and psychological outcomes for athletes undergoing injury rehabilitation.

References

Andersen, M. B. (1992). Sport psychology and procrustean categories: An appeal for synthesis and expansion of service. *Association for the Advancement of Applied Sport Psychology Newsletter, 7*(3), 8–9.

Andersen, M. B., Denson, E. L., Brewer, B. W., & Van Raalte, J. L. (1994). Disorders of personality and mood in athletes: Recognition and referral. *Journal of Applied Sport Psychology, 6*, 168–184.

Bianco, T. M., & Orlick, T. (1996). Social support influences on recovery from sport injury [Abstract]. *Journal of Applied Sport Psychology, 8*, S57.

Bobele, M., & Conran, T. J. (1988). Referrals for family therapy: Pitfalls and guidelines. *Elementary School Guidance, 22*, 192–198.

Bordin, E. S. (1979). The generalizability of the psychanalytic concept of the working alliance. *Psychotherapy: Theory, Research, and Practice, 16*, 252–260.

Brewer, B. W. (1993). Self-identity and specific vulnerability to depressed mood. *Journal of Personality, 61*, 343–364.

Brewer, B. W. (in press). Adherence to sport injury rehabilitation programs. *Journal of Applied Sport Psychology.*

Brewer, B. W., Daly, J. M., Van Raalte, J. L., Petitpas, A. J., & Sklar, J. H. (1994). A psychometric evaluation of the Rehabilitation Adherence Questionnaire [Abstract]. *Journal of Sport & Exercise Psychology, 16*, S34.

Brewer, B. W., Jeffers, K. E., Petitpas, A. J., & Van Raalte, J. L. (1994). Perceptions of psychological interventions in the context of sport injury rehabilitation. *The Sport Psychologist, 8*, 176–188.

Brewer, B. W., Linder, D. E., & Phelps, C. M. (1995). Situational correlates of emotional adjustment to athletic injury. *Clinical Journal of Sport Medicine, 5*, 241–245.

Brewer, B. W., Petitpas, A. J., & Van Raalte, J. L. (in press). Referral of injured athletes for counseling and psychotherapy. In R. R. Ray & D. M. Wiese-Bjornstal (Eds.), *Psycho-social interaction in sports medicine: A counseling approach.* Champaign, IL: Human Kinetics.

Brewer, B. W., Petitpas, A. J., Van Raalte, J. L., Sklar, J. H., & Ditmar, T. D. (1995). Prevalence of psychological distress among patients at a physical therapy clinic specializing in sports medicine. *Sports Medicine, Training and Rehabilitation, 6*, 138–145.

Brewer, B. W., & Petrie, T. A. (1995). A comparison between injured and uninjured football players on selected psychosocial variables. *Academic Athletic Journal, 10*, 11–18.

Brewer, B. W., Van Raalte, J. L., Petitpas, A. J., Sklar, J. H., & Ditmar, T. D. (1995). Predictors of perceived sport injury rehabilitation status. In R. Vanfraechem-Raway & Y. Vanden Auweele (Eds.), *IXth European Congress on Sport Psychology proceedings: Part II* (pp. 606–610). Brussels: European Federation of Sports Psychology.

Byerly, P. N., Worrell, T., Gahimer, J., & Domholdt, E. (1994). Rehabilitation compliance in an athletic training environment. *Journal of Athletic Training, 29*, 352–355.

Chan, C. S., & Grossman, H. Y. (1988). Psychological effects of running loss on consistent runners. *Perceptual and Motor Skills, 66*, 875–883.

Crossman, J., & Jamieson, J. (1985). Differences in perceptions of seriousness and disrupting effects of athletic injury as viewed by athletes and their trainer. *Perceptual and Motor Skills, 61*, 1131–1134.

Crossman, J., Jamieson, J., & Hume, K. M. (1990). Perceptions of athletic injuries by athletes, coaches, and medical professionals. *Perceptual and Motor Skills, 71*, 848–850.

Culpepper, W. L., Masters, K. S., & Wittig, A. F. (1996, August). *Factors influencing injured athletes' adherence to rehabilitation.* Paper presented at the annual meeting of the American Psychological Association, Toronto, Ontario, Canada.

Daly, J. M., Brewer, B. W., Van Raalte, J. L., Petitpas, A. J., & Sklar, J. H. (1995). Cognitive appraisal, emotional adjustment, and adherence to rehabilitation following knee surgery. *Journal of Sport Rehabilitation, 4*, 23–30.

Danish, S. J. (1986). Psychological aspects in the care and treatment of athletic injuries. In P. E. Vinger & E. F. Hoerner (Eds.), *Sports injuries: The unthwarted epidemic* (pp. 345–353). Littleton, MA: PSG.

DeFrancesco, C., Miller, M., Larson, M., & Robinson, K. (1994, October). *Athletic injury, rehabilitation, and psychological strategies: What do the athletes think?* Paper presented at the annual meeting of the Association for the Advancement of Applied Sport Psychology, Incline Village, NV.

Derscheid, G. L., & Feiring, D. C. (1987). A statistical analysis to characterize treatment adherence of the 18 most common diagnoses seen at a sports medicine clinic. *Journal of Orthopaedic and Sports Physical Therapy, 9*, 40–46.

DiMatteo, M. R., Sherbourne, C. D., Hays, R. D., Ordway, L., Kravitz, R. L., McGlynn, E. A., Kaplan, S., & Rogers, W. H. (1993). Physicians' characteristics influence patients' adherence to medical treatment: Results from the Medical Outcomes Study. *Health Psychology, 12,* 93–102.

Duda, J. L., Smart, A. E., & Tappe, M. K. (1989). Predictors of adherence in rehabilitation of athletic injuries: An application of personal investment theory. *Journal of Sport & Exercise Psychology, 11,* 367–381.

Durso-Cupal, D. D. (1996). *Can mental practice enhance recovery for ACL patients?* Unpublished manuscript, Utah State University, Logan.

Eichenhofer, R. B., Wittig, A. F., & Balogh, D. W., & Pisano, M. D. (1986, May). *Personality indicants of adherence to rehabilitation treatment by injured athletes.* Paper presented at the Annual Meeting of the Midwestern Psychological Association, Chicago, IL.

Fields, J., Murphey, M., Horodyski, M., & Stopka, C. (1995). Factors associated with adherence to sport injury rehabilitation in college-age recreational athletes. *Journal of Sport Rehabilitation, 4,* 172–180.

Fisher, A. C., Domm, M. A., & Wuest, D. A. (1988). Adherence to sports-injury rehabilitation programs. *The Physician and Sports Medicine, 16,* 47–52.

Fisher, A. C., & Hoisington, L. L. (1993). Injured athletes' attitudes and judgments toward rehabilitation adherence. *Journal of Athletic Training, 28,* 48–54.

Fisher, A. C., Mullins, S. A., & Frye, P. A. (1993). Athletic trainers' attitudes and judgments of injured athletes' rehabilitation adherence. *Journal of Athletic Training, 28,* 43–47.

Flint, F. A., & Weiss, M. R. (1992). Returning injured athletes to competition: A role and ethical dilemma. *Canadian Journal of Sport Sciences, 17,* 34–40

Ford, I. W., & Gordon, S. (1993). Social support and athletic injury: The perspective of sport physiotherapists. *The Australian Journal of Science and Medicine in Sport, 25,* 17–25.

Gordon, S., & Lindgren, S. (1990). Psycho-physical rehabilitation from a serious sport injury: Case study of an elite fast bowler. *Australian Journal of Science and Medicine in Sport, 22,* 71–76.

Gordon, S., Milios, D., & Grove, J. R. (1991). Psychological aspects of the recovery process from sport injury: The perspective of sport physiotherapists. *Australian Journal of Science and Medicine in Sport, 23,* 53–60.

Grove, J. R., Hanrahan, S. J., Stewart, R. M. L. (1990). Attributions for rapid or slow recovery from sports injuries. *Canadian Journal of Sport Sciences, 15,* 107–114.

Hall, J. A., Roter, D. L., & Katz, N. R. (1988). Meta-analysis of correlates of provider behavior in medical encounters. *Medical Care, 26,* 1–19.

Heil, J. (1993). *Psychology of sport injury.* Champaign, IL: Human Kinetics.

Henderson, J., & Carroll, W. (1993). The athletic trainers' role in preventing sport injury and rehabilitating injured athletes: A psychological perspective. In D. Pargman (Ed.), *Psychological bases of sport injuries* (pp. 15–31). Morgantown, WV: Fitness Information Technology.

Heyman, S. R. (1993). When to refer athletes for counseling of psychotherapy. In J. Williams (Ed.), *Applied sport psychology: Personal growth to peak performance* (2nd ed., pp. 299–308). Palo Alto, CA: Mayfield.

Hokanson, R. G. (1994). *Relationship between sports rehabilitation practitioners' communication style and athletes' adherence to injury rehabilitation.* Unpublished master's thesis, Springfield College, MA.

Ivey, A. E., Ivey, M. B., & Simek-Morgan, L. (1993). *Counseling and psychotherapy: A multicultural perspective* (3rd. ed.). Boston: Allyn and Bacon.

Izzo, C. M. (1994). *The relationship between social support and adherence to sport injury rehabilitation.* Unpublished master's thesis, Springfield College, MA.

Johnson, S. B. (1993). Chronic diseases of childhood: Assessing compliance with complex medical regimens. In N. A. Krasnegor, L. Epstein, S. B. Johnson, & S. J. Yaffe (Eds.), *Developmental aspects of health compliance behavior* (pp. 157–184). Hillsdale, NJ: Erlbaum.

Kahanov, L., & Fairchild, P. C. (1994). Discrepancies in perceptions held by injured athletes and athletic trainers during the initial evaluation. *Journal of Athletic Training, 29,* 70–75.

Kiesler, D. J., & Watkins, L. M. (1989). Interpersonal complementarity and the therapeutic alliance: A study of relationship in psychotherapy. *Psychotherapy, 26,* 183–194.

Kivlighan, D. M., & Schmitz, P. J. (1992). Counselor technical activity in cases with improving working alliances and continuing-poor working alliances. *Journal of Counseling Psychology, 39,* 32–38.

Kleiber, D. A., & Brock, S. C. (1992). The effect of career-ending injuries on the subsequent well-being of elite college athletes. *Sociology of Sport Journal, 9,* 70–75.

Lampton, C. C., Lambert, M. E., & Yost, R. (1993). The effects of psychological factors in sports medicine rehabilitation adherence. *Journal of Sports Medicine and Physical Fitness, 33,* 292–299.

Larson, G. A., Starkey, C. A., & Zaichkowsky, L. D. (1996). Psychological aspects of athletic injuries as perceived by athletic trainers. *The Sport Psychologist, 10,* 37–47.

Laubach, W. J., Brewer, B. W., Van Raalte, J. L., & Petitpas, A. J. (1996). Attributions for recovery and adherence to sport injury rehabilitation. *Australian Journal of Science and Medicine in Sport, 28,* 30–34.

Leddy, M. H., Lambert, M. J., & Ogles, B. M. (1994). Psychological consequences of athletic injury among high-level competitors. *Research Quarterly for Exercise and Sport, 65,* 347–354.

Linder, D. E., Brewer, B. W., Van Raalte, J. L., & DeLange, N. (1991). A negative halo for athletes who consult a sport psychologist: Replication and extension. *Journal of Sport & Exercise Psychology, 13,* 133–148.

May, S., & Taylor, A. H. (1994). The development and examination of various measures of patient compliance, for specific use with injured athletes. *Journal of Sports Sciences, 12,* 180–181.

McDonald, S. A., & Hardy, C. J. (1990). Affective response patterns of the injured athlete: An exploratory analysis. *The Sport Psychologist, 4,* 261–274.

Meani, E., Migliorini, S., & Tinti, G. (1986). La patologia de sovraccarico sportivo dei nuclei di accrescimento apofisari [The pathology of apophyseal growth centres caused by overstrain during sports]. *Italian Journal of Sports Traumatology, 8,* 29–38.

Meichenbaum, D. (1985). *Stress inoculation training.* Elmford, NY: Pergamon Press.

Meichenbaum, D., & Turk, D. C. (1987). *Facilitating treatment adherence.* New York: Plenum.

Nideffer, R. M. (1983). The injured athlete: Psychological factors in treatment. *Orthopedic Clinics of North America, 14,* 373–385.

Nixon, H. L. II. (1994). Social pressure, social support, and help seeking for pain and injuries in college sports networks. *Journal of Sport & Social Issues, 18,* 340–355.

Noyes, F. R., Matthews, D. S., Mooar, P. A., & Grood, E. S. (1983). The symptomatic anterior cruciate-deficient knee. Part II: The results of rehabilitation, activity modification, and counseling on functional disability. *Journal of Bone and Joint Surgery, 65-A,* 163–174.

Orlinsky, D. E., & Howard, K. I. (1986). Process and outcome in psychotherapy. In S. L. Garfield & A. E. Bergin (Eds.), *Handbook of psychotherapy and behavior change* (pp. 311–381). New York: Wiley.

Pearson, L., & Jones, G. (1992). Emotional effects of sports injuries: Implications for physiotherapists. *Physiotherapy, 78,* 762–770.

Petitpas, A., & Danish, S. J. (1995). Caring for injured athletes. In S. M. Murphy (Ed.), *Sport psychology interventions* (pp. 255–282). Champaign, IL: Human Kinetics.

Potter, M. J. (1995). *Psychological intervention during rehabilitation case studies of injured athletes.* Unpublished master's thesis, University of Western Australia, Nedlands, Australia.

Satterfield, M. J., Dowden, D., & Yasamura, K. (1990). Patient compliance for successful stress fracture rehabilitation. *Journal of Orthopaedic and Sports Physical Therapy, 11,* 321–324.

Sexton, T. L., & Whiston, S. C. (1994). The status of the counseling relationship: An empirical review, theoretical implications, and research directions. *The Counseling Psychologist, 22,* 6–78.

Shaffer, S. M. (1992). *Attributions and self-efficacy as predictors of rehabilitative success.* Unpublished master's thesis, University of Illinois at Urbana-Champaign, Urbana-Champaign.

Shelbourne, K. D., & Wilckens, J. H. (1990). Current concepts in anterior cruciate ligament rehabilitation. *Orthopaedic Review, 19,* 957–964.

Smith, A. M., Scott, S. G., O'Fallon, W. M., & Young, M. L. (1990). Emotional responses of athletes to injury. *Mayo Clinic Proceedings, 65,* 38–50.

Smith, A. M., Stuart, M. J., Wiese-Bjornstal, D. M., Milliner, E. K., O'Fallon, W. M., & Crowson, C. S. (1993). Competitive athletes: Preinjury and postinjury mood state and self-esteem. *Mayo Clinic Proceedings, 68,* 939–947.

Smith, A. M., Young, M. L., & Scott, S. G. (1988). The emotional responses of athletes to injury. *Canadian Journal of Sport Sciences, 13,* 84P–85P.

Taylor, A. H., & May, S. (1995a). Physiotherapist's expectations and their influence on compliance to sports injury rehabilitation. In R. Vanfraechem-Raway, & Y. Vanden Auweele (Eds.), *IXth European Congress on Sport Psychology proceedings: Part II* (pp. 619–625). Brussels: European Federation of Sports Psychology.

Taylor, A. H., & May, S. (1995b). Development of a Sports Injury Clinic Athlete Satisfaction Scale for auditing patient perceptions. *Physiotherapy Theory and Practice, 11,* 231–238.

Taylor, A. H., & May, S. (1996). Threat and coping appraisal as determinants of compliance to sports injury rehabilitation: An application of protection motivation theory. *Journal of Sports Sciences,14,* 471–482.

Taylor, S. E. (1995). *Health psychology* (3rd ed.). New York: McGraw-Hill.

Udry, E. (1996). Social support: Exploring its role in the context of athletic injuries. *Journal of Sport Rehabilitation, 5,* 151–163.

Van Raalte, J. L. & Andersen, M. B. (1996). Referral processes in sport psychology. In J. L. Van Raalte & B. W. Brewer (Eds), *Exploring sport and exercise psychology* (275–284). Washington, DC: American Psychological Association.

Van Raalte, J. L., Brewer, B. W., & Petitpas, A. J. (1992, October). *Correspondence between athlete and trainer appraisals of injury rehabilitation status.* Paper presented at the annual meeting of the Association for the Advancement of Applied Sport Psychology, Colorado Springs, CO.

Webborn, A. D. J., Carbon, R. J., & Miller, B. P. (1997). Injury rehabilitation programs: "What are we talking about?" *Journal of Sport Rehabilitation, 6,* 54–61.

Wiese, D. M., Weiss, M. R., & Yukelson, D. P. (1991). Sport psychology in the training room: Implications for the treatment team. *The Sport Psychologist, 5,* 15–24.

Wiese-Bjornstal, D. M., Smith, A. M., & LaMott, E. E. (1995). A model of psychologic response to athletic injury and rehabilitation. *Athletic Training: Sports Health Care Perspectives, 1,* 17–30.

Wise, A., Jackson, D. W., & Rocchio, P. (1979). Preoperative psychologic testing as a predictor of success in knee surgery. *American Journal of Sports Medicine, 7,* 287–292.

Wittig, A. F., & Schurr, K. T. (1994). Psychological characteristics of women volleyball players: Relationships with injuries, rehabilitation, and team success. *Personality and Social Psychology Bulletin, 20,* 322–330.

11

Social Support and Injury: A Framework for Social Support-Based Interventions With Injured Athletes

Charles J. Hardy

Kevin L. Burke
Georgia Southern University

R. Kelly Crace
College of William & Mary

Social support has far-reaching implications for dealing with sport injuries. This chapter reviews the research literature on social support, with particular emphasis given to an understanding of the role that social support can play in facilitating recovery from sport injuries. The chapter has two major thrusts: (a) definitional, conceptual, and empirical information on the social support construct and (b) strategies for providing the different dimensions of social support and for creating and maintaining the injured athlete's social support network.

After stressful events people turn to those closest to them as a source of strength. It is those closest to us who carry our burdens when we are incapable; who offer a shoulder on which to cry, shelter from adversity, and solace from grief. Significant others share their resources to help those for whom they care through these most difficult periods of life. (Hobfoll & Stephens, 1990, p. 459)

The Stress of Injury

Although athletes confront numerous challenges within the competitive environment, one of the most common and most stressful is dealing with injury. Danish (1986) stated that injury can be highly stressful because it not only threatens physical well-being "but acts as a threat to the athlete's self-concept, belief system, social and occupational functioning, values, commitments, and emotional equilibrium" (p. 346). Injury can force athletes to (a) accept a new definition of their abilities, (b) redefine their role on the team, (c) withdraw from or change the current level of involvement, and (d) redirect future career opportunities, both within and outside of sport (Hardy & Crace, 1990; Silva & Hardy, 1991).

Even though athletes react to injury in many different ways, Gordon (1991) argued that "every athlete who experiences an injury that renders him or her even temporarily inactive or disabled will experience a painful loss, and the subsequent physical and emotional significance of this loss is likely to be equivalently great" (p. 15). Hobfoll (1988, 1989) suggested that psychological stress occurs (a) when there is a threat of a net loss of resources, (b) when there is an actual loss of net resources, or (c) when coping strategies, the investment of resources, yield no net resource gain. Hobfoll (1989) defined resources as "those objects, personal characteristics, conditions, or energies that are valued by the individual or group or that serve as a means for attaining these objects, personal characteristics, conditions, or energies" (p. 516). For the injured athlete, the loss can involve a loss of independence, social mobility, capacity to perform, and exposure to pain, and the threat of disfigurement, permanent disability, and death (Hobfoll & Stephens, 1990). Thus, dealing with injury involves coping with the stress of perceived losses in personal resources (McDonald & Hardy, 1990), and is one of the toughest opponents an athlete may have to face (Silva & Hardy, 1991).

The Role of Social Support in Dealing with the Stress of Injury

When confronted with the stress of injury, athletes will attempt to minimize net resource losses. In order to offset this loss, athletes will employ their personal resources. When an athlete is injured, a loss in personal resources can be experienced. In the absence of effective personal resources, athletes will seek the support of others to help them cope with the injury, thereby extending their resource pool (Hobfoll & Stokes, 1988). Social support provides resources that can assist in dealing with the stress of injury by (a) providing a feeling of attachment to others; (b) directly preventing or limiting resource loss; (c) providing for resources that are lost; and/or (d) activating latent coping resources (Hobfoll & Stephens, 1990).

Research has demonstrated that support provided by others is helpful in coping with life stress, crisis, mental and physical illness, unemployment, job stress, bereavement, childbirth, mortality risk, burnout, AIDS, feelings of loss, loneliness, problems related to academic performance, adolescent depression, behavioral problems, and other stressors (cf., Albrecht & Adelman, 1984; Albrecht & Hall, 1991; Barrera & Garrison-Jones, 1992; Billings & Moos, 1981; Blanchard, Albrecht, Ruckdeschel, Grant, & Hemmick, 1995; Broadhead et al., 1983; Caplan, 1976; Cobb, 1976; Cohen, 1988; Cohen & Syme, 1985; Cutrona & Suhr, 1994; Dubow, Tisak, Causey, & Hryshko, 1991; Ford & Sutphen, 1996; Ganster & Victor, 1988; Goldsmith & Albrecht, 1993; Gore, 1978; Hammer, 1981; Hobfoll & Stephens, 1990; House, 1981; Jones & Moore, 1987; Lackovic-Grgin, Dekovic, Milosavljevic, 1996; Leavy, 1983; Lovell & Richey, 1991; Pines, Aronson, & Kafry, 1981; Richman & Rosenfeld, 1987; Rounds, Galinsky, & Stevens, 1991; I. G. Sarason & Sarason, 1986; Schaefer, Coyne, & Lazarus, 1981; Tracy, 1990; Zigler, Taussig, & Black, 1992). Recently, research has shown social support to be an even more robust factor. Woodward, Rosenfeld, and May (1996) found that "at risk of school failure" students who do not receive social support report several differences from those who receive an average amount of social support. Those students receiving no social support report more moves from their neighborhood, less time studying, lower school satisfaction, fewer close friends, less acceptance by their peer groups, less interest from their caretakers, poorer health, and lower self-esteem. In nontraditional students, satisfaction with social support has been found to be related to students who viewed themselves as being high in communication competence (Query, Parry, & Flint, 1992).

Supported individuals are generally more mentally and physically healthy than are unsupported individuals, perhaps due to the *health-sustaining* and *stress-reducing* functions of social support (Shumaker & Brownell, 1984). Moreover, it is reported that the treatment and recovery process is often enhanced by social support (Wallston, Alagna, DeVellis, & DeVellis, 1983), an effect extended to injured athletes (Gordon & Lindgren, 1990; Ievleva & Orlick, 1991; Silva & Hardy, 1991; M. R. Weiss & Troxel, 1986; Wiese & Weiss, 1987). Other findings of social support in athletics show that coach and parental support was positively associated with higher self-esteem and enjoyment for young athletes (Leff & Holye, 1995; Smoll, Smith, & Barnett, 1993). Social support may also be indirectly related to the rate of injury to athletes

(Blackwell & McCullagh, 1990; Lavalle & Flint, 1996). Recent injury research indicates that athletes who report satisfaction with social support tend to have lower levels of tension/anxiety, with the latter being positively correlated with injury rates. Coping resources, therefore, may play a part in injury occurrence (Andersen & Williams, 1988).

It appears, therefore, that there is ample evidence for the use of social support-based interventions in dealing with sport injury. Rotella and Heyman (1986) and Silva and Hardy (1991) have argued that social support is critical in the rehabilitation of the injured athlete and, therefore, should be a concern of those who are directly involved in the care and treatment of injured athletes. According to Gottlieb (1988), however, the mobilization of social support reflects the "impulses and natural activities of ordinary citizens striving to secure the resources they need to grapple with changing life circumstances" rather than to the efforts of professional practitioners (p. 519). What is needed is a framework for professionals interested in translating the research on social support into practical strategies for developing and nurturing support as well as ways of assisting individuals in the use and delivery of social support (Gottlieb, 1988; I. G. Sarason, Sarason, & Pierce, 1990a). This is particularly relevant for the injured athlete, because numerous authors have suggested that social support is an effective *psychological technique* that can be used to motivate injured athletes during rehabilitation (c.f. Hardy & Crace, 1990; Wiese & Weiss, 1987). This chapter will provide (a) an introduction to the construct of social support and (b) a framework for social support-based interventions, including practical strategies for maximizing the therapeutic properties of social support when dealing with the injured athlete.

What Is Social Support?

Durkheim (1952) argued that the loss of social ties or *anomie* was antithetical to psychological well-being. In his seminal study of suicide, Durkheim found that suicides were more prevalent among those with few close social ties. Although the importance of interpersonal relationships for promoting health holds intuitive appeal, "the concept of social support has been operationalized in a somewhat bewildering assortment of ways"(Wilcox, 1981b, p. 98).

In its broadest sense, social support is the essence of being *social*. Simplistic definitions view social support as the number of friendships, relatives nearby, and organizational involvement (Eckenrode & Gore, 1981). Wilcox (1981a) defined social support as having a "confidant" or spouse. Kaplan, Cassel, and Gore (1977) viewed social support as the "metness" or gratification of basic social needs, approval, esteem, succor, and belonging. Moss (1973) defined social support as "the subjective feeling of belonging, of being accepted or being loved, of being needed all for oneself and for what one can do" (p. 237).

Although theorists differ on specifics, there is now wide agreement that social support is a multidimensional construct. For example, Caplan (1974) defined social support as assistance from significant others in completing tasks, in the provision of instrumental aid (money, tools, advice) to deal with particular situations, and in mobilizing psychological resources to deal with emotional problems. Cobb (1976) viewed social support as informational aid belonging to one or more of three categories: (a) information leading individuals to believe that they are cared for or loved, (b) information leading individuals to believe that they are esteemed and valued, and (c) information leading individuals to believe that they belong to a network of communication and mutual obligation in which others can be counted on in time of need. Thus, it is appropriate to conceptualize social support as a form of *social commerce* (Gottlieb, 1988). This commerce represents an exchange of resources between at least two people, with the outcome being the enhancement of the recipient's well-being (Richman, Rosenfeld, & Hardy, 1992; Shumaker & Brownell, 1984). These resources include providing *emotional, informational* and *tangible support* (Albrecht & Adelman, 1984; Cohen & Hoberman, 1983; Cohen & Wills, 1985; Conrad, 1985; House, 1981; Kahn & Antonucci, 1980; Pines et al., 1981; I .G. Sarason & Sarason, 1985; R. Weiss, 1974).

The Dimensions of Social Support

Richman et al. (1993) have argued that the social support process involves four elements: (a) a support provider; (b) a support recipient; (c) the transaction between the provider and the recipient; and (d) the outcomes of the transaction. Members of one's social network offer emotional, informational, and tangible support by enacting various behaviors. Some support behaviors require expertise on the part of the provider, whereas others do not (Rosenfeld, Richman, & Hardy, 1989).

Recipients are perceived to be proactive elements of the support process. Recipients have personal characteristics that affect how they interact with others and how they access the needed support. The transaction between provider and recipient allows for an exchange of resources to take place. The recipient transmits a need for a specific type of support to potential providers who have to recognize the request for help and then be willing and capable of offering the type of support requested (Albrecht & Adelman, 1984). The recipient must perceive the behaviors of providers to be helpful in meeting expressed needs (I. G. Sarason et al., 1990a). Finally, the outcome is the enhancement of the recipient's physical and psychological well-being.

Behaviors that fulfill support functions include expressing emotional support (e.g., affection), providing appraisal support (e.g., performance feedback), giving information (e.g., advice and role clarification), offering emotionally sustaining behaviors (e.g., empathy), and listening to the concerns and feeling of others (Albrecht & Adelman, 1984). These behaviors represent three general dimensions of social support: (a) emotional, (b) informational, and (c) tangible social support. Based upon the work of Pines et al. (1981) and Richman et al. (1993), Hardy and Crace (1991) proposed that such behaviors can be grouped into eight distinguishable dimensions of social support (see Table 1).

Table 1. Dimensions of Social Support

Dimension	Definition
Listening Support	Behaviors that indicate people listen to you without giving advice or being judgmental.
Emotional Support	Behaviors that comfort you and indicate that people are on your side and care for you.
Emotional Challenge	Behaviors that challenge you to evaluate your attitudes, values, and feelings.
Task Appreciation	Behaviors that acknowledge your efforts and express appreciation for the work you do.
Task Challenge	Behaviors that challenge your way of thinking about your work in order to stretch you, motivate you, and lead you to greater creativity, excitement, and involvement in your work.
Reality Confirmation	Behaviors that indicate that people are similar to you—see things the way you do—helps you confirm your perceptions and perspectives of the world and helps you keep things in focus.
Material Assistance	Behaviors that provide you with financial assistance, products, or gifts.
Personal Assistance	Behaviors that indicate a giving of time, skills, knowledge, and/or expertise to help you accomplish your tasks.

The Measurement of Social Support

B. R. Sarason, Sarason, and Pierce (1990) have reported that social support can be assessed by examination of *social networks, received support,* or *perceived support.* Social networks analyses provide information on the individual's social integration into and interconnectedness within a group. Network support type measures include the network size, relationship, density, quality of relationship intensity, frequency and desirability of contact. Received support examines what individuals obtain from others. Received support type measures include enacted support—actions of others to assist a particular individual—and received support—the recipient's account of the support given to them by others. Perceived support focuses on the perceptions of both the need for and availability of social support. Perceived support type measures include availability, satisfaction, general status, specific status, general factor, and structural/ multidimensional questionnaires.

Heitzmann and Kaplan (1988) maintained that the measurement of social support has been problematic. Although numerous scales, questionnaires and other assessment tools purport to measure this construct, the psychometric properties of the majority of these measures have not been convincingly documented. For example, a two-part social support measure, the Social Support Questionnaire for Transactions (SSQT) and the Social Support Questionnaire for Satisfactions (SSQS) (Doeglas, Suurmeijer, & Briancon, 1996), has recently been introduced but needs to be further tested. Additionally, the measures differ substantially in length, focus, approach, and the nature of the support that is evaluated (see Bruhn & Phillips, 1984; Heitzmann & Kaplan, 1988; House & Kahn, 1985; Tardy, 1988, for a review of the measures). According to B. R. Sarason et al. (1990), "the main problem with the measurement of social support has been that although the measures have multiplied like rabbits, relatively little work has been done to establish their comparability or lack of it" (p. 20). Moreover, relatively few measures of social support have published validity and reliability data (Heitzmann & Kaplan, 1988).

However, Heitzmann and Kaplan (1988) suggest that the state of social support measurement is not necessarily bleak, despite the lack of comparability and psychometric data. Because meaningful conclusions from research studies depend on the valid and reliable measurement of social support, research on social support must be viewed critically, with careful attention to the measurement instrument employed. In spite of the methodological concerns, the available evidence suggests that social support is an important variable in sustaining health and in mitigating life stress (Shumaker & Brownell, 1984). Consistent with the framework of this paper, we recommend the Social Support Survey—SSS (Richman et. al., 1993). The SSS presents respondents with operationalizations of the eight types of social support—Listening Support, Task Appreciation Support, Task Challenge Support, Emotional Support, Emotional Challenge Support, Reality Confirmation Support, Tangible Assistance Support, and Personal Assistance Support—and requires them to indicate the support providers, satisfaction with the support, difficulty of obtaining more of each type of support, and their perception of the importance of each type of support for their overall well-being. The SSS is grounded in contemporary research and has received empirical support (e.g., Woodward et al., 1996).

The Functions and Mechanisms of Social Support

The overall function of social support is to enhance the recipient's well-being. The assumption underlying all models and empirical investigations is that supported individuals are more mentally and physically healthy than nonsupported individuals. This is thought to be due to the health-sustaining and stress-reducing functions of social support (Shumaker & Brownell, 1984). The more effective the social support an individual receives, the better his or her mental and physical health. Conversely, ineffective or low quantities of social support reduce mental and physical well-being.

Social support can also moderate or buffer the impact of stress on the individual and, thus, indirectly affect well-being. At low levels of social support, the relationship between stress and psychological and physiological well-being should be strong and direct; as social support increases, the relationship should weaken. Under conditions of maximal support, the relationship between stress and well-being should be nonexistent.

Explanations for these two functions have yet to be established; however, it has been suggested that effective social support networks alter the organism's cognitions, affect, immune system function, and/or behavior. Gottlieb (1988) concluded that

> by examining changes in the parties' causal and control attributions, their self esteem and self-conceptions, feelings of deviance, and their sense of hopefulness and meaning attached to their predicaments, significant advances can be made in our understanding of the pathways whereby social support promotes adaptation and impacts health. (p. 539)

I. G. Sarason et al. (1990a) have argued that although support may be communicated through specific behaviors, the active ingredient of social support is an individual's belief that others value and care about the individual and that others are willing to assist if the person needs support. The primary effect of these beliefs is that they "foster the feeling that we are worthwhile, capable, and valued members of a group of individuals"(I. G. Sarason et al., 1990a, p. 121). When individuals perceive the world as supportive, they feel that the resources necessary for the attainment of their goals are available to them, either from within themselves or from their support network. That is, a sense of personal agency is enhanced by the feeling that one's well-being is the concern of others. Thus, although social support may have unique dimensions, the dimensions share some common variance.

Hardy, Richman, & Rosenfeld (1991) have argued that it is possible that the perception of the availability of social support undergirds the buffering function, whereas one's linkages and social integration support the direct function (for a review see Cohen, 1988; Cutrona & Russell, 1990; B. R. Sarason et al., 1990; I. G. Sarason et al., 1990a).

It should be noted, however, that social support can have negative effects on both the recipient and the provider. The amount (too much or too little) of social support may not match the needs of the individual who needs the support (Rook, 1992; I. G. Sarason, Sarason, & Pierce, 1990b). For the recipient, social support may lead to increased pressure to conform. Such pressure might cause people to behave in unhealthy ways. Moreover, recipients may feel smothered and controlled, may "lose face" because of the need for social support (Goldsmith, 1994), and may feel indebted to support providers (Shumaker & Brownell, 1984). Providing support can drain one's resource pool (i.e., emotions, time, finances), alter one's attitude toward the recipient, and increase the provider's sense of personal vulnerability (Hobfoll & Stephens, 1990; Perrine, 1993; Shumaker & Brownell, 1984).

A Framework for Social Support-Based Interventions With Injured Athletes

Are we able to apply our understanding of social networks to ourselves? In so doing we may be able to escape our own isolation as professionals . . . If we cannot model the benefits of work among supportive networks, then we are not likely to influence others with our findings. What is worse, without such support in our lives, our own health and well being may suffer before we can influence anyone. In no other activity . . . would the means by which we proceed appear to be so important as in the activity of nuturance of life-sustaining networks of social support. (Pilisuk, 1982, p. 29)

Hobfoll and Stephens (1990) have indicated that the following factors should be considered when designing social support-based interventions: (a) evaluation of loss, (b) intensity of support-based interventions, (c) evaluation of other resources, (d) timing, (e) emotions and cognitions versus action, (f) drain of resources, and (g) environmental versus individual intervention.

The first step is to determine the nature of the stress. Injury can be categorized as a negative, uncontrollable event that involves the loss of or a threat to physical assets, relationships, achievement, and social roles (Cutrona & Russell, 1990). The next step is to determine the most effective type of social support to counter the stress of injury. Because specific types of social support facilitate coping with particular types of life stress (Cutrona & Russell, 1990; R. Weiss, 1974), social support will have a beneficial effect to the extent that the support actually received is appropriately matched to the specific needs activated by the stressor (I. G. Sarason et al., 1990a). Because perception of one's needs is a subjective process, this matching process can be rather difficult. *Who* provides *what* is a crucial element for determining the utility of social support as well as in designing effective social support-based interventions.

Emotional support is essential because emotion-focused coping is important in reducing the intensity of emotions as a result of the injury (Cutrona & Russell, 1990; Hobfoll & Stephens, 1990). The longer the effects of the injury last, the more emotional support will be required. For some injuries, physical limitations may necessitate tangible support to compensate for the assets lost as a result of the injury. Thus, although emotional support appears to play a key role in coping with injury, the degree that the injury affects the athlete's capacity to function in a variety of life roles will create a broad range of support needs. Because injury can adversely affect numerous life roles, a broad range of support needs will most likely need to be provided for effective healing to occur.

Another factor to consider is the intensity of the support that is available. The limited research on natural support systems indicates that effective support is intensive and provided by the closest loved ones. Thus, the *source* of support appears to be an important factor for determining intensity of support-based interventions. I. G. Sarason et al. (1990a) suggested that when the recipient perceives that the support provider is interested, empathic, and committed, the intended support provisions will be helpful and used.

It is important to realize that social support is but one resource, and its utility clearly is dependent upon its interaction with other resources that can be harnessed during the rehabilitation process. To facilitate the rehabilitation process, it is important to include other resources (i.e., personal characteristics and injury characteristics) that might interact with social support.

An additional important consideration is the timing of support behaviors. The stress of injury and the effectiveness of social support are dynamic processes. Whereas initial support efforts will need to focus primarily on emotional support, the type of support needed will change as a function of the stress sequence experienced. Emotional, tangible, and informational support are all important types of support for the injured athlete. However, the type of support that is emphasized will vary with the type of stress experienced throughout the rehabilitation process.

It is also important to remember that the use of resources is not without costs. Over time, support recipients may find it increasingly difficult to ask for the type of support needed, and providers may feel increasingly strained when summoned for assistance. It is important to provide ways to control for the drain in resources so that the support system will not become overtaxed, for example, having a professional supervise the support process, making psychological and medical expertise easily accessible to the providers, and developing a mulitplex network of support providers (Hobfoll & Stephens, 1990).

Consideration may need to be given to the gender of the athlete who is experiencing the injury. Although it may be too early to be certain, some recent research (Woodward et al., 1996) suggests that same-gender groups experience different levels and types of social support. This study suggests that male groups need to provide more "emotional" and "listening" social support. Female groups need to provide additional support in the areas of "technical challenge" and "emotional challenge" social support.

Finally, consideration should be given to alter the environment in ways that facilitate providing effective social support. The context of social support can be a critical factor because the stress of injury involves the loss of many tangible resources (Hobfoll & Stephens, 1990).

Based upon the work of Hardy and Crace (1991), Hobfoll and Stephens (1990), and Richman, Hardy, Rosenfeld, & Callanan (1989), the following strategies are offered to assist in the creation, provision, and maintenance of effective social support for injured athletes. It is important to remember, however, that "no one intervention effort is suitable for all situations, even if they concern similar stressors, because the interaction of persons, resources, and environments is too varied" (Hobfoll & Stephens, 1990, p. 474).

The Provision of Support Needs for Injured Athletes

Providing Emotional Support

Providing support that is primarily emotional in nature includes (a) emotional support, (b) emotional challenge, and (c) listening.

Listen carefully. Active listening involves focusing on the *what* as well as the *how* of the communication (Rosenfeld, Wilder, Crace, & Hardy, 1990). One

and openness. An open-door type policy indicates that the injured athlete can comfortably discuss personal thoughts and feelings. Undoubtedly, this contributes to the injured athlete's commitment to the rehabilitation process. Athletes who receive high levels of emotional support from their coaches have been observed to be more highly motivated in comparison to those who receive low levels of support (Ungerleider & Golding, 1991).

Providing Informational Support

Providing support that is primarily informational in nature includes (a) task appreciation, (b) task challenge, and (c) reality confirmation.

Develop your injury knowledge base. One of the prerequisites for providing task-related support is that the provider must have context expertise. He or she must be viewed by the athlete as a credible and knowledgeable person. Expertise requires not only an understanding of the technical aspects of the injury, but also the mental and emotional challenges of the rehabilitation process.

Deliver effective instructional feedback. Feedback that affirms effort and task mastery should be delivered in a sincere and personalized manner utilizing the *sandwich principle* (Kirkpatrick, 1982; Quick, 1977; 1980; Smoll & Smith, 1979). In this approach, the technical instruction is sandwiched between affirming and encouraging statements. For example, "you're putting a lot of effort into that exercise. You may want to concentrate on getting a full range of motion so that the strength and flexibility of that muscle group will be more extensive."

In addition, the feedback should be focused on daily rehabilitation process goals rather than upon desired rehabilitation outcomes. The preferred time, place, and manner in which the recipient wants the task-related support delivered should be determined. Often, athletes desire to have this type of support delivered immediately—as soon as possible so that appropriate adjustments can be made.

Utilize technical modalities. An increasingly popular medium to deliver task support is through the use of physiological, biomechanical, and psychological tools. For example, mood inventories, biofeedback units, and computerized isokinetic strength testing equipment provide data that the athlete can use to track the progress of the rehabilitation. This technology allows injured athletes to receive the task-related support they need in a unique and objective manner. It is important to remember, however, that such technology is best used as an adjunct to interpersonal interaction rather than as a replacement.

Do not be afraid to challenge and confront. Injured athletes should be challenged in an honest and straightforward manner. Through personal conferences, injured athletes should be encouraged to objectively assess their rehabilitation progress. Such self-assessments by injured athletes are more likely to be received in a nondefensive manner when trust and respect have been secured. When confronting the injured athlete, the support provider should be (a) accurate, (b) sensitive, (c) concrete, and (d) respectful. Modeling confrontation with these elements will likely increase athletes' receptivity to task challenge support. Perhaps the most important thing to remember is that confrontation must be delivered in a supportive manner. According to Egan (1973), "confrontation without support is disastrous; support without confrontation is anemic" (p. 132).

Provide reality touchstones. This can be accomplished in several effective ways: (a) Create sharing opportunities between injured athletes; (b) have injured athletes who have successfully rehabilitated from similar injuries share their experiences with currently injured athletes; and (c) arrange small group meetings or support groups where injured athletes can openly discuss their thoughts and feelings about issues related being injured (M. R. Weiss & Troxell, 1986; Wiese & Weiss, 1987). Athletes with similar experiences (i.e., injury) profit from small group meetings where they can connect with people who understand how they feel and empathize with what they are experiencing. In addition, this type of support can facilitate the transition from sport to other life roles.

Providing Tangible Support

Providing support that is primarily material in nature includes (a) material assistance and (b) personal assistance.

Beware of boundaries. Beware that certain governing bodies within sport such as the National Collegiate Athletic Association may prohibit you from providing this type of support to athletes. Read the rules and regulations of the governing bodies for the sport you are involved with. If you are still unclear as to what the boundaries are, contact your athletic administrators for clarification. Make sure that athletes understand the rules and regulations regarding whom they can count on to provide this type of support. We are all familiar with cases where the inappropriate provision of this type of support by coaches and alumni has resulted in punishments and expulsions.

Define your boundaries. It may be helpful to establish a personal philosophy about providing this type of support. In developing this philosophy examine your motives, your past behavior, your qualifications, and the rules and expectations of your administration as well as the rules and regulations of the governing bodies of the sport. Once you have developed your philosophy, communicate it to injured athletes. Let them know exactly what you can and will do as well as what you cannot and will not do. If you choose to be a provider, you may find it helpful to establish "windows of time" to assist injured athletes. This has the advantage of assuring them that you are available and focused on meeting their specific need.

Trying to please everybody all the time leads to failure. Moreover, giving to every injured athlete who needs material support can lead to *resource bankruptcy*. Rather than alleviating the stress of injury, support interventions that bankrupt the social network actually increase stress. A simple rule of thumb is to give within your means. Do not overextend yourself.

Deliver on time. Tangible support, whether it be the provision of some material product or personal assistance, is best received at the time it is requested. We do not mean to suggest that you drop everything you are doing to provide for others; however, such a request usually is time limited. Thus, a timely response on your part will increase the likelihood of the support need is being met. It should be noted, however, that severely injured athletes may require long-term tangible support. Thus, the use of a multiplex network is necessary to avoid a depletion of provider resources.

Offer tangible support interest-free. When you give tangible support, refrain from putting the recipient in a state of indebtedness to you, especially psychologically. Such a relationship, although supportive, is not social support. Give freely and unconditionally. Do not attach strings to your support and do not feel pressured into giving because you feel indebted to the recipient.

Creating and Maintaining an Effective Support System

Danish and D'Augelli (1983) suggested that although the ongoing support of caring others is essential, ultimately the individual must assume the responsibility of creating and maintaining the support he or she needs. Athletes should first be encouraged to assess the structure and efficacy of their social support system. This involves identification of (a) the types of support they feel they need, (b) the nature of their current network, and (c) the level of satisfaction they have with their network in meeting their needs.

It is also beneficial to determine the type-provider match. In other words, it is important to determine *who* provides *what* type of social support. The research by Rosenfeld et al. (1989) indicates that, for athletes, support that requires sport expertise is provided primarily by coaches, whereas other forms of support are provided by friends and parents. This indicates that athletes have two type-provider match systems: (a) those requiring expertise on the part of the provider and (b) those not requiring such expertise.

The next step is to actually locate and determine the availability of potential support providers. Danish and D'Augelli (1983) offer the following guidelines when looking for support providers: (a) They must be someone with whom the athlete has frequent contact—someone who is available when needed; (b) they must understand athlete's potential as well as limitations; (c) they must be someone on whom the athlete can rely; and (d) they should be someone to whom the athlete can give something in return. Athletes need to understand that people who are in supportive roles will not be able to provide *all* the support they need. For example, although parents may provide them with emotional support, parents may not be able to provide injured athletes with the task-challenge support they need to successfully recover from the injury. In a similar manner, a member of the sports medicine staff may be able to provide the tangible and informational support, but may not be able to provide emotional support. Moreover, it appears that reciprocity is an important element in the development of a support network.

Athletes should also be advised to invest some energy in developing new networks and utilizing *natural helpers,* such as coaches, trainers and physical therapists, and parents. These natural helpers can help the athlete in staying motivated during the rehabilitation process, making them feel a part of the team, and directing their energies toward recovery.

Coaches. Coaches can be helpful by providing emotional and informational support during recovery from injury. Coaches can serve an important social support function by encouraging the injured athlete to stay involved in team activities and meetings. In addition, injured athletes can serve as an assistant coach by monitoring their position during practice and competition in order to develop more effective strategies. Another commonly employed strategy is to assign the injured athlete the task of collecting game statistics. Unfortunately, this task is typically less successful because it is viewed by the athlete as a token gesture. "If this is so important, why isn't one of the noninjured athletes doing this?" It is important for the athlete's involvement to be a necessary and valued function for the team.

Perhaps the coach can schedule a weekly meeting with the injured athletes to get their feedback on what they have observed throughout the week at practice and to discuss game strategy with them. Coaches can also be most helpful by continually reinforcing the notion that the most important team function injured athletes can perform is to commit to an effective rehabilitation training program, thus facilitating a timely return to the team.

Teammates. Teammates can be helpful by providing emotional, informational, and tangible support during recovery from injury. Every effort should be made to keep injured athletes involved with the team. This involvement should include both on- and off-the-field activities. On of the best sources for this type of support is the injured athletes' teammates. According to Silva and Hardy (1991) when injured athletes are not allowed to isolate themselves from the team, feelings of letting the team down are minimized, important "family" ties are maintained, and fears of being replaced and forgotten are decreased.

Injury may cause the injured person to no longer see him- or herself as an athlete. Moreover, injured athletes may no longer be perceived as athletes by their teammates. This may severely impact the interpersonal dynamics within a team. Rotella and Heyman (1986) have argued that injury has the potential to rupture friendships between teammates. To decrease this potential, teammates should work toward expanding the relationship beyond the athletic role. To the extent that athletes derive their identity through the athletic role this can be difficult. Rather than relating to them in terms of how the injury will affect their future as an athlete, teammates should be encouraged to expand their focus to how the injury impacts other life roles.

Finally, teammates can serve an important function by giving of their time and talents to assist injured athletes in meeting the demands of roles outside of sport. Moreover, they may wish to give injured athletes gifts and/or tokens of appreciation for their contribution to the team.

Athletic trainers and physical therapists. Trainers and PTs can be helpful by providing emotional, informational, and tangible support throughout the rehabilitation process. Trainers and PTs can serve an important function by networking and coordinating *peer modeling.* Peer modeling involves connecting an injured athlete with another athlete who has recovered successfully from a similar injury (Wiese & Weiss, 1987). Through the interaction, it is believed that informational, emotional, and tangible support can be provided. Although the athletes do not have to come from the same sport, it is important that someone be found with as close to the same experience as possible. Because trainers and PTs are often aware of athletes with similar injuries, they are the logical linking agent. Trainers and PTs can start creating a *peer model bank* of athletes who have agreed to talk with injured athletes about the rehabilitation experience. By remaining the go-betweens, trainers and PTs can facilitate selecting the most appropriate peer model as well as preventing the model from being bombarded with requests from injured athletes.

In addition, trainers and PTs can assist in increasing the injured athlete's involvement with team activities by coordinating the rehabilitation training around team activities. For example, physical therapy could be scheduled concurrently with team taping to encourage communication with teammates, or scheduled around team meetings so that athlete would have a chance to attend. It is very easy for an athlete to withdraw into physical therapy in order to avoid any uncomfortable feelings associated with being with teammates or attending team functions. The more the athlete can openly discuss such feelings and be encouraged to gradually become more involved with the team, the quicker an athlete will be able to readopt the role of a teammate.

Trainers and PTs can also be helpful in establishing support groups for injured athletes (Wiese & Weiss, 1987). Although these groups are normally led by a mental health professional, the natural helpers can be quite helpful in the coordination process. Support groups represent a forum for injured athletes to discuss thoughts and emotions with similar others. The group can provide a sense of universality, a realization that they are not alone in having experienced injury or the psychological reaction to the event, as well as instruction on coping strategies for dealing with the stress of injury.

Parents. Parents can be helpful by providing emotional support during the rough times of rehabilitation. In addition, it is crucial to use this opportunity to foster other roles that form a child's identity. If the athlete views him- or herself as primarily an athlete, you can imagine the devastating impact an injury will have on the athlete's identity and self-worth. Parents can gradually bring focus toward other important roles to indicate how positive aspects of one's life can still occur during setbacks in other areas of life.

Have the athlete list the potential supporters for each type of support and then describe what he or she would like the person to do. Next, have the athlete list the steps to be taken in requesting these behaviors from the person(s) the athlete has identified. Finally, have the athlete identify a time frame for requesting the support he or she feels is necessary. Instruct athletes to continue this process until they feel that they have received the type of support they need. As with all plans, it is suggested that the athletes prepare a back-up plan or strategy.

In order to maintain the athlete's support system it is advised that he or she remain in regular contact with the members of the athletic network. Encourage athletes to record and evaluate the effectiveness of each provider as well as the type-provider match. In addition, have them discuss with their providers any adjustments that need to be made as well as ways to nurture the provider's involvement in the athlete's network and vice versa.

In addition, encourage the athlete to find ways that will allow the provider to feel appreciated and valued. Material and verbal rewards can be offered in a reciprocal manner, thereby building a sense of mutual caretaking. Caution should be employed, however, against developing co-dependent relationships that harm rather than help as well as those that decrease the personal agency of the people within the network.

It is important for athletes to realize that they can use their own resources as a support system for themselves and others. Although it is important to utilize the resources of others, to become totally dependent upon external support could immobilize the athlete. According to Hanson and Lubin (1986) the goal support interventions is to "overcome the need to depend too much on environmental support by developing ourselves as a support system" (p. 63). Developing self-support involves increasing awareness of yourself, keeping agreements with yourself and others, and exercising more effective problem solving (Hanson & Lubin, 1986). To become self-supportive, therefore, the injured athlete must set clear goals about the recovery process, establish clear and specific behavioral agreements/contracts with him- or herself, and bring to closure all unfinished business surrounding the injury. These actions can lead to enhanced feelings of personal agency, the foundation of continuing self-support. The point is that the injured athlete cannot be totally dependent upon others for support, but should attempt to use the support provided by others as a base for developing a self-support system.

Points to Ponder

Research indicates that our social ties are the foundation of our interpersonal interactions and that the formation, maintenance, and severance of effective social support systems is fundamental to our well-being (Hammer, Makiesky-Barrow, & Gutwirth, 1978). More specifically, research in a variety of fields supports the conclusion that the sense of being supported may facilitate athletes' coping with the stress of injury. However, because research has demonstrated that social support can have negative health effects (Hardy et al., 1991; Hobfoll, 1985; Hobfoll & London, 1986) it is important to remember that social support is not a panacea for dealing with injury or the demands stemming from the stress of modern life. Moreover, it is important to remember that not all social ties are supportive (Hobfoll & Stokes, 1988).

Although it is unlikely that one can exist without any social support, the degree as well as the type of support needed varies as a function of both personal as well as environmental factors. Moreover, recent research indicates that the need for social support is an individual disposition (I. G. Sarason et. al., 1990b) and that we can engage in behaviors that may facilitate, debilitate, and/or functionally substitute for social support (Golding & Ungerleider, 1991).

Even though the evidence to date is collectively more promising than definitive, there appears to be ample warrant for intense interest in the concept of social support, both theoretically and clinically. Indeed, it is fundamentally obvious that social support is an integral part of the quality of human life (Albrecht & Adelman, 1984). Social support is much more than a coping skill for the victims of extreme stress, like injured athletes; it is a life skill. As stated by Gottlieb (1988), "the enterpri[s]e of building supportive ties and networks of mutual aid is inextricably tied to the larger challenge of learning to nurture and be nurtured by our human attachments" (p. 541).

References

Albrecht, T. L., & Adelman, M. B. (1984). Social support and life stress: New directions for communications research. *Human Communication Research, 11*, 3–22.

Albrecht, T. L., & Hall, B. J. (1991). The role of personal relationships in organizational innovation. *Communication Monographs, 58*, 273–288.

Andersen, M. B., & Williams, J. M. (1988). A model of stress and athletic injury: Prediction and prevention. *Journal of Sport and Exercise Psychology, 11*, 294–306.

Barrera, M., & Garrison-Jones, C. (1992). Family and peer social support as specific correlates of depressive symptoms. *Journal of Abnormal Clinical Psychology, 20 (1)*, 1–16.

Billings, A. G., & Moos, R. H. (1981). The role of coping responses and social resources in attenuating the stress of life events. *Journal of Behavioral Medicine, 4*, 139–157.

Blackwell, B., & McCullagh, P. (1990). The relationship of athletic injury to life stress, competitive anxiety and coping resources. *Athletic Training, 25 (1)*, 23–27.

Blanchard, C. G., Albrecht, T. L., Ruckdeschel, J. C., Grant, C. H., & Hemmick, R. M. (1995). The role of social support in adaptation to cancer and to survival. *Journal of Psychosocial Oncology, 13*, 75–95.

Broadhead, W. E., Kaplan, B. H., James, S. A., Wagner, E. H., Schoenbach, V. J., Grimson, R., Heyden, S., Tibblin, G., & Gehlbach, S. H. (1983). The epidemiologic evidence for a relationship between social support and health. *American Journal of Epidemiology, 117*, 521–537.

Bruhn, J. G., & Phillips, B. U. (1984). Measuring social support: A synthesis of current approaches. *Journal of Behavioral Medicine, 7*, 151–169.

Caplan, G. (1974). *Support systems and community mental health.* New York: Behavioral Publications.

Caplan, G. (1976). The family as a support system. In G. Caplan & M. Killilea (Eds.), *Support systems and mutual help* (pp. 19–36). New York: Grune and Stratton.

Cobb, S. (1976). Social support as a moderator of life stress. *Psychosomatic Medicine, 38*, 300–314.

Cohen, S. (1988). Psychosocial models of the role of social support in the etiology of physical disease. *Health Psychology, 7*(3), 269–297.

Cohen, S., & Hoberman, H. M. (1983). Positive events and social supports as buffers of life change stress. *Journal of Applied Social Psychology, 13*, 99–125.

Cohen, S., & Syme, L. (Eds.). (1985). *Social support and health.* New York: Academic Press.

Cohen, S., & Wills, T. A. (1985). Stress, social support, and the buffering hypothesis. *Psychological Bulletin, 98*, 310–357.

Conrad, C. (1985). *Strategic organizational communication: Cultures, situations, and adaptations.* New York: Holt, Rinehart, and Winston.

Cutrona, C. E., & Russell, D. W. (1990). Type of social support and specific stress: Toward a theory of optimal matching. In B. R. Sarason, I. G Sarason, & G. R. Pierce (Eds), *Social support: An interactional view* (pp. 319–366). New York: John Wiley & Sons.

Cutrona, C. E., & Suhr, J. A. (1994). Social support communication in the context of marriage: An analysis of couples' supportive interactions. In B. R. Burleson, T. L. Albrecht, & I. G. Sarason (Eds.), *Communication of social support: Messages, interactions, relationships, and community* (pp. 113–135). Thousand Oaks, CA: Sage.

Danish, S. (1986). Psychological aspects in the care and treatment of athletic injuries. In P. F. Vinger & E.F. Hoerner (Eds.), *Sports injuries: The unthwarted epidemic* (2nd ed., pp. 345–353). Littleton, MA: PSG Publishing.

Danish, S., & D'Augelli, A. (1983). *Helping skills II: Life development intervention.* New York: Human Sciences.

Doeglas, D., Suurmeijer, T., & Briancon, S. (1996). An international study on measuring social support: Interactions and satisfaction. *Social Science & Medicine, 43 (9)*, 1389–1397.

Dubow, E. F., Tisak, J., Causey, D., & Hryshko, A. (1991). A two-year longitudinal study of stressful life events, social support, and social problem-solving skills: Contributions to children's behavioral and academic adjustment. *Child Development, 62*, 583–599.

Durkheim, E. (1952). *Suicide*. New York: Free Press.

Eckenrode, J., & Gore, S. (1981). Stressful events and social supports: The significance of context. In B. H. Gottlieb (Ed.), *Social networks and social support* (pp. 43–68). Beverly Hills, CA: Sage.

Egan, G. (1973). *Face to face: The small group experience and interpersonal growth*. Pacific Grove, CA: Brooks/Cole.

Ford, J., & Sutphen, R. D. (1996). Early intervention to improve attendance in elementary school for at-risk children: A pilot program. *Social Work in Education, 18*, 95–102.

Ganster, D. C., & Victor, B. (1988). The impact of social support on mental physical health. *British Journal of Medical Psychology, 61*, 17–36.

Golding, J. M., & Ugerleider, S. (1991). Social resources and mood among masters track and field athletes. *Journal of Applied Sport Psychology, 3*,142–159.

Goldsmith, D. J. (1994). The role of facework in supportive communication. In B. R. Burleson, T. L. Albrecht, & I. G. Sarason (Eds.), *Communication of social support: Messages, interactions, relationships, and community* (pp. 29–49). Thousand Oaks, CA: Sage.

Goldsmith, D., & Albrecht, T. L. (1993). The impact of supportive communication networks on test anxiety and performance. *Communication Education, 42*, 142–158.

Gordon, S. (1991, Summer). Sport psychology and the professional training of health care professionals. *AAASP Newsletter*, pp. 15.

Gordon, S., & Lindgren, S. (1990). Psycho-physical rehabilitation from a serious sport injury: Case study of an elite fast bowler. *The Australian Journal of Science and Medicine in Sport, 22*, 71–76.

Gore, S. (1978). The effect of social support in moderating the health consequence of unemployment. *Journal of Health and Social Behavior, 19*, 157–165.

Gottlieb, B. H. (1988). Support interventions: A typology and agenda for research. In S.W. Duck (Ed.), *Handbook of personal relationships: Theory, research and interventions* (pp. 519–541). New York: John Wiley & Sons.

Hammer, M. (1981). Social supports, social networks, and schizophrenia. *Schizophrenia Bulletin, 7*, 45–57.

Hammer, M., Makiesky-Barrow, S., & Gutwirth, L. (1978). Social networks and schizophrenia. *Schizophrenia Bulletin, 4* 522 545.

Hanson, P. G., & Lubin, B. (1986, Winter). Support systems: Understanding and using them effectively. *Organization Development Journal, 39–00*.

Hardy, C. J., & Crace, R. K. (1990). Dealing with injury *Sport PsychologyTraining Bulletin 1, 6*, 1–8.

Hardy, C. J., & Crace, R. K. (1991). Social support within sport. *Sport Psychology Training Bulletin, 3*, 1, 1–8.

Hardy, C. J., Richman, J. M., & Rosenfeld, L. B. (1991). The role of social support in the life stress/injury relationship. *The Sport Psychologist, 5*, 128–139.

Heitzmann, C. A., & Kaplan, R. M. (1988). Assessment of methods for measuring social support. *Health Psychology, 7* (1) 75–109.

Hobfoll, S. E. (1985). The limitations of social support in the stress process. In I. G. Sarason & B. R. Sarason (Eds.), *Social support: Theory, research, and application* (pp. 391–414). The Hague: Martinus Nijhoff.

Hobfoll, S. E. (1988). *The ecology of stress*. Washington, DC: Hemisphere.

Hobfoll, S. E. (1989). Conservation of resources: A new attempt at conceptualizing stress. *American Psychologist, 44*, 513–524.

Hobfoll, S. E., & London, P. (1986). The relationship of self-concept and social support to emotional distress among women during war. *Journal of Social and Clinical Psychology, 12,* 87–100.

Hobfoll, S. E., & Stephens, M. A. P. (1990). Social support during extreme stress: Consequences and intervention. In B. R. Sarason, I. G Sarason, & G. R. Pierce (Eds.), *Social support: An interactional view* (pp. 454–481). New York: John Wiley & Sons.

Hobfoll, S. E., & Stokes, J. P. (1988). The process and mechanics of social support. In S. W. Duck (Ed.), *Handbook of personal relationships: Theory, research and interventions* (pp. 497–517). New York: John Wiley & Sons.

House, J. (1981). *Work stress and social support.* Reading, MA: Addison-Wesley.

House, J. S., & Kahn, R. L. (1985). Measures and concepts of social support. In S. Cohen & S. L. Syme (Eds.), *Social support and health* (pp. 83–108). New York: Academic Press.

Ievleva, L., & Orlick, T. (1991). Mental links to enhanced healing: An exploratory study. *The Sport Psychologist, 5,* 25–40.

Jones, W., & Moore, T. (1987). Loneliness and social support. Special issue: Loneliness: Theory, research, and applications. *Journal of Social Behavior and Personality, 2,* 145–156.

Kahn, R. L., & Antonucci, T. C. (1980). Convoys over the life course: Attachment, roles and social support. In P. B. Baltes & O. Brim (Eds.), *Life span development and behavior* (Vol. 3, pp. 253–286). Boston: Lexington Press.

Kaplan, B. H., Cassel, J. C., & Gore, S. (1977). Social support and health. *Medical Care, 15* (5), 47–58.

Kirkpatrick, D. L. (1982). *How to improve performance through appraisal and coaching.* New York: AMACOM.

Lackovic-Grgin, K., Dekovic, M., & Milosavljevic, B. (1996). Social support and self-esteem in unemployed university graduates. *Adolescence, 31,* 701–707.

Lavallee, L., & Flint, F. (1996). The relationship of stress, competitive anxiety, mood state, and social support to athletic injury. *Journal of Athletic Training, 31 (4),* 296–299.

Leavy, R. L. (1983). Social support and psychological disorder: A review. *Journal of Community Psychology, 11,* 3–21.

Leff, S. S., & Hoyle, R. H. (1995). Young athletes' perceptions of parental support and pressure. *Journal of Youth and Adolescence, 24,* 187–203.

Lovell, M. L., & Richey, C. A. (1991). Implementing agency-based social-support skill training. *Families in Society: The Journal of Contemporary Human Services, 72 (9),* 563–572.

McDonald, S. A., & Hardy, C. J. (1990). Affective response patterns of the injured athlete: An exploratory analysis. *The Sport Psychologist, 4,* 261–274.

Moss, G. (1973). *Illness, immunity and social interaction,* New York: John Wiley & Sons.

Perrine, R. M. (1993). On being supportive: The emotional consequences of listening to another's distress. *Journal of Social and Personal Relationships, 10,* 371–384.

Pilisuk, M. (1982). Delivery of social support: The social inoculation. *American Journal of Orthopsychiatry, 52,* 20–31.

Pines, A. M., Aronson, E., & Kafry, D. (1981). *Burnout.* New York: Free Press.

Query, J., Parry, D., & Flint, L. J. (1992). The relationship among social support, communication competence, and cognitive depression for nontraditional students. *Journal of Applied Communication Research, 20 (1),* 78–94.

Quick, T. L. (1977). *Person to person managing: An executive's guide to working effectively with people.* New York: St. Martin's Press.

Quick, T. L. (1980) *The quick motivation method: How to make your employees happier, harder working, and more productive.* New York: St Martin's Press.

Richman, J. M., Hardy, C. J., Rosenfeld, L. B., & Callanan, R. A. E. (1989). Strategies for enhancing social support networks in sport: A brainstorming experience. *Journal of Applied Sport Psychology, 1,* 150–159.

Richman, J. M., & Rosenfeld, L. B. (1987). Stress reduction for hospice workers: A support group model. *Hospice Journal, 3*, 205–221.

Richman, J. M., Rosenfeld, L. B., Hardy, C. J. (1993). The Social Support Survey: An initial evaluation of a clinical measure and practice model of the social support process. *Research on Social Work Practice, 3*, 288–311.

Rook, K. S. (1992). Detrimental aspects of social relationships: Taking stock of an emerging literature. In H. O. F. Veiel & U. Baumann (Eds.), *The meaning and measurement of social support* (pp. 157–169). New York: Hemisphere Publishing.

Rosenfeld, L. B., Richman, J. M., & Hardy, C. J. (1989). Examining social support networks among athletes: Description and relationship to stress. *The Sport Psychologist, 3*, 23–33.

Rosenfeld, L. B., Wilder, L., Crace, R. K., & Hardy, C. J. (1990). Communication fundamentals: Active listening. *Sport Psychology Training Bulletin, 1*, 5, 1–8.

Rotella, R. J., & Heyman, S. R. (1986). Stress, injury, and the psychological rehabilitation of athletes. In J. M. Williams (Eds.), *Applied sport psychology; Personal growth to peak performance* (pp. 343–364). Palo Alto, California: Mayfield.

Rounds, K., Galinsky, M., & Stevens, S. (1991). Linking people with AIDS in rural communities: The telephone group. *Social Work, 36*, 13–18.

Sarason, B. R., Sarason, I. G., & Pierce, G. R. (1990). Traditional views of social support and their impact on assessment. In B. R. Sarason, I. G Sarason, & G. R. Pierce (Eds.), *Social support: An interactional view* (pp. 9–25). New York: John Wiley & Sons.

Sarason, I. G., & Sarason,B. R. (1985). *Social support: Theory, research, and applications.* Boston: Martinus Nijhoff International.

Sarason, I. G., & Sarason, B. R. (1986). Experimentally provided social support. *Journal of Personality and Social Psychology, 50*, 122–125.

Sarason, I. G., Sarason, B. R., & Pierce, G. R. (1990a). Social support, personality and performance. *Journal of Applied Sport Psychology, 2*, 117–127.

Sarason, I. G., Sarason, B. R., & Pierce, G. (1990b). Social support: The search for theory. *Journal of Social and Clinical Psychology, 9*, 133–147.

Schaefer, C., Coyne, J. C., & Lazarus, R. S. (1981). The health-related functions of social support. *Journal of Behavioral Medicine, 4* (4), 381–406.

Shumaker, S. A., & Brownell, A. (1984). Toward a theory of social support: Closing conceptual gaps. *Journal of Social Issues, 40*, 11–36.

Silva, J. M., & Hardy, C. J. (1991). The sport psychologist: Psychological aspects of injury in sport. In F. O. Mueller & A. Ryan (Eds.), *The sports medicine team and athlete injury prevention* (pp. 114–132). Philadelphia, PA: F. A. Davis.

Smoll, F. L., & Smith, R. E. (1979). *Improving relationship skills in youth sport coaches.* East Lansing: Michigan Institute for the Study of Youth Sports.

Smoll, F. L., Smith, R. E., & Barnett, N. P. (1993). Enhancement of children's self-esteem through social support training for youth sport coaches. *Journal of Applied Psychology, 78*, 602–610.

Tardy, C. (1988). Social support: Conceptual clarification and measurement options. In C. H. Tardy (Ed.), *A handbook for the study of human communication: Methods and instruments for observing, measuring, and assessing communicatin processes* (pp. 347–364). Norwood, NJ: Albex.

Tracy, E. (1990). Identifying social support resources of at-risk families. *Social Work, 35*, 252–258.

Ungerleider, S., & Golding, J. (1991). Beyond strength: Psychological profiles of Olympic athletes. *Track Technique, 116*, 3704–3709.

Wallston, B. S., Alagna, S. W., DeVellis, B. M., & DeVellis, R. F. (1983). Social support and health. *Health Psychology, 2*, 367–391.

Weiss, M. R., & Troxel, R. K. (1986). Psychology of the injured athlete. *Athletic Training, 21* (2), 104–109, 154.

Weiss, R. (1974). The provision of social relationships. In Z. Rubin (Ed.), *Doing unto others* (pp. 17–26). Englewood Cliffs, NJ: Prentice Hall.

Wiese, D. M., & Weiss, M. R. (1987). Psychological rehabilitation and physical injury: Implication for the sportsmedicine team. *The Sport Psychologist, 1,* 318–330.

Wilcox, B. L. (1981a). Social support, life stress, and psychological adjustment: A test of the buffering hypothesis. *American Journal of Community Psychology, 9,* 371–387.

Wilcox, B. L. (1981b). Social support in adjusting to marital disruption: A network analysis. In B. Gottlieb (Ed.), *Social networks and social support* (pp. 97–115). Beverly Hills, CA: Sage Publications.

Woodward, M. S., Rosenfeld, L. B., & May, S. K. (1996). Sex differences in social support in sororities and fraternities. *Journal of Applied Communication Research, 24,* 260–272.

Zigler, E., Taussig, C., & Black, K. (1992). Early childhood intervention. *American Psychologist, 47,* 997–1006.

12

Mental Paths to Enhanced Recovery From a Sports Injury

Lydia Ievleva
University of New South Wales

Terry Orlick
University of Ottawa

The greatest discovery of my generation is that human beings, by changing the inner attitudes of their minds, can change the outer aspects of their lives. . . . It is too bad that more people will not accept this tremendous discovery and begin living it. (James, 1950, p. 258)

Drawing from the authors' extensive field experience, as well as from results of a comprehensive study which examined a number of psychosocial factors related to sports injury rehabilitation using subjects diagnosed with the same degree of ankle or knee injuries, this chapter discusses mental strategies for enhancing recovery from sports injury (Ievleva & Orlick, 1991). A survey format was used in the study, and the scores between those identified as either fast- or slow-healing subjects based on recovery time were compared. The rate of recovery was found to be significantly related to the extent to which certain mental activities were engaged in, most notably, goal setting, healing mental imagery, and positive self-talk.

Given the demands of contemporary sport and the high rate of sports injuries, virtually all high-performance athletes experience some sort of injury at some time during their athletic career. Depending on the sport, an athlete can expect to endure at least one significant interruption, and often several interruptions, to training and competition due to injury. Although much of the attention of coaches and sport psychology consultants is focused on preparing athletes for competition, this attention is often cut off completely when an athlete becomes injured. Because of this, an injured athlete may feel excluded, neglected, or of little importance. Many athletes feel abandoned or alone when they are injured. This is partly because they are out of the limelight, inactive, and watching from a distance and partly because the prior support and reinforcement from important people in their sport are often directed elsewhere, to those still actively competing. It is particularly difficult for injured athletes when the coaching staff and the organization fail to demonstrate any concern or genuine interest in that individual. For example, some coaches do not call, visit, write, or maintain contact for extended periods of time. Many athletes are left feeling they are on their own when trying to cope with debilitating and sometimes career-ending injuries, unless they are fortunate enough to have a strong support base. Much of this depends upon the treatment, approach, and attention that an injured athlete receives from the outset from coaches, doctors, physiotherapists, and sport psychologists. It is important that each of these professionals recognizes that there is a person connected to this leg, arm, and body. The extent to which each of these people can make the athlete feel positive, optimistic, and in control of his or her own healing greatly influences the extent to which the athlete will heal fully and efficiently.

Fortunately, attention to the mental side of healing has been gaining greater recognition among sports medicine practitioners as highlighted by the following comments appearing in sports injury journals. Ron Dunn, former head Athletic Trainer at Western Kentucky University at Bowling Green, Kentucky, asserts that despite all the highly sophisticated resources in expertise and equipment "designed to cure the injured athlete, most trainers would agree that correcting the physical malfunctioning is only half the battle" (Dunn, 1983, p. 34). Richard Steadman, Chairman, Medical Group of the U.S. Alpine Ski Team, divides rehabilitation into three categories: "psychological rehabilitation, physiologic rehabilitation, and rehabilitation of the injured area" (Steadman, 1982, p. 289). Gary Faris, a certified trainer and staff psychologist at the Fort Collins Sports Medicine Clinic in Colorado, agrees that in order to attain the goals of rehabilitation, one must address the emotional state as well as the physical:

> To treat a knee and ignore the brain and emotions that direct the choreography of that knee is not consistent with total care of the patient. Any

comprehensive rehabilitation plan will want to interface the proper **external** rehabilitation procedures with proper **internal** state of mind of the patient. When these two factors come together, successful results are tremendously enhanced. A positive state of mind promotes better attendance and attentiveness to, and more intensity toward the external rehabilitation procedures, which yield successful results. (Faris, 1985, p. 546)

More recent advances in attention to psychological aspects of rehabilitation in the medical profession are the inclusion of an entire chapter in a major new sports injury rehabilitation text devoted to the issue (Botterill, Flint, & Ievleva, 1996), as well as Dr. Richard Steadman's keynote address to the 1997 AAASP Conference.

This current trend in sports injury rehabilitation in particular, and the health care community in general, towards a greater integration of mind and body in the treatment of illness and injury has a very long history. Although it may represent a new wave in contemporary medical thinking, the ideas that have spawned the fields of behavioral medicine, health psychology, and psychoneuroimmunology are far from new. In fact, the role of visualization and belief in healing—psychological tools that are gaining increasing acceptance for enhancing physical healing—are considered the most ancient healing techniques ever used by humans (Achterberg, 1985; Samuels & Samuels, 1975).

It is clear that psychological factors play a vital role in injury rehabilitation. Which are the most important factors and how they function in the recovery process, however, have yet to be determined. Nevertheless, there is much anecdotal as well as empirical evidence to suggest that certain psychological characteristics either enhance or retard healing. This is based on a classic mind-body principle posited by pioneers in biofeedback research, Green, Green, and Walters (1970):

Every change in a physiological state is accompanied by an appropriate change in the mental-emotional state, conscious or unconscious; and conversely, every change in the mental-emotional state, conscious or unconscious, is accompanied by an appropriate change in the physiological state. (p. 3)

Considerable support for the mind-body relationship is found in contemporary behavioral medicine literature (Achterberg, 1985; Borysenko, 1987; Cousins, 1989a, 1989b; Goleman & Gurin, 1995; Gordon, Jaffe, & Bresler, 1984; Locke & Colligan, 1986; Peper, Ancoli, & Quinn, 1979; Rossi, 1986; Siegel, 1986, 1989; Simonton, Matthews-Simonton, & Creighton, 1978).

For instance, in those studies investigating biofeedback benefits and placebo effects, it has been found that the triggering mechanism for personal control and healing lies totally within the subject. With biofeedback training one becomes aware of direct control over one's body. A placebo produces only an *awareness* that the healing process has begun, because of the belief that it has begun.

Mental imagery plays a leading role in directing the physical changes produced by biofeedback training and placebos. It is believed that healing may be triggered or accelerated through positive, constructive, and goal-directed imagery (Barabasz & McGeorge, 1978; Cousins, 1989a, 1989b; Green & Green, 1977; Korn & Johnson, 1983; Simonton et al., 1978; Schwartz, 1984; Siegel, 1986, 1989). Similarly, it is the symbolic or imagined processes in action that determine the placebo effect. The placebo, a symbol of healing, triggers a healing visualization in the patient (Borkovec, 1985; Brody, 1985; Frank, 1961). The placebo has been shown to be effective even while patients are fully cognizant of the inert property of the placebo (Park & Covi, 1965; Vogel, Goodwin, & Goodwin, 1980). This indicates that the mere suggestion that healing should take place may spontaneously result in a healing image.

Psychological Considerations in Recovery

Certain attitudes and psychological factors may either hinder or enhance the effectiveness of a particular treatment, as well as an injured athlete's ability to cope. Among these are the athlete's belief in his or her own self-healing capacity, the nature of emotional support available, faith in the physician's or physiotherapist's skill, and the degree to which the athlete wants to heal.

The support an athlete receives from family, teammates, friends, etc., can have a significant impact on the ability to cope. How this support system responds to the athlete's injury can affect the athlete's response. It is, therefore, important to understand the nature of these influences that occur outside the officially recognized therapeutic environment.

It is important for anyone working with an injured athlete to allow for full expression of feeling, to listen, and to show empathy. With the unburdening, the injured athlete may then feel freer to focus on moving forward. As Faris (1985) asserts, "It is time well spent, for if the athlete's mental attitude is sour, the outcome will be retarded" (p. 549). It can also be helpful to remind athletes that it is normal to have ups and downs during the recovery process. Some days are better than others. Sometimes there are doubts. Moving forward generally occurs in a series of waves. Encourage athletes to *hang in there*—all great athletes experience this. Persistence is important here, just like in practice, games, and competitions.

The best physical and psychological care is no guarantee of a speedy and successful rehabilitation. In the final analysis, it is the athlete who is responsible for the success of his or her own recovery. As Arnheim (1985) states, "Trainers must educate all of their injured charges to understand that rehabilitation and full recovery are a cooperative venture, with major responsibility resting on the athletes' shoulders" (p. 207). This is no different from striving to improve and excel in sports. The athlete alone is ultimately responsible for making it happen.

A commonly cited factor mediating injury rehabilitation is "secondary gain." This term refers to an injury's providing such benefits as attention from trainers and sympathy from peers, an honorable way of disengaging from the pressures of living up to high expectations, or freeing up time and energy to pursue other personal goals. This type of gain has been a relatively rare occurrence with national team athletes with whom we have worked. Most are highly motivated to get back to active training and competing as quickly as possible. Some athletes who are unable to acquire time off to rest or to balance their lives in any other way, however, may see some value in an injury in that it lessens the expectations placed upon them and may give them an honorable way out.

An example of this occurred with a top collegiate athlete. *Patty* found herself faced with enormous demands being placed on her time and energy. In her senior year, she desperately sought to balance a difficult academic course load while performing as the #1 player on her team. There were numerous time-consuming team-related demands that included not only those activities inherent with practice and competing, for instance, traveling to tournaments, but also team social events, such as a camping trip, which left her with only one weekend of the entire semester to herself. Despite feeling increasingly distressed and overwhelmed, she did not feel herself to be in a position to make the decision to take time off from either the team social or practice activities to keep up with her studies, as this would have been frowned upon by her coach as well as her teammates. The coach felt she should just "tough it out." It was not long before Patty sustained an ankle injury, which finally excused her from enough practices to regain control and stability over her school and personal life. In fact, in her own words, she described the injury as a "Godsend." It was the only way that she was able to seize control over her life. Balancing the demands of training, traveling, classwork, and social life is a common problem for college athletes. When their lives become too unbalanced for too long, we can lose people psychologically, or physically.

In some cases, therefore, an injury or illness may provide a valuable *time-out* that the athlete may not have initiated on his or her own. As such, the injury may be perceived as an opportunity to bring one's life back into balance and improve one's quality of life.

Mental Paths to Recovery From Injury

This section discusses specific mental activities that have the capacity to enhance injury recovery, in much the same way that they enhance sport performance. They are as follows:

* Commitment
* Seeing the Opportunities
* Goal Setting
* Attitude and Belief
* Positive Self-Talk
* Relaxation
* Mental Imagery
* Coping with Fear of Reinjury

Commitment

The first element critical to rapid recovery is one's *commitment* to heal. The athlete must want to fully recover and fully commit to doing so. Persistence and patience are necessary when confronting any challenge, and this applies to full recovery from injury as well (Orlick, 1996).

Seeing the Opportunities

The process of recovering from an injury also involves personal learning and growth. Just as the word for *crisis* in Chinese has two characters—one meaning *danger,* the other meaning *opportunity*—an injury may be viewed as a chance to learn and to grow, as a challenge to overcome, rather than as a catastrophe.

In the applied behavioral medicine community it is strongly held that if one treats only the physical symptoms, and neglects the psychological component of health and healing, an underlying problem will likely resurface in some other form or symptom until the original issue is addressed and resolved satisfactorily. In fact, for most forms of illness, a health crisis is viewed as a "wake-up call." Our bodies are constantly sending us messages. Some are benign, happy, and joyful, whereas others are indicative of stress, conflict, and imbalance. Often, personal lifestyle, health habits, or intra- or interpersonal conflicts may be the problem sources. If we choose to ignore early warning signs, the body may require more drastic measures to get our attention. It is said that first we get a whisper in the ear, then a tap on the shoulder, and if that doesn't do the trick, then a knock on the head! This is exemplified by injuries and illnesses resulting from overtraining, overworking, and overfatigue, as, for example, in the Epstein-Barr Syndrome.

An illness may indeed serve as a signal of something in the psychological domain that has been neglected. Positive psychological perspectives are needed to promote faster recovery—health and well-being. This is supported by a great deal of evidence shared at a recent conference (The 2nd National Conference on The Psychology of Health, Immunity and Disease, sponsored by The National Institute for the Clinical Application of Behavioral Medicine, Orlando, 1990) on the application of behavioral medicine, where there was consensus that all dramatic improvement and recovery from serious, if not terminal, illness are coincident with a major psychological or spiritual insight and positive transformation. This implies that in order for a health breakthrough to occur, a psychological one needs to precede it. It is, therefore, important to listen to our bodies and heed those *inner* voices conducive to wellness. This may be accomplished as a preventive measure, as well as be directed towards enhanced healing and enhanced performance. Commonly suggested methods for cultivating inner awareness are such practices as meditation, progressive relaxation, and yoga.

Athletes in our study were asked whether the time-out from their sport accompanying their injury resulted in any valuable lessons or new perspectives that contributed to their future achievement. Subjects in the fast healing group derived greater benefits in the form of enhanced insight and enjoyment in their sport, whereas those in the slow-healing group found no benefits at all. In addition, those athletes who learned from the experience and accepted it as a challenge and opportunity fared better in terms of their recovery time. In other words, these athletes made the most of a bad situation. They turned crises into blessings. This is consistent with the findings from world-class athletes where there was always a substantial gain in insight or approach to training that subsequently substantially improved the athlete's training and/or performance.

Following are examples of valuable lessons learned from the injury experience by some athletes with whom we have worked.

Ann, while ranked in the top five in the world in her sport, learned about the importance for rest by experiencing recurring injuries. For most developing athletes, the need to train is paramount. Having reached certain heights of competitive success, however, it then becomes more important to discipline oneself to rest. It was Ann's tenacity and drive that led to her success, but these very same qualities applied to her training made her increasingly at risk to overtraining and injury. She discovered that she was most likely to become injured during a lull in the competitive season, when she would find herself bored and with an excessive drive to train harder and recklessly. Whereas her willingness to train hard had been her strength on her rise in the world rankings, she now had to learn to *back off* training and focus on remaining well in order to maintain or advance her position. Initially, this notion went directly way to improve your skills is to employ both supportive and confirming behaviors while you listen. Supportive and confirming behaviors communicate the message that the injured athlete is acknowledged, understood, and accepted.

Another important aspect of effective listening is patience. Often, people are somewhat reluctant to jump right into a conversation about personal and/or emotional topics. They wish to be assured that their confidence will be protected before self-disclosure takes place. The listener may be obliged to demonstrate trustworthiness and an understanding of the particular demands placed upon the athlete in his or her sport. Active listening without giving advice or being judgmental is an excellent way to earn this type of trust.

In addition, emotionality to your messages may provide them the support the injured athlete needs. This does not mean throwing out your own emotions. Empathic listeners focus on the feeling as well as the content of what the others say. By reflecting the feeling you are observing, you indicate a truer level of understanding. This tends to create a relationship that will also allow for emotional challenges where attitudes, values, and feelings are explored and evaluated.

Know thyself. When strategizing the provision of emotional support for injured athletes, be aware of your emotional needs as well as your reactions to those who are distressed. The frequency with which people seek emotional support from you is often a good indication of your ability to manage your own anxiety associated with interacting with the "victim" of injury. Gottlieb (1988) maintained that providers could benefit from becoming more aware of the impact that their coping strategies have on the support process as well as adopting more palatable strategies.

Switch hats occasionally. Often we use only one type of social support because it seems exclusively suited to the support providers, our personality, or professional role. This can result in neglect of, or hesitancy toward, other support approaches. Unfortunately, the most underdeveloped, yet most needed, form of support is emotional support. Allow yourself to be open to providing emotional support. Gradually, you will find others turning to you for this type of support and may find this becoming a more natural part of your personality or role.

Involve the "natural helping network." Regular, informal contact with the *natural helping network* within sport—coaches, teammates, athletic trainers and physical therapists, and parents—should be encouraged. Injury involves rather intense emotional reactions and heightened needs that may be ameliorated by this network.

Create an open environment. As much as possible, structure the physical environment wherein you meet the athlete so that it communicates acceptance what is is normally prescribed, that is, he has set out to master lucid dreaming. Furthermore, he is now using his dreams to facilitate his recovery and foster his hopes to return to play in time for the playoffs.

To enhance the recovery process, exceptional athletes accept the injury and do everything in their power to initiate a positive and complete recovery. They also take advantage of what can be learned from the experience (e.g., about oneself or one's relationship to one's sport). This is depicted in a comment made by an exceptionally fast, self-directed healer—a professional dancer who experienced a knee injury due to overuse/overtraining: "I would have a conversation with my other self and ask myself why I had created this situation, where it stemmed from in me, what it made me realize about me and how to go about it to make the most of what could be done."

Caregivers should help athletes to explore the benefits and insights permitted by a time-out, and personal commitment to recovery, which may ultimately prove fruitful and healthy for the athlete in the longrun.

Goal Setting

Setting specific relevant goals for each session, day, week, month, etc., is an important element in any training program, including programs for regaining optimal health. Goals translate commitment into specifically relevant action. Minimal and ideal targets can be set, listing the specific steps required to reach them. The results from our study with injured athletes clearly showed that the fast healers were much more involved in goal setting than were the slow healers, especially where daily goals were concerned (Ievleva & Orlick, 1991).

End result or affirmation imagery, in which athletes imagine themselves accomplishing their goals, as well as process imagery, in which athletes imagine themselves engaged in their daily goals, is recommended. The procedure for end result imagery, described in *Getting Well Again* by Simonton et al. (1978), is adapted here for recovery from sports injury.

1. Select a goal.
2. Relax.
3. See yourself with goal already met.
4. Imagine, with as many details as possible, the feelings you would have having reached your goal.
5. See the response of others close to you regarding your achievement.
6. Go over the steps it took to reach your goal and experience satisfaction at each level.
7. Allow yourself to feel happy about reaching your goal.
8. Gradually come back to the present.
9. Then open your eyes and commence action on that first step.

For those who have difficulty seeing or feeling their goals being achieved, or who get negative images, it is suggested they stop, acknowledge their doubts and fears, and then make a list of all the positive attributes that will enable reaching the goal, for example, talent, treatment, and tenacity. This is done to help them believe or to recognize that they have the tools necessary to meet the goals and that they are in control.

A beneficial feature of goal setting is that it usually involves some form of imagery. When one thinks of a goal or thinks through a plan to accomplish a goal, some mental images normally flash through one's mind. Goal setting, therefore, may be an indirect link to the extent of mental imagery taking place. Setting a goal in itself is a statement of expectation, and hence a conceptualization of success is likely to occur. It is highly probable that once a goal is set, a person will periodically re-contemplate, or re-imagine, achieving that goal. This may serve to conjure up an image of success, control, or those activities in which one can engage that are consistent with achieving that goal. It also follows that daily goals are the most effective means towards this end. The results from our study confirm this, in that daily goal setting was found to be more related to recovery time than either the long-term or returning to sport goals (Ievleva & Orlick, 1991).

Attitude and Belief

Belief in one's capacity to influence personal healing and attain full recovery greatly influences the healing process. Once one has set goals, it is important to believe that they may be accomplished. This requires persistence and ongoing positive reminders in longer rehabilitations in which the end may seem so distant. It is important for the athlete to realize that the quality of his or her continued recovery depends on maintaining a positive attitude to allow the physiological healing processes to take place. Although one cannot control the fact that one is injured, and may be facing a lengthy rehabilitation process, one **can** direct and control the way he or she thinks about it. In other words, rather than thinking about all that has gone wrong, and how one's life is disrupted due to the injury, it is more conducive to focus on the positive and what *can* be done. In tune with this view, Dunn suggests the following prescription for achieving goals that he adapted from *The Magic of Thinking Big* (D. Schwartz, 1978):

1. Refuse to talk negatively about health. A person may receive a little sympathy but will never get respect or loyalty by complaining. This is particularly true in athletics.
2. Refuse to worry about poor health. Worry is a negative emotion and fear of ill health or injury in athletics often results in injury or illness due to unconscious adjustment in activity.

3. Be genuinely grateful for good health. This will help keep a person's thoughts focused on the positive aspects of her or his health.

Finally, a person should understand that the body responds to its own needs. Very gradual exercise, not in excess, is an important tool in rehabilitation. (Dunn, 1983, p. 34)

Positive Self-Talk

The degree of optimism injured athletes display is indicative of their coping style. A positive outlook indicates adjustment to the new condition and an orientation towards improvement. In contrast, a negative outlook indicates preoccupation with the implication of the injury, which leads to little effort towards improvement. Outlook may, therefore, have an important impact on recovery time. This is supported by the results about self-talk in our study (self-talk being reflective of one's attitude, belief, and outlook). Those whose self-talk was positive, self-encouraging, and determined, healed much more rapidly than did those whose self-talk can best be described as whining and self-pitying—that is, it tended to be totally negative, self-deprecatory, and unforgiving. See Table 1 for representative examples.

Table 1. Examples of Positive Self-Talk From the Fast-Healing Group and Examples of Negative Self-Talk From the Slow-Healing Group

Positive Self-Talk:
- How can I make the most out of what I can do now?
- I can beat this thing.
- I can do anything.
- I told myself, "I can do it. I can beat the odds and recover sooner than normal."
- I want to go spring skiing. I'll be totally healed by then.
- I have to work to get my leg as strong as the other one.
- It's feeling pretty good.
- It's getting better all the time.

Negative Self-Talk:
- It's probably going to take forever to get better.
- I'll never make up for the lost time.
- What a stupid thing to do. Dumb mistake.
- What a useless body.
- It will never be as strong again.
- Stupid fool! Stupid injury. Stupid leg.
- I talked to myself about how frustrated I was. There is nothing good about this, and there is nothing I can do about it.
- Why me?

Positive thinking can influence one's belief and perspective, and belief is often translated into action through positive self-talk. Monitoring internal dialogue can be effective in taking control, guiding positive thoughts, and reducing negative thoughts. This is done first by planning to think in positive terms and, secondly, by responding to negative thoughts that may still occur, as a cue to switch to a positive thought.

Thinking and acting in positive ways contribute to personal well-being and enhanced health. Focusing on the positive, on what is within personal control and what can be done to enhance the situation and your recovery, is much more effective than dwelling on the negative. Kabat-Zinn (1990) emphasizes in his book *Full Catastrophe Living* that there is usually much more **right** with one's body than there is ever **wrong**. It therefore pays to focus on, and appreciate more, what is going well, than to focus on what is not. It is also very helpful to carry on a positive dialogue with one's body, particularly in those areas on which one is focused on rehabilitating.

Injured athletes invariably have moments when they make disparaging remarks to their injured body part (e.g., "You stupid, useless knee."). Ask them to reflect on how they would feel and respond if spoken to in such terms, and then invite them to consider speaking positively, kindly, and lovingly to the injured part, much as one might speak to one's injured child, for instance, "It's ok, knee. I'm going to take care of you. You're going to take care of me. You're getting stronger all the time; together we're going to make you as good as new . . . "

Relaxation

Relaxation practice in any of its various forms, whether it be physical relaxation, meditation, progressive relaxation, breath control, yoga, etc., plays an integral role in behavioral medicine and stress reduction programs. The health benefits accrued from engaging in relaxation on a regular basis have been well documented. Relaxation helps open avenues in our minds that regulate our bodies. Through relaxation practice we can become more aware of, and connected, to our bodies and thereby more able to direct their activities. Using relaxation in combination with imagery, one can also initiate physical and behavioral change.

It is common for one's tension level to increase due to the stress of being injured, especially in the injured area. Regularly practicing a relaxation routine can be effective in relaxing the area and relieving the tension, thereby also reducing any pain. Staying loose and relaxed facilitates recovery by increasing blood circulation. The greater the blood flow, the faster injured tissues are repaired (Benson, 1975; Bresler, 1984a, 1984b). Relaxation is now generally recognized to be effective for treating pain as well (Benson, 1995; Kabat-

Zinn, 1995; Turk & Nash, 1995). A leading panel of medical experts assembled by the the NIH are reported in the *Journal of the American Medical Association* (July 24–31, 1996) to have embraced relaxation treatment for pain management (NIH Technology Assessment Panel on Integration of Behavioural and Relaxation Approaches Into the Treatment of Chronic Pain and Insomnia, 1996).

Swearingen, an orthopedic surgeon and clinical instructor at the University of Colorado School of Medicine, has seen many skiing injuries that tend to fall into the "severe" category. He employs mental techniques to lower activation and tension level right in the emergency room in the attempt to couple the injury with a state "conducive to body rest and healing" (Swearingen, 1984, p. 102). Following treatment at the hospital, Swearingen then instructs his patients in relaxation and meditation. He draws upon the work of Benson (1975) for relaxation, believing that the state of rest generated is beneficial to healing (Swearingen, 1984).

Mental Imagery

Positive images of healing, as well as images of being fully recovered, are useful in enhancing one's belief and mobilizing one's own healing powers both within and outside of sport. The value of imagery in healing has a long history in Eastern philosophies and is currently gaining increasing acceptance in the West.

There are many clinical reports of therapeutic benefits that result from imagery. Although most are anecdotal, there is increasing documentation of cases to support the healing benefits of engaging in healing imagery (Achterberg, 1989; Cousins, 1989a, 1989b; Epstein, 1986, 1989; Krippner, 1985; Olness, 1995; Rossman, 1984, 1995).

Simonton et al. (1978) have reported positive findings as a result of implementing a relaxation and imagery program with patients diagnosed as having medically incurable cancer. Forty-one percent showed improvement, whereas 22.2% demonstrated total remission, and 19.1%, tumor regression. It was their contention that the practice of relaxation and imagery enhanced the immune system (Simonton et al., 1978). A subsequent study by Hall (1983) supports the above conclusion. His study tested the effects of hypnosis plus imagery on lymphocyte function. The results showed an increased immune response, but only for those who scored high on hypnotizability.

In our own study on recovery from athletic injuries (Ievleva & Orlick, 1991), it was found that athletes used three types of imagery. These included healing imagery in which athletes tried to see and feel the body parts healing; imagery during physiotherapy when they imagined the treatment promoting recovery;

and total recovery imagery in which they imagined being totally recovered, returning to their sport, and performing well again. Athletes felt that all three types of imagery were helpful; however, healing imagery evidenced the greatest relationship to recovery time. Case studies with athletes have been reported (Foster & Porter, 1987), in which negative images (e.g., of the injury as it occurred, inflamed, torn, etc.) have interfered with positive imagery of healing and recovery and hence impeded recovery. This trend for negative imagery to have the opposite effect of positive imagery was supported in our study.

It is generally considered more effective to use healing imagery after first eliciting some form of "relaxation response" to *quiet* and enhance the receptivity of the mind. According to Jaffe and Bresler (1984), "Attaining a state of bodily relaxation is a prerequisite for all work with therapeutic guided imagery, for it provides inhibition of somatic muscle activity and verbal thoughts and allows mental images to become dominant" (p. 61). The usual procedure is to engage in some form of progressive muscle relaxation or meditation before beginning the healing imagery. Other methods involve hypnosis, and some have even taken advantage of a patient's being under anesthesia. It was originally thought that while anesthetized, patients are totally oblivious to events around them including casual conversation. It has since been discovered that patients, when later hypnotized, can recall all that was said during and/or following surgery. Apparently, what is said can significantly influence the patient's recovery in either a positive or negative way, depending on what was said (Green & Green, 1977; Korn & Johnson, 1983). Pearson (1961) demonstrated that patients receiving positive suggestions about a quick recovery while "unconscious," that is, under anesthesia, had an average hospitalization stay of 2.4 days less than did the control group.

Green and Green (1977) have reported the successful results of a doctor who used postsurgical suggestions:

> After testing reflexes to make certain that the patient was coming to consciousness, he would begin talking in a very low voice, telling the patient how well the operation had gone, how nicely the body had responded, how well the repairs were made. He planted the idea that there would be little pain, and possibly none at all; the tissues would recover very quickly; there would be no infection; the patient would be walking in a very short time. Nurses in intensive care soon noticed that his patients recovered more rapidly than others and asked him to work with other patients too. (p. 327)

The preceding evidence supports the programmability of the unconscious mind for promoting the healing process. Although anesthesia and hypnosis may be efficient in accessing the unconscious in certain cases, a much more

Table 2. Basic Components Involved in Self-Directed Healing

- Relaxing mentally and physically.
- Maintaining a positive attitude.
- Mentally connecting with the injured body part and imagining healing taking place within—seeing, feeling, and experiencing healing, using as much detail as possible.
- Seeing and feeling the body exactly as one would like it to be.
- Imagining the body fully functioning and performing well at desired activities.
- Reminding oneself that one is feeling good and improving more and more each day.

practical method that offers similarly effective results involves self-directed relaxation and imagery. Table 2 outlines the basic components involved in self-directed healing.

Daily practice is recommended to attain best results. What precisely is to be imagined is determined individually. An image that works for one person may not be as effective for someone else. For example, among the Simonton et al. (1978) cancer patients, one patient saw her white cells as "killer sharks" attacking the cancer cells, whereas another saw the white cells as white knights. The important feature is that one see one's own bodily resources as being powerful and effectual. Simonton et al. also included suggestions of chemotherapy or radiation treatment's being effective, although the emphasis is on one's own body leading the battle towards recovery. This can be applied to the physiotherapy setting, for example, seeing/feeling the treatment minimizing scar tissue, increasing blood flow, or strengthening the muscle or tissue. Athletes should be clearly informed about what the treatment is designed to do so they can imagine those effects taking place.

Arnheim (1985) and Swearingen (1984), both medical practitioners who draw upon the mind's capacity to heal, explain healing imagery as follows:

It is important that the athlete be educated about the physiological process of healing. Once the healing process is understood, the athlete is instructed to imagine it taking place during therapy and throughout the day. If an infection is being fought, the body's phagocytes can be imagined as "Pac Men" gobbling up infectious material. When tissue is torn, clot formation and organization can be imagined, followed by tissue regeneration and healing. . . . [This] helps the athlete psychologically to be part of the process and to take major responsibility for rehabilitation. (Arnheim, 1985, p. 217)

[Swearingen draw] pictures depicting the four stages of the healing process—clot formation around the fracture, the change of the clot into fibrous tissue lattice, calcium crystallization on the latticework, and re-structuring of new bone around the fracture site. . . . My impression is that since I adopted this approach [i.e. meditation and visualization], the necessary time in the cast and the morbidity during the healing process have both been significantly reduced. (Swearingen, 1984, p. 104)

Imagining the healing process can be enhanced by knowing precisely what it looks like physiologically. It is not essential that it be realistic, but it must symbolize positive change (Green & Green, 1977; Jaffe & Bresler, 1984; Simonton et al., 1978).

Because injured athletes are unable to practice physically, mental practice becomes that much more important if they are to maintain a certain skill level. Performance imagery can also be a powerful tool in this regard. Not only does it provide a medium by which to rehearse sport skills, but it also helps preparation for situations that are infrequently encountered in physical practice or competition. Imagery practice can be effective in preparing injured athletes for any number of competitive or practice situations and thus helps them to retain confidence in their ability and to dissipate any lingering fears they may have of reinjury upon return to competition.

When one approaches return to training and competition, it is important to incorporate details in the performance imagery of the use of such protective devices as taping or braces as would be required for actual activity. An omission of such detail in the imagery may result in the kind of pain, soreness, or discomfort that would typically occur if physically performing the activity without the protective device. This occurred with a university basketball player with whom we worked who habitually taped his previously injured ankles before every practice and game to avoid soreness. He had, however, inadvertently neglected to do so in his imagery. Once the taping was included in subsequent imagery, the soreness did not recur.

Timing is an important consideration concerning the athlete's readiness to practice certain forms of imagery. For example, it may be advisable to focus solely on relaxation and pain management immediately following knee reconstruction surgery, before commencing with healing imagery. It may not be feasible to practice performance imagery until enough healing has taken place for the athlete to feel ready to contemplate being active and performing again. In some cases, the injury may have been so dramatic or traumatic that it would be unreasonable to expect the athlete to have sufficiently recovered psychologically, let alone physically, to apply the mental energy required to implement self-directed healing, if there has not been enough opportunity for rest. Table 3 summarizes how imagery may be used in rehabilitation.

Table 3. Summary of Imagery Applications During Rehabilitation

1. **Healing Imagery:** Visualizing and feeling the healing taking place to the injured area internally.
   Examples: seeing the bone mending, or ligaments knitting together, or broken-down tissues being washed away and being replaced with healthy ones.

2. **Recovery Imagery:** Visualizing full recovery of strength and mobility, effectively moving through specific motions and situations that put the most demand on the injured area. Engaging in imagery that involves feeling positive, enthusiastic, and confident about returning to training and competition.
   Examples: imagining full range of motion in one's knee or shoulder; ankle supporting all of one's weight; return of full strength and flexibility of a muscle.

3. **Performance Imagery:** Re-experiencing or imagining individual skills and calling up feelings associated with one's best performances. Visualizing returning to competition and performing at one's best again.
   Examples: Imagining making that winning shot or crossing the finish line first or performing a Personal Best in your event, and how that would feel—emotionally as well as physically.

4. **Pain Management Imagery:** Imagining the pain being washed away or seeing cool colors soothing and reducing any inflammation and pain.
   Examples: seeing cool blues running through the area; imagining an ice pack; or imagining the pain leaving one's body.

5. **Treatment Imagery:** Being fully engaged mentally during a physio session, imagining what the treatment is designed to do, working efficiently and powerfully.
   Examples: imagining the ultrasound treatment flushing away any scar tissue; feeling muscles loosening and releasing tension during massage.

Coping With Fear of Reinjury

Once full recovery has been attained, fear of reinjury may hold back some athletes. Such fear can result in additional muscular tension that can contribute to the increased possibility of reinjury. Regular practice of the mental skills outlined above throughout the rehabilitation period, however, tends to prevent such fears from arising. Maintaining a relaxed, positive attitude, and regularly envisioning successful recovery and return to sport tend to pre-empt any negative images or fears. This is confirmed by what is reported by the fast healers in our study, who were generally less fearful or worrisome about reinjury as compared to the slower healers. Where fears of reinjury did surface in the faster healers, they were modified by a desire to look for positive lessons, exercise greater caution, and exert greater personal control in the future. Respondents in the slow-healing group tended just to dwell on the negative possibilities.

A combination of relaxation and imagery (systematic desensitization) has been reported useful in counteracting any residual fears of reinjury (Nideffer, 1976; Rotella & Campbell, 1983). It is based on the principle that it is impossible to be both relaxed and anxious at the same time. First the athlete is asked to identify the fear. Then a relaxed state is elicited using a relaxation technique, following which the athlete is asked to visualize the situation they are fearful of. In this way the anxiety-provoking scenario is associated with the relaxed state.

Physical Activity

When possible, the athlete should be encouraged to remain physically active in an alternative activity (providing it does not impede the recovery process). Aside from the fitness aspect, staying active has several benefits: Dissipating the excess energy resulting from the sudden inability to train, maintaining a sense of control, reducing stress, and keeping up self-image (Crossman, 1986; Salisbury, 1984; Steadman, 1982; Willis, 1983). For those whose injury precludes any form of physical activity, meditation or relaxation training may assist coping with anxiety or depression that accompanies exercise deprivation (Massimo, 1985).

Recommendations

Athletes who are very determined and positive about rehabilitation, as well as those who imagine or *see* and *feel* their recovery and successful resumption of their sport activity, fare much better than do those with negative outlooks. The following is a summary of practical suggestions for use with recovering athletes:

For the injured athlete:

◆ Stay involved with the sport as much as possible.
◆ Set daily goals for healing and improvement as well as long-term goals for recovery.
◆ Develop a physiotherapy plan and plan to mentally prepare for optimal healing each day.
◆ Do mental imagery of healing and of achieving goals.
◆ Emphasize positive aspects of the recovery.
◆ If the injury must be described, always attempt to follow it with a positive statement or image about recovery (if not out loud, at least to yourself).
◆ Say positive things to yourself about your rehabilitation and your future performance possibilities, every day.

- Be alert to any negative thoughts, imagery or 'replays' of the injury. Change the image to a positive, healing one.
- Take advantage of the "time out" as an opportunity to rest and reflect.
- Practice relaxation techniques, particularly if under stress.
- Use audiotapes designed to promote relaxation, healing imagery, and performance imagery, such as on *Inner Sports* by Ievleva & Stillwell (1997), and on *In Pursuit of Personal Excellence* by Orlick (1988).

For those helping an injured person to enhance recovery:

- Maintain contact and involvement with the injured person (e.g., coaches can make a point in their agenda to call once a week).
- Show compassion while encouraging and supporting progress.
- Point out the opportunities the "time out" may provide.
- Speak of possibilities as opposed to limitations.
- Point out and name other athletes who have had similar injuries who are now at the top of their game again.
- Reinforce the fact that the athlete has the capacity to directly influence his or her own healing.
- Encourage the athlete to set specific daily recovery goals for rehabilitation (in conjunction with his or her physiotherapist or trainer), to *think into* his or her body in helpful ways, to use relaxation and mind/body imagery strategies to enhance recovery.
- Mention the fact that the same mental skills that enabled the athlete to excel in sport can be applied to excel at healing (e.g., commitment, belief, positive imagery, full focus, mental readiness, refocusing and constructive evaluation)
- Listen closely to the athlete's concerns
- Adapt your program according to individual input and needs.
- Be flexible in your attitude and approach and encourage athletes to be flexible while on the path to recovery.
- When you provide committed athletes the psychological principles and concepts related to healing they can play with, they are likely to develop creative and imaginative ways of implementing them to enhance their own healing.

To guard against injury and illness:

- Avoid overtraining athletes (consider individual recovery times required).
- Avoid overloading athletes (consider overall schedule and demands the athlete is facing).

◆ Provide athletes with adequate time to rest and recover between practice, workouts, and games.

◆ Encourage good nutritional habits.

◆ Teach athletes good stress reduction and stress control strategies and perspectives.

It is our hope that healers and healees alike will begin to make greater use of their inner mental resources to enhance injury rehabilitation and personal well-being.

References

Achterberg, J. (1985). *Imagery and healing: Shamanism and modern medicine*. Boston, MA: New Science Library.

Achterberg, J. (1989). Mind and medicine: The role of imagery in healing. *Journal of the American Society for Psychical Research, 83*(2), 93–100.

Arnheim, D. D. (1985). *Modern principles of athletic training*. St. Louis: Times Mirror/Mosby College Publishing.

Barabasz, A. F., & McGeorge, C .M. (1978). Biofeedback, mediated biofeedback and hypnosis in peripheral vasodilation training. *American Journal of Clinical Hypnosis, 21,* 28–37.

Benson, H. (1975). *The relaxation response*. New York: William Morrow.

Benson, H. (1984). *Beyond the relaxation response*. New York: Berkeley Books.

Benson, H. (1995). The relaxation response. In D. Goleman & J. Gurin (Eds.), *Mind body medicine* (pp. 233–258). Marrickville, New South Wales: Choice Books.

Borkovec, T. D. (1985). Placebo: Defining the unknown. In L. White, B. Tursky, G. E. Schwartz (Eds.), *Placebo: Theory, research, and mechanisms* (pp. 59–64). New York: The Guilford Press.

Borysenko, J. (1987). *Minding the body, mending the mind*. Reading, MA: Addison-Wesley Publishing Company, Inc.

Botterill, C., Flint, F., & Ievleva, L. (1996). Psychology of the injured athlete. In J. E. Zachezewski, D. J. Magee, & W. S. Quillen (Eds.), *Athletic injuries and rehabilitation* (pp. 791–805). Philadelphia, PA: W. B. Saunders.

Bresler, D. E. (1984a). Conditioned relaxation: The pause that refreshes. In J. S. Gordon, D. T. Jaffe, & D. E. Bresler (Eds.), *Mind, body, and health: Toward an integral medicine* (pp. 19–36). New York: Human Sciences Press, Inc.

Bresler, D. E. (1984b). Mind-controlled analgesia: The inner way to pain control. In A. A. Sheikh (Ed.), *Imagination and healing* (pp. 211–230). Farmingdale, NY: Berkley Books.

Brody, H. (1985). Placebo effect: An examination of Grunbaum's definition. In L. White, B. Tursky, G. E. Schwartz (Eds.), *Placebo: Theory, research and mechanisms* (pp. 37–58). New York: The Guilford Press.

Coue, E. (1974). *Self-mastery through autosuggestion*. New York: Samuel Weiser.

Cousins, N. (1989a). *Head first: The biology of hope and the healing power of the human spirit*. New York: Penguin Books.

Cousins, N. (1989b). Belief becomes biology. *Advances, 6*(3), 20–29.

Crossman, J. E. (1986). Psychological and sociological factors supporting athletic injury. *Coaching Review, May/June,* 54–58.

Dunn, R. (1983). Psychological factors in sports medicine. *Athletic Training, 18*(1), 34–35.

Epstein, G. (1986). The image in medicine: Notes of a clinician. *Advances, 3*(1), 22–31.

Epstein, G. (1989). *Healing visualizations: Creating health through imagery*. New York: Bantam Books.

Faris, G. J. (1985). Psychologic aspects of athletic rehabilitation. *Clinics in Sports Medicine, 4*(3), 545–551.

Foster, J., & Porter, K. (1987). *Mental training for healing athletic injury.* Unpublished manuscript.

Frank, J. (1961). *Persuasion and healing.* Baltimore, MD: Johns Hopkins Press.

Goleman, D., & Gurin, J. (Eds.) (1995). *Mind body medicine.* Marrickville, New South Wales: Choice Books.

Gordon, J. S., Jaffe, D. T., & Bresler, D. E. (1984). *Mind, body, and health: Toward an integral medicine.* New York: Human Sciences Press, Inc.

Green, E. E., & Green, A. M. (1977). *Beyond biofeedback.* New York: Delacorte Press/Seymour Lawrence.

Green, E. E., Green, A. M., & Walters, E. D. (1970). Voluntary control of internal states: Psychological and physiological. *Journal of Transpersonal Psychology, 2,* 1–26.

Green, E. E., Green, A. M., & Walters, E. D. (1979). Biofeedback for mind/body self-regulation: Healing and creativity. In E. Peper, S. Ancoli, & M. Quinn (Eds.), *Mind/body integration: Essential readings in biofeedback* (pp. 125–140). New York: Plenum Press.

Hall, H. R. (1983). Hypnosis and the immune system: A review with implications for cancer and the psychology of healing. *American Journal of Clinical Hypnosis, 25*(3), 92–103.

Ievleva, L., & Decent, B. (1997, September). *Application of mental skills to sports injury rehabilitation.* Presentation to the annual meeting of The Association for the Advancement of Applied Sport Psychology, San Diego, CA.

Ievleva, L. (Voice), & Stillwell, L. (Music) (1997). *Inner sports: Mental skills for peak performance* [Audiocassette set]. Champaign, IL: Human Kinetics.

Ievleva, L., & Orlick, T. (1991). Mental links to enhanced healing: An exploratory study. *The Sport Psychologist, 5*(1), 25–40.

Jaffe, D. T., & Bresler, D. E. (1984). Guided imagery. In J. S. Gordon, D. T. Jaffe, & D. E. Bresler (Eds.), *Mind, body, and health: Toward an integral medicine* (pp. 56–69). New York: Human Sciences Press, Inc.

James, W. (1950). *The principles of psychology* (Vol. I). New York: Dover Publications. (Original publication date 1890.)

Kabat-Zinn, J. (1995). Mindfulness meditation: Health benefits of an ancient Buddhist practice. In D. Goleman & J. Gurin (Eds.), *Mind body medicine* (pp. 259–276). Marrickville, New South Wales: Choice Books.

Kabat-Zinn, J. (1990). *Full catastrophe living: Using the wisdom of your body and mind to face stress, pain, and illness.* New York: Delacorte Press.

Korn, E. R., & Johnson, K. (1983). *Visualization: The uses of imagery in the health professions.* Homewood, IL: Dow Jones-Irwin.

Krippner, S. (1985). The role of imagery in health and healing: A review. *Saybrook Review, 5*(1), 32–41.

Locke, S., & Colligan, D. (1986). *The healer within: The new medicine of mind and body.* New York: New American Library.

Massimo, J. (1985). Psychological recovery from injury. *International Gymnast, April,* 42–43, 58.

NIH Technology Assessment Panel. (1996). Integration of behavioral and relaxation approaches into the treatment of chronic pain and insomnia. *Journal of the American Medical Association, 276*(4), 313–318.

Nideffer, R. (1976). *The inner athlete.* San Diego, CA: Enhanced Performance Associates

Olness, K. (1995). Hypnosis: The power of attention. In D. Goleman & J. Gurin (Eds.), *Mind body medicine* (pp. 277–290). Marrickville, New South Wales: Choice Books.

Orlick, T. (1996). The wheel of excellence. *Journal of Performance Education, 1*(1), 3–18.

Orlick, T. (1988). *In pursuit of personal excellence* [Audiocassette]. Ottawa, ON: Coaching Association of Canada.

Park, L. C., & Covi, L. (1965). Nonblind placebo trial: An exploration of neurotic outpatients response to placebo when its inert content is disclosed. *Archives of General Psychiatry, 12*, 336–345.

Patterson, D. M. (1979). Progressive relaxation training: Overview, procedure and implication for self-regulation. In E. Peper, S. Ancoli, & M. Quinn (Eds.), *Mind/body integration: Essential readings in biofeedback* (pp. 187–200). New York: Plenum Press.

Pearson, R. E. (1961). Response to suggestions given under general anesthesia. *American Journal of Clinical Hypnosis, 4,* 106–114.

Peper, E., Ancoli, S., & Quinn, M. (1979). *Mind/body integration: Essential readings in biofeedback*. New York: Plenum Press.

Porter, K., & Foster, J. (1986). *The mental athlete: Inner training for peak performance*. New York: Ballantine Books.

Rossi, E. L. (1986). *The psychobiology of mind-body healing*. New York: W.W. Norton & Company, Inc.

Rossman, M. L. (1995). Imagery: Learning to use the mind's eye. In D. Goleman & J. Gurin (Eds.), *Mind body medicine* (pp. 291–300). Marrickville, New South Wales: Choice Books.

Rossman, M. L. (1984). Imagine health! Imagery in medical self-care. In A. Sheikh (Ed.), *Imagination and healing* (pp. 231–258). Farmingdale, NY: Berkley Books.

Rotella, R. J., & Campbell, M. S. (1983). Systematic desensitization: Psychological rehabilitation of injured athletes. *Athletic Training, 18*(2), 140–142; 151.

Salisbury, N. (1984). The comeback trail. *New Body, 3*(6), 56–58.

Samuels, M., & Samuels, N. (1975). *Seeing with the mind's eye*. New York, NY: Random House/Berkeley: The Bookworks.

Schwartz, D. (1978). *The magic of thinking big*. New York: Prentice-Hall, Inc.

Schwartz, G. E. (1981). Disregulation and systems theory: A biobehavioral framework for biofeedback and behavioral medicine. In D. Shapiro, J. Stoyva, J. Kaniya, T. X. Barber, N. E. Miller, & G. Schwartz (Eds.), *Biofeedback and behavioral medicine* (pp. 27–29). New York: Aldine.

Schwartz, G. E. (1984). Psychophysiology of imagery and healing: A systems perspective. In A.A. Sheikh (Ed.), *Imagination and healing* (pp. 35–50). Farmingdale, NY: Berkeley Books.

Siegel, B. S. (1986). *Love medicine & miracles*. New York: Harper & Row.

Siegel, B. S. (1989). *Peace, love and healing*. New York: Harper & Row.

Simonton, O. C., Matthews-Simonton, S., & Creighton, J. L. (1978). *Getting well again*. New York: Bantam Books.

Steadman, J. R. (1982). Rehabilitation of skiing injuries. *Clinics in Sports Medicine, 1*(2), 289–294.

Swearingen, R. L. (1984). The physician as the basic instrument. In J. S. Gordon, D. T. Jaffe, & D. E. Bresler (Eds.), *Mind, body, and health: Toward an integral medicine* (pp. 101–106). New York: Human Sciences Press Inc.

Turk, D. C., & Nash, J. M. (1995). Chronic pain: New ways to cope. In D. Goleman & J. Gurin (Eds.), *Mind body medicine* (111–130). Marrickville, New South Wales: Choice Books.

Vogel, A. V., Goodwin, J. S., & Goodwin, J. M. (1980). The therapeutics of placebo. *American Family Physician, 22,* 105–109.

Willis, H. (1983). Some psychological effects of athletic injuries. *Physiotherapy in Sport, 5*(3), 16–17.

13

Seeing Helps Believing: Modeling in Injury Rehabilitation

Frances A. Flint
York University

Modeling has been used extensively within sport as an instructional tool for the learning of motor skills and social behavior. The extension of this technique into the realm of sport injury rehabilitation affords motivation, injury-rehabilitation information, and behavioral cues for recovering athletes. For athletes who have never experienced a major injury, a key component of a successful recovery involves learning how to cope with the process of rehabilitation and return to competition. Thus, athletes who have already effected a complete recovery from injury are ideal models. Seeing someone similar successfully overcome the obstacle of an injury can help an injured athlete believe that recovery is possible. In this sense, "seeing helps believing."

"I thought I was invincible until this happened." Such were the words of a highly recruited, first-year university basketball player as she recounted her reactions to a season-ending knee injury. Never having experienced a major injury before, she suffered through the loss of the image she held of being a physically active, elite-level athlete. In addition, the daily exercise and competitive pursuits to which she was accustomed were now replaced with dependency and physical disability. Consequently, in the hours and days immediately postinjury, despair and depression dominated the psyche of this injured athlete.

Certainly with the current surgical techniques and rehabilitation programs available, this kind of injury scenario no longer need be considered devastating and potentially career ending, but what of the psychological trauma sustained by the injured athlete? How can therapists, coaches, and teammates support the injured athlete through the difficult periods of depression and despondency that may result from injury, and how can these people aid in the recovery process? It has been suggested that psychological skills such as goal setting, visualization, relaxation training, and negative thought stopping be used to provide psychological rehabilitation in conjunction with physical recovery protocols (Feltz, 1984; Gordon, 1986; Weiss & Troxel, 1986; Wiese & Weiss, 1987). One technique that has been given minimal attention in the psychological rehabilitation of athletic injuries is the use of modeling or observational learning.

Modeling has been described as an ideal way to communicate skills, attitudes, and behaviors through the observation of behavioral or verbal cues provided by a model (Bandura, 1986a). Modeling has been used extensively in sport, and teachers and coaches have often relied on this teaching tool for the transmission of knowledge in motor skill learning (McCullagh, Weiss, & Ross, 1989; Weiss & Klint, 1987). Thus, athletes are familiar with observing models in either a live or filmed format for the purpose of motor skill learning or the transmission of psychological information (e.g., motivation). In order to understand the potential beneficial effects of modeling in a therapeutic context, it is important to understand common affective reactions to injury and the psychological needs of recovering injured athletes.

Psychological Reactions to Athletic Injury

When a university-level basketball player was asked how she felt after suffering a major knee injury she responded,

> That week between the time of the injury and surgery, . . . if you excuse it—it was hell—because I didn't know what to think . . . That was the worst week I can ever comprehend in my life . . . my school suffered and I was trying to get around campus on crutches. My social life suffered with respect to relationships with other people, because I was so confused and I was angry . . . I had so many emotions running through my head. (quoted in Flint, 1991, p. 142)

The athlete also remarked that she was having to contend with an overload of medical information on injury and surgery that she didn't understand, while trying to deal with the reality of the sudden end to her playing season. In addition, because she was only a freshman, doubts about whether she would be able to complete a university athletic career were evident.

When a severe injury occurs, it is common that the injured athlete must cope with an excess of medically based information, the loss of physical capability, the emotions of withdrawing from a desired activity, and a dependency on others to fulfill daily needs. At the same time, anxiety about the uncertainty of the future may be exacerbated by the severity of the injury and the limitations imposed by the injury (Lynch, 1988; Purtilo, 1978). All of these experiences and emotions may flood the injured athlete and create confusion and feelings of helplessness (McDonald & Hardy, 1990; Yukelson, 1986). The athlete may over- or under-exaggerate the extent of the injury and draw unwarranted conclusions as to the implications of the injury. In addition to irrational thoughts, affective reactions can become influential and may partially determine the actions and behavior of the injured athlete (Rotella, 1988; Yukelson, 1986). Anger, depression, and despair emanating from this sense of loss and confusion may become overwhelming and interfere with the recovery process (Feltz, 1984; Yukelson, 1986).

Thus, the athlete who becomes injured may experience a myriad of emotions that may be detrimental to the recovery process. Helping the athlete deal with these emotions is an important component in the psychological rehabilitation program.

Psychological Needs During Recovery

For athletes who are accustomed to seeking control over opponents and game situations, their own helplessness due to injury can be overwhelming. Specific psychological needs of injured athletes must be satisfied and strategies developed to promote a complete healing process. In the same way that the athlete requires technical information from coaches in order to develop skill, so too the injured athlete needs guidance from physicians, therapists, and others so that the recovery process can be as comprehensive as possible.

Yukelson (1986) has suggested that athletes can overcome injury by employing the same psychological qualities that helped them to excel in their athletic endeavors (e.g., pride, determination, and hard work). Bev Smith, a former Canadian National Women's Basketball team member and All-American, provides an excellent example of this transfer of athletic excellence determination to injury recovery. Bev had sustained several knee injuries and surgery in her illustrious career and remarked that

> if you keep your perspective on it and look one day at a time, then that'll come, but, I mean, you have to get up every morning and you have to do

your leg weights. It's the most unromantic thing in the morning . . . a lot of people think comebacks . . . they see TV documentaries on these athletes who have come back and it's all really spectacular and romantic . . . but it's not—it's drudgery, it's getting up every morning and doing these small little things, doing the leg weights, doing them at night before you go to bed even though you're tired—those things really pay off. (quoted in Flint, 1991, p. 151)

Bev's dedication to her injury recovery consisted of the same psychological factors (i.e., goal setting, persistence) as those applied to her basketball skill development.

With this in mind, an identification of the specific psychological needs and strategies for recovery must be the first step in the rehabilitation process. Athletes who have recovered from injury consistently identify the same emotions, needs, and factors as helpful in overcoming injury. For instance, taking an active role and responsibility for the recovery process is perceived as being vital (Ievleva & Orlick, 1991; McDonald & Hardy, 1990). Also, having a social support structure through family, peers, and coaches, other injured athletes, or therapists, provides a valuable foundation on which to tackle the hardships of recovery from injury (Flint, 1991; McDonald & Hardy, 1990; Smith, 1980; Wiese & Weiss, 1987).

Fisher (1990) concurred with the importance of psychological factors in injury rehabilitation and identified self-confidence as a primary component in this process. According to Fisher, three aspects of self-confidence that become important in the recovery process include competence, control, and commitment. *Competence* relates to the feeling that a task can be accomplished successfully, and in the instance of an injured athlete, this means a successful return to competition. The *control* aspect describes the athlete's feeling that he or she has the ability to take command of a certain situation, such as the rehabilitation program. The last aspect, *commitment,* refers to the athlete's willingness and capability to stay with a task. Fisher (1990) indicated that "any strategy that promotes any of these 3 ends will increase the likelihood of treatment adherence" (p. 154). Thus, pertinent injury and rehabilitation information and strategies for coping become critical components for increasing the athlete's confidence in a successful recovery from injury.

Much of the information needed by the injured athlete to promote the psychological aspects of recovery can be gained through the use of modeling. Listening to someone like Bev Smith talk about setting daily goals for recovery and dedication to the small details of rehabilitation, seeing another athlete struggle through reconditioning, or hearing a similar other talk about the frustration of injury and the joy related to returning to play can all be influential for the recently injured athlete. This is especially true if the athlete has never experienced a major injury before and has no experience on which to base hopes for recovery. Not knowing what to expect, how to behave under injury conditions, or how to tackle the challenges of recovery may present a problem for the injured athlete.

Modeling—What Is It?

Modeling has long been regarded as a powerful instructional tool for the learning of motor skills and social behaviors (McCullagh et al., 1989). The theoretical strength and empirical support for the effects of modeling make it a viable intervention strategy, particularly in the area of sport and exercise.

A number of theories have been forwarded to explain the modeling-behavior relationship. The most consistent efforts have been made by Bandura (1969, 1977, 1986a, 1986b), with social-cognitive theories of modeling being the most popular. This theory proposes that modeling or observational learning is one of the primary modes used by individuals to gain socialization information and cognitive skills. Behaviors, attitudes, and skills can be learned through modeling via behavioral and verbal cues provided by the model (Bandura, 1986a). As the observer views a model, symbolic representation or verbal coding takes place, and these cues are placed in memory. Through this vicariously gained information, judgment criteria are established, and new behavioral patterns can be learned. Judgments about capabilities are often comparative; therefore, seeing someone similar to oneself perform a novel task or particular behavior can enhance the perception about the observer's capacity to recreate the action (Bandura, 1986a).

A number of significant factors help to determine the effectiveness of a modeling experience and whether the observer will have incentive to copy the modeled behavior. These factors may include physical characteristics of the model (e.g., physique, age, sex), model type (e.g., mastery vs. coping), and number of models. By presenting multiple, diversified models, it is hoped that at least one of the models will demonstrate characteristics similar to the observer's and will capture the attention of the observer, thus creating a common bond.

The importance of model-observer characteristics has been stressed by Bandura (1977) and McCullagh et al. (1989). It is proposed that the observer will form a bond with the model through the identification of similarities and, thus, the observer will be more motivated to pay attention to the message the model is conveying (McCullagh et al., 1989). In sport these similarities may relate to playing position, level of competition, or style of play. Therefore, the selection of specific characteristics of the model, creating a "similar other," is critical for effecting behavioral change in observers.

Model similarity is a particularly salient aspect of the observer-model relationship because it may determine if the observer will pay attention to the model. A perfect example of the effect of model-observer similarity was provided by an injured female basketball player who had just undergone anterior cruciate ligament (ACL) surgery. While watching a videotape of other female basketball players who had experienced the same surgery, she described one of the models who caught her attention and her reasons for noticing the model: "One of the girls who talked about the pain after coming out of surgery, I had it too. Because I could relate completely to what she was talking about, I understood it" (quoted in Flint, 1991, p. 246). Obviously this model had an impact on the observer through the shared experience of pain. This common bond, which had been formed between the two, may have been influential in encouraging the observer to pay attention to the verbal and behavioral cues provided by the model.

Another important aspect of the model-observer relationship is the type of model presented. Model similarity is established through the level of expertise displayed by the model, such as a mastery or expert model as compared to a coping model. *Mastery* or *exemplary models* demonstrate errorless task execution and show tasks as they are to be performed perfectly (Schunk, Hanson, & Cox, 1987). On the other hand, *coping models* initially demonstrate negative cognitions and affects and an imperfect performance. Gradually, the coping model demonstrates positive thoughts, high self-efficacy, and strategies needed to overcome problems and improve performance. The use of coping models is particularly pertinent to injury rehabilitation because the injured observer can relate to the stages of recovery demonstrated by the model who is overcoming an injury.

The last factor, the use of multiple, diversified models, has also been demonstrated as effective in the learning of new behaviors and motor skills (Thelen, Fry, Fehrenbach, & Frautschi, 1979). This modeling strategy entails the use of at least two, but possibly more, persons who demonstrate the target behavior. The models should be diverse, however, in terms of personal characteristics (e.g., sex, age) and physical attributes (e.g., size, physical abilities) to increase the likelihood that the observer will be able to identify with at least one of the models. The visible characteristics of the model may result in a psychological bonding effect by the observer because a similarity with the model is recognized. This aspect of bonding may have a motivational effect on the observer and may prompt the observer to expend more effort to "be like" the model. The use of multiple models also provides the observer with more than one exposure to the target behavior, which enhances the opportunity for learning.

against her grain, but she soon realized the wisdom of rest, to the point where she found delight in her newfound discipline to take days off and enjoy and express herself in other healthier ways. She discovered that, indeed, sometimes less is more. She learned to focus and appreciate herself not only as a human *doing* but also as a human *being*.

Alison, a member of a World Cup championship team, broke her ankle the week before selections were being made to the national team. Initially, it appeared that she would be denied any chance of participating in the World Cup championships just months away. After much discussion, she resolved to seize the opportunity and rise to the challenge. Alison was not known for her discipline in training—she relied on her exceptional natural ability to carry her through. With the increased caliber of competition, however, she reluctantly understood, that sooner or later, she was going to have to train if she was going to maintain and advance in her position. She was now faced with committing to arduous rehabilitation training in order to have any chance of pursuing her dream of a World Cup championship. Alison risked the possibility of great disappointment and chose to view the injury as an opportunity to grow both as a player and as a person. It was an opportunity to slow down the hectic pace of her work life and focus inward—to appreciate and allow herself to be a human *being* (rather than a human *doing*), to address certain personal issues, to acquire the training discipline—both mentally and physically. She also found that once she made the commitment to a speedy and full recovery, she was surrounded by many who were quick to assist her. For the first time, she discovered the extent to which others cared about her and her progress. Her rehabilitation became a gratifying experience. Patty also grew to enjoy her mental training, which included relaxation and performance and healing imagery. She began availing herself of these strengthening mental tools that she then carried with her after recovering from the injury. In the end, her outcome was very fulfilling in that she was not only ready to play but also able to lead her team to victory.

Another case where injury led to valuable lessons involved an Olympic 10k runner. Due to an injury, Lynn was forced to train in a swimming pool, which she soon discovered to be more efficient than road training, for water training enhanced both her technique and her concentration, as well as prevented the wear and tear on her body that roadwork inevitably entails. She subsequently implemented pool training even while healthy, a method to which she attributes her successful performance at the Olympics.

In a more recent case in the currently running study *Mental Skills Applied to Sports Injury Rehabilitation* (Ievleva & Decent, 1997), a first-grade player from a top rugby league team in Australia has taken the opportunity of his rehabilitation to catch up on reading and developing his mental skills beyond

When modeling is used as a psychological intervention in therapeutic situations, it is felt that the model-observer relationship will act as a catalyst to effecting a positive approach to the rehabilitation process. By watching the model, the injured athlete gains knowledge about rehabilitation, strategies for handling setbacks, and the confidence that, if others can recover from injury, so can he or she. Feltz (1988) suggests that the effect of modeling resides in experience with the task or behavior: "The less experience one has had with a task or situation, the more one will rely on others to judge one's own capabilities" (p. 427). Thus, athletes injured severely for the first time would be considered extremely naive in terms of what is required to accomplish a complete recovery.

In summary, strong empirical evidence exists for the powerful effects of modeling on performance, cognitions, and emotional responses in observers. In particular, the use of specific strategies, such as similar, diversified, and coping modeling, has been shown to have enduring beneficial effects in anxiety-producing, clinical, and therapeutic settings. The provision of coping models via videotape presentation may be particularly salient to athletes as they pursue physical rehabilitation postinjury. The psychological benefits of watching a similar other recover from injury could have far-reaching effects on effort and persistence in adherence to rehabilitation programs.

Informal and Formal Modeling in the Medical Context

Both informal and formal modeling techniques have been used within a medical context to bolster the observer's sense that recovery from a serious health threat is possible. In many cases, these observer-model situations occur informally and naturally within a rehabilitation setting as a therapist points out another person with the same injury who is progressing with the rehabilitation process. Often, an athlete who has returned to competition after recovering from a serious injury is identified by coaches or therapists as an example for the injured athlete. This is a form of informal modeling in which the main benefit to the observer is a motivational boost and very little hard data on psychological strategies or ways of overcoming obstacles to recovery are conveyed.

An excellent example of informal modeling was provided by Kerrin Lee-Gartner at the 1992 Winter Olympics, when she won the gold medal in women's downhill skiing. The head coach of the Canadian women's ski team remarked, "It'll make us believe again. It'll make injured skiers like Kate Pace and Lucie LaRoche say, 'I can win again'" (quoted in Byers, 1992, p. E18). Kerrin became a model for injured skiers because, despite five knee surgeries and a broken ankle, she was able to recover and win Olympic gold. This is an instance of informal modeling because strategies for recovery were not provided by Kerrin, but rather, a motivational example was set for others to follow.

In order to ensure that pertinent, useful information and strategies for a complete rehabilitation process are being displayed by the model, the modeling process should be formalized. In formal modeling, a situation is created whereby one or more models present specific verbal or visual cues that expose the observer to vicarious experiences, verbal persuasions, and emotional exhortations. Depending on how the modeling experience is structured, all three of these sources of self-confidence information can be presented, or one specific source can be isolated and highlighted. In formal modeling, the model-observer situation is created to gain the maximum benefit from the exposure.

For instance, in order to reduce preoperative anxiety, increase postoperative ambulation, and decrease the number of days in the hospital after surgery, newly hospitalized patients can be exposed to postsurgical roommates who demonstrate various coping behaviors (Kulik & Mahler, 1987). The exposure to postoperative sensations and events through a coping model better prepares the observer by providing accurate information on which cognitive appraisal of the situation can be made (Kulik & Mahler, 1987). According to Lazarus (1966), the observer will experience less stress in these situations because the events are now interpreted as less threatening due in a large part to the newly acquired cognitive and behavioral responses. In other words, because of the modeling experience, the preoperative patient now knows what to expect, and this may help alleviate fear.

In order to provide the observer with a maximal amount of pertinent information regarding medical procedures and outcomes, videotape or film modeling may be used to augment therapy in clinical settings (Thelen et al., 1979; Melamed & Siegel, 1975). Recently, videotape modeling was used as a psychological intervention within an athletic population (Flint, 1991). Female athletes who had just undergone a surgical repair of the ACL in the knee watched a videotape of several coping models. The videotape consisted of interviews with seven basketball players who had all recovered from knee ligament surgery. Six of the players in the videotape were interviewed at various stages of recovery from ACL surgery extending from 2 weeks to 7 years postsurgery. The seventh player was an example of complete progress of a full recovery from a few weeks postsurgery to 16 months postsurgery. These players were interviewed in a question-and-answer format describing the playing situation when they were injured, the problems and fears they experienced during their recovery from surgery, and various aspects of their rehabilitation. Heavy emphasis was placed on how they had overcome the problems they faced during recovery and on a positive outlook with respect to their return to a basketball career. At the end of each interview, there were scenes of the recovered player during practice and game sessions demonstrating a total capability to participate.

The modeling videotape was seen by the injured athletes on three separate occasions: immediately postsurgery, at 2 months postsurgery, and at 4 months postsurgery. Pertinent insights into the needs of the recovering athletes were provided, and this information affords us a guideline for the designing of modeling interventions for athletic injury rehabilitation.

In general, immediately postsurgery, the injured athletes tended to notice things that related to the emotions associated with the injury and the surgery. For example, one subject picked out a specific model in the videotape as similar to herself " . . . because when she injured it she said 'F____' and I knew exactly what she was going through because the same thing was going through my mind too" (quoted in Flint, 1991, p. 243). Another recovering athlete commented that she felt comforted knowing "that other basketball players had some of the same feelings about the injury. Even though I feel a lot of support from parents and teammates it is good to know that other injured athletes have similar feelings and that I'm not going crazy" (quoted in Flint, 1991, p. 246). Most of the comments initially noticed by the injured athletes who watched the videotape were in some way connected to affective responses to the injury and surgery that were verbalized by the models.

Later, at 2 and 4 months postsurgery, the verbal statements and actions of the models that attracted more notice tended to change as the rehabilitation process continued. One injured athlete summed this up perfectly when she said, "Everybody in the tape said something that I could relate to, but it has changed as my rehab. progressed" (quoted in Flint, 1991, p. 246). Several of the injured athletes remarked about their recovery and said that some of the statements made by the models meant more to them now that they were experiencing the struggles of rehabilitation. One injured athlete commented that the model who was cycling with one leg and then both legs caught her attention because "I remember how frustrated I was when I couldn't do a single rotation and finally being able to cycle without any pain and actually sweating" (quoted in Flint, 1991, p. 241). In general, there was an overwhelmingly positive response to the verbalizations and actions of the models, and it appears that a bonding effect did occur between models and observers.

Injured athletes who watched the videotape also provided insight and qualitative information on their perceptions relative to their rehabilitation progress. They were asked to outline the factors that had helped them adhere to the rehabilitation program or the reasons they had not persisted in their physical rehabilitation. They were also asked to reflect on their experience and discuss what assistance would have been helpful to them in their recovery (i.e., more social support, more advice). It was interesting to note that the injured athletes who watched the videotape appeared to be motivated to adhere to their rehabilitation programs, had knowledge about what had helped them throughout rehabilitation, and were definitive with their needs during the recovery period (e.g., goal setting). The videotaped modeling experience appeared to have a positive effect on the perceptions of the injured athletes in terms of their ability to handle a physical rehabilitation program.

When combined with the use of the videotape medium, coping models can be effective in reducing fears and anxiety in therapeutic settings. Thelen et al. (1979) supported the efficacy of videotape or film modeling over live modeling because the opportunity to present naturalistic modeling sequences would be difficult or unrealistic to create in a clinical setting. The videotape format also allows for the reconstruction of the most desirable scenes and the multiple viewing of specific situations or conditions (L. A. Anderson, DeVellis, & DeVellis, 1987). This format is versatile in that it affords self-administration by the injured athlete at times when the need is greatest, such as when setbacks occur in the recovery process. In terms of costs, after an initial relatively high expenditure, the videotape becomes an inexpensive tool for augmenting the rehabilitation process. Much support exists in the literature for the use of videotape modeling in therapeutic settings (L. A. Anderson et al., 1987; Kendall & Watson, 1981; Thelen et al., 1979).

Information Provided Through Modeling: The Specifics

What information should be provided through formalized modeling experiences? Is there information that would be of prime benefit to the observer and other information that could be harmful? These questions and others related to the modeling experience have been posed in the medical psychology literature (Weinman & Johnston, 1988). Within the dimensions of sport psychology and sports medicine, however, the use of multiple coping models to demonstrate behavior and attitudes conducive to the rehabilitation of athletic injuries is a relatively new strategy. Thus, it is important that direction be sought from allied medical and health fields in order to discern valid content and composition guidelines for modeling interventions in rehabilitation.

In addition to injury and rehabilitation information, common questions asked by injured athletes, parents, and coaches relate to the procedures of surgery, its potential disfiguring effects, and the prospects for complete recovery. Often, the shock of a major injury and fear of possible surgery creates a mental obstruction and the injured athlete is unable to be receptive to injury information. In some cases, too much information or medical technicalities creates an overload situation and details of the injury are forgotten or misunderstood (Flint, 1991; Samples, 1987). If a videotaped presentation by a former injured athlete, outlining some pertinent injury information, was available through either the physician or therapist's office, then the injured athlete could refer to it as needed.

Van der Ploeg (1988) provides us with useful information on the perceptions of hospital patients relative to stressful medical situations, and this furnishes guidance on the development of modeling experiences. He found that hospital patients described the most stressful medical situations and events to include pain, the inability to discuss one's problems, and the lack of sufficient information on medical conditions. Thus, information provided to medical patients should be designed to ameliorate these stressful situations. In terms of athletes, the only concrete guidelines concerning patient information comes from Heil (cited in Samples, 1987, p. 174). He stated that the information should include the exact nature of the injury, the procedures and rationale for rehabilitation, the potential obstacles that lie ahead and how to overcome them, and the feelings the athlete may experience through the recovery period. Thus, Heil's recommendations concerning injured athletes are in concert with Van der Ploeg's (1988) research.

Kulik and Mahler (1987) suggest that, in general, the more information a patient has preoperatively about what to expect, the better are the chances of recovery being facilitated. Two concerns with this approach of full injury and surgery disclosure are the aspects of fear and the impression of control. If the information provided to the injured athlete is too detailed and graphic, then the fear experienced may be overwhelming, and the athlete will suffer from a feeling of loss of control over the situation. In this case, the stress and fear created by explicit details of the injury and surgery may be greater than the perception that the athlete has of his or her ability to overcome the injury. It is vital that any information provided or psychological interventions applied help injured athletes gain more confidence that they are capable of performing activities that may benefit overall recovery. Gaining insight from a similar other who has successfully rehabilitated an athletic injury could help reduce fear and increase confidence for a complete recovery.

The concept of fear reduction and perceptions of control are two important aspects of information provided to the injured athlete. Few guidelines exist for the composition or content of information designed to reduce stress in medical settings (Johnson, 1984; Wilson, 1981). According to K. O. Anderson and Masur (1983), the best kind of information is a combination of sensory and procedural details that can help foster accurate expectations and allow for correct cognitive interpretations of sensations to be experienced. Through this information, both procedural stress (immediate aspects) and outcome stress (long-term factors) can be alleviated (Weinman & Johnston, 1988). The procedural stress relates to details of the surgery (pain, disfigurement), and outcome stress is associated with the prognosis for a complete recovery. Perhaps in this situation, a previously injured athlete who has recovered from a similar injury can provide valuable information on the immediate effects of injury and surgery, obstacles to be expected, strategies to encourage adherence to rehabilitation, and realistic expectations for future recovery.

Athletes sustaining injury for the first time have no experience on which to base their expectations for a full recovery. Fear of the unknown may result in dysfunctional attitudes on the part of the injured athlete and may delay the recovery process (Rotella & Heyman, 1986). This situation creates the perfect opportunity for vicarious learning from a similar other who can provide an accurate account of the road ahead (Kulik & Mahler, 1987; Weiss & Troxel, 1986; Wiese & Weiss, 1987). Models who provide cues to coping behavior and effective strategies for dealing with challenging or threatening situations are an untapped resource in the rehabilitation of athletic injuries.

Conclusion

The old adage, "treat the person, not the injury" has specific implications in the rehabilitation of athletic injuries. As we know, the injured athlete will experience a psychophysiological response to trauma, and this dictates that both the physical and psychological needs of the athlete must be considered when designing a rehabilitation protocol (Lynch, 1988; Weiss & Troxel, 1986; Wiese & Weiss, 1987). It is inappropriate to treat tissue damage, but not to treat trauma to the psyche. As Chesterfield remarked, "I find by experience, that the mind and the body are more than married, for they are most intimately united; and when one suffers, the other sympathizes" (cited in Frost, 1971, p. 191).

Recovery from major injury, both physically and psychologically, is a long and arduous process requiring adherence to a comprehensive rehabilitation program. As we know, "compliance may currently be one of the greatest challenges facing the health professions" (Cerkoney & Hart cited in Turk, Meichenbaum, & Genest, 1983, p. 177). Any strategies that are effective in encouraging persistence in the face of obstacles to recovery are vital components of any rehabilitation protocol. One of the most effective means of conveying information and psychological strategies for injury rehabilitation that may be helpful to the recovering athlete is modeling and, after all, "now that I have seen that others can recover from serious injury, then so can I!"

References

Anderson, K. O., & Masur, F. T. (1983). Psychological preparation for invasive medical and dental procedures. *Journal of Behavioral Medicine, 6,* 1–40.

Anderson, L. A., DeVellis, B. M., & DeVellis, R. F. (1987). Effects of modeling on patient communication, satisfaction, and knowledge. *Medical Care, 25,* 1044–1056.

Bandura, A. (1969). *Principles of behavior modification.* New York: Holt, Rinehart & Winston.

Bandura, A. (1977). Self-efficacy: Toward a unifying theory of behavioral change. *Psychological Review, 84,* 191–215.

Bandura, A. (1986a). *Self-efficacy mechanism in psychological activation and health-promoting behavior*. Stanford University, Department of Psychology, Stanford, CA.

Bandura, A. (1986b). *Social foundations of thought and action: A social cognitive theory*. Englewood Cliffs, NJ: Prentice-Hall.

Byers, J. (1992, February 16). Canadian ski gold an inspiration to others. *The Toronto Star*, p. E18.

Feltz, D. L. (1984). The psychology of sports injuries. In P. F. Vinger & E. F. Hoerner (Eds.), *Sports injuries: The unthwarted epidemic* (2nd ed., pp. 336–344). Littleton, MA: PSG.

Feltz, D. L. (1988). Self-confidence and sports performance. In K. B. Pandolf (Ed.), *Exercise and sport sciences reviews* (Vol. 16, pp. 423–457). New York: Macmillan.

Fisher, C. A. (1990). Adherence to sports injury rehabilitation programmes. *Sports Medicine, 9*, 151–158.

Flint, F. A. (1991). *The psychological effects of modeling in athletic injury rehabilitation*. (Doctoral dissertation, University of Oregon, 1991). (Microform Publications No. BF 357).

Frost, R. B. (Ed.). (1971). *Psychological concepts applied to physical education and coaching*. Reading, MA: Addison-Wesley.

Gordon, S. (1986, March). Sport psychology and the injured athlete: A cognitive-behavioral approach to injury response and injury rehabilitation. *Science Periodical on Research and Technology in Sport, BU-1*, pp. 1–10.

Iveleva, L., & Orlick, T. (1991). Mental links to enhanced healing: An exploratory analysis. *The Sport Psychologist, 4*, 25–40.

Johnson, M. (1984). Dimensions of recovery from surgery. *International Review of Applied Psychology, 33*, 505–520.

Kendall, P. C., & Watson, D. (1981). Psychological preparation for stressful medical procedures. In C. K. Prokop & L. A. Bradley (Eds.), *Medical psychology: Contributions to behavioral medicine* (pp. 198–218). New York: Academic Press.

Kulik, J. A., & Mahler, H. I. (1987). Effects of preoperative roommate assignment on postoperative anxiety and recovery from coronary-bypass surgery. *Health Psychology, 6*, 525–543.

Lazarus, R. S. (1966). *Psychological stress and the coping process*. New York: McGraw-Hill.

Lynch, G. P. (1988). Athletic injuries and the practicing sport psychologist: Practical guidelines for assisting athletes. *The Sport Psychologist, 2*, 161–167.

McCullagh, P., Weiss, M. R., & Ross, D. (1989). Modeling considerations in motor skill acquisition and performance: An integrated approach. In K. B. Pandolf (Ed.), *Exercise and sport sciences reviews* (Vol. 17, pp. 475–513). Baltimore: Williams & Wilkins.

McDonald, S. A., & Hardy, C. J. (1990). Affective response patterns of the injured athlete: An exploratory analysis. *The Sport Psychologist, 4*, 261–274.

Melamed, B. G., & Siegel, L. J. (1975). Reduction of anxiety in children facing hospitalization and surgery by use of filmed modeling. *Journal of Consulting and Clinical Psychology, 43*, 511–521.

Purtilo, D. T. (1978). *Health professional/patient interaction* (2nd ed.). Philadelphia: Saunders.

Rotella, R. J., & Heyman, S. R. (1986). Stress, injury and the psychological rehabilitation of athletes. In J. M. Williams (Ed.), *Applied sport psychology: Personal growth to peak performance* (pp. 343–364). Palo Alto, CA: Mayfield.

Samples, P. (1987). Mind over muscle: Returning the injured athlete to play. *The Physician and Sportsmedicine, 15*(10), 172–180.

Schunk, D. H., Hanson, A. R., & Cox, P. D. (1987). Peer-model attributes and children's achievement behaviors. *Journal of Educational Psychology, 79*, 54–61.

Smith, R. (1980). Development of an integrated coping response through cognitive-affective stress management training. In C. H. Nadeau, W. R. Halliwell, K. M. Newell, & G. C. Roberts (Eds.), *Psychology of motor behavior and sport: 1979* (pp. 54–72). Champaign: Human Kinetics.

Thelen, M. H., Fry, R. A., Fehrenbach, P. A., & Frautschi, N. M. (1979). Therapeutic videotape and film modeling: A review. *Psychological Bulletin, 86*, 701–720.

Turk, D. C., Meichenbaum, D., & Genest, M. (1983). *Pain and behavioral medicine*. New York: Guilford Press.

Van der Ploeg, H. M. (1988). Stressful medical events: A survey of patients' perceptions. In S. Maes, C. D. Spielberger, P. B. Defares, & I. G. Sarason (Eds.), *Topics in health psychology* (pp. 193–203). New York: Wiley.

Weinman, J., & Johnston, M. (1988). Stressful medical procedures: An analysis of the effects of psychological interventions and of the stressfulness of the procedures. In S. Maes, C. D. Spielberger, P. B. Defares, & I. G. Sarason (Eds.), *Topics in health psychology* (pp. 205–217). New York: Wiley.

Weiss, M. R., & Klint, K. A. (1987). "Show and tell" in the gymnasium: An investigation of developmental differences in modeling and verbal rehearsal of motor skills. *Research Quarterly for Exercise and Sport, 58,* 234–241.

Weiss, M. R., & Troxel, R. K. (1986). Psychology of the injured athlete. *Athletic Training, 21,* 104–109, 154.

Wiese, D. M., & Weiss, M. R. (1987). Psychological rehabilitation and physical injury: The role of the sports medicine team. *The Sport Psychologist, 1,* 318–330.

Wilson, J. F. (1981). Behavioural preparation for surgery: Benefit or harm. *Journal of Behavioural Medicine, 4,* 79–102.

Yukelson, D. (1986). Psychology of sport and the injured athlete. In D. B. Bernhardt (Ed.), *Clinics in physical therapy* (pp. 175–195). New York: Churchill Livingstone.

14

The Use of Imagery in the Rehabilitation of Injured Athletes

Lance B. Green
Tulane University

The purpose of this chapter is to provide an educational text that (a) cites existing literature supporting a mind-body paradigm for rehabilitation from psychophysiological and psychomotor perspectives, (b) demonstrates the application of imagery techniques within the chronology of an athletic injury, and (c) describes the performance-related criteria to which an athlete can compare his or her progress during rehabilitation. The chronology includes the period of time preceding the injury, the attention given to the athlete immediately following the injury, and the subsequent rehabilitation program leading to the return of the athlete to practice and competition. Examples of imagery experientials are used to illustrate the application of imagery throughout the chronology.

A recent study conducted by Wiese, Weiss, and Yukelson (1991) reported that athletic trainers support the use of psychological strategies when dealing with injury rehabilitation of athletes. Listening to coaches and trainers, Wiese et al. identified intrinsic motivation on the part of the athlete and social support as key strategies and skills in the recovery process. It was also reported that the use of imagery was not perceived as important relative to the other techniques.

Wiese et al. (1991) indicated that the reluctance on the part of trainers to advocate the use of imagery techniques may have resulted from their not feeling qualified to use such techniques and/or not believing in their efficacy. It may be important to educate health professionals involved with the rehabilitation of injured athletes about the "why" and "how to" of imagery techniques.

Perspectives on Mind-Body Integration

In most cases, athletes are currently left with a rehabilitation program housed in the traditional confines of a medical model that does not include a mind-body orientation. That the athlete may have the capacity to expedite his or her own recovery with the use of cognitive strategies such as imagery does not seem to be recognized to the degree that it should be.

Psychophysiological Perspectives

Substantial evidence exists that speaks to the credibility of using a mind-body approach in explaining human existence and the intricacies of the healing process. By viewing the human being as an organism that contains a constant interchange between mental and physiological functions, one recognizes the interdependence of one's actions. Historically, patients' beliefs about the efficacy of the treatment they received and their own input into the process have been at the forefront of both Chinese and Navajo practices (Porkert, 1979; Sandner, 1979). Indeed, Gardner (1985) speaks of multiple intelligences that an individual possesses to varying degrees. One of these is the "body-kinesthetic intelligence . . . the ability to use one's body in highly differentiated and skilled ways" (p. 206). These skilled ways include "the body being trained to respond to the expressive powers of the mind" (p. 206).

At the cornerstone of this position, however, lies the principle of homeostasis advanced by Cannon (1932, cited in Ievleva & Orlick, 1991) which establishes "a process of interaction between the brain and the body toward maintaining internal stability."

Green, Green, and Walters (1979) adhere to what they call the psychophysiological principle. It suggests that for every physiological change that occurs in the body, there is an appropriate change in the mental-emotional state. They also suggest that the converse of this phenomenon is equally true. Others have established that imagery triggers similar neurophysiological functions as does actual experience (Leuba, 1940; Perky, 1910; Richardson, 1969).

Surgent (1991) suggests that there is a mind-body connection that facilitates the healing process. He indicates that your immune system doesn't work alone. . your mind also has a voice in what goes on. There is a communication network between your brain and your immune system, like telephone lines between a general and his field commanders. . . . Feelings, attitudes, and beliefs are organized in your brain and communicated to your immune system by chemical messengers. These can have an effect on the healing process which can be either positive or negative. (pp. 4–5)

This claim has been substantiated by findings reported by Hall (1983), who revealed an increased immune response when he tested the effects of hypnosis and imagery on lymphocyte function. The most recent support for the interplay between the use of imagery and immune system responses has been reported by Achterberg (1991), AuBuchon (1991), and Post-White (1991). They have provided evidence that describes the positive effects the immune system experiences when triggered by imagery.

Literature pertaining to psychoneuroimmunology further establishes the plausibility of the mind-body paradigm during rehabilitation. Achterberg, Matthews-Simonton, and Simonton (1977), as well as Fiore (1988), have reported that certain psychological characteristics of patients influenced recovery from cancer. Simonton, Matthews-Simonton and Creighton (1978) provide evidence that supports the use of imagery in the treatment for cancer. Others have reported positive effects of the use of imagery during the rehabilitation of various illnesses and injuries, such as psoriasis (Gaston, Crombez, & Dupuis, 1989); stress management (Hanley & Chinn, 1989); ulcers, paraplegia, fractures, hip disarticulations, and intra-abdominal lesions (Korn, 1983).

In addition, a large number of studies have indicated that the use of imagery produces physiological responses, such as salivation (Barber, Chauncey, & Winer, 1964), increase in pupillary size (Simpson & Paivio, 1966), increased heart rate (May & Johnson, 1973), changes in electromyograms (Sheikh & Jordan, 1983), increases in blood-glucose, inhibition of gastrointestinal activity, and changes in skin temperature (Barber, 1978).

When these findings are taken to their logical end, it may be worth considering that when one takes physiologic measurements, one is in fact taking corresponding psychological indicators simultaneously. The results reported may depend entirely on what category of measurement is being taken and the perspective from which the investigator originates, for instance, psychology, physiology, and psychophysiology.

The possibility exists that the specialization in professional orientation prevalent in today's scientific community is merely part of the lasting ripple effect created by the Cartesian medical model and does nothing but perpetuate an all too narrow perspective from which to draw conclusions concerning the human condition. As a consequence, the thoughts of Diderot from the middle 18th century may be applicable today. He spoke of the intention at that time of scholars to reinstate holism as an appropriate perspective for medicine so that it "may be advanced to the point of where it was two thousand years ago" (McMahon & Sheikh, 1986, p. 12).

Psychomotor Perspectives

From a sport psychology perspective, it appears that there is, at the very least, a logical leap from the relationship of imagery and sport performance to the impact of imagery on the healing process of injuries. The concept that the use of mental rehearsal facilitates the execution of certain motor skills under certain conditions is well documented (for reviews see Corbin, 1972; Feltz & Landers, 1983).

In addition, Hecker and Kaczor (1988) have summarized existing theoretical models that have been advanced to explain the processes involved with mental imagery and its influence on athletic performance, for example, motor skill development. These include (a) the symbolic learning theory, which posits that symbolic rehearsal advances the development of skills requiring cognitive processes (Sackett, 1935); (b) the psychoneuromuscular theory associated with Jacobsen's work (1938), which identified muscular innervations during imagery that are similar to those occurring during actual performance; (c) the attention-arousal set, which integrates cognitive and physiological aspects of rehearsal in order to distinguish between relevant and irrelevant cues (Feltz & Landers, 1983; Vealey, 1987); and (d) the bioinformational theory of Lang (1979) in which imagery processes the stimulus characteristics of an imagined scenario and the physiological/behavioral responses that accompany them.

Other models, such as Greene's (1972) multilevel hierarchical control of motor programs and Pribram's (1971) two-process model of imagery, have been applied to the development of motor programs and further describe the interdependence of mind and body. Greene maintains that a motor movement is the result of a mind-body system composed of a number of levels. The higher levels initiate a ballpark motor response to environmental input, which is then refined by lower levels of neuromuscular processing. The end result is the appropriate motor movement that meets the requirements of the task.

Pribram's (1971) two-process model of imagery includes neuropsychological processes identified as TOTE and TOTEM systems. The TOTE system refers to the exchange of feedback and feedforward mechanisms between the environment and the organism in order to produce movement. The TOTEM system is an application of these processes in which images conduct TOTE operations on each other exclusively within the mental environment.

It seems viable to suggest, therefore, that the same models used to explain psychophysiological and psychomotor processes used in athletic performance can be applied when describing the place of imagery during the rehabilitation associated with the healing of athletic injuries, for instance, the reestablishing of fine and gross motor movements, the reestablishing of psychoneurological pathways. However, as Hecker and Kaczor (1988) have indicated, when each of these theories is taken alone, it proves to be inadequate in explaining the complex, mind-body process of imagery. Therefore, a more encompassing approach must be advanced, such as a "systems theory" suggested by Schwartz (1984).

He maintains that systems theory "has the potential to provide a metatheoretical framework for integrating the biological, psychological, and social consequences of imagery on health and illness" (Schwartz, 1984, p. 35). In describing the synthesis attained by implementing systems theory, he elaborates on the metaprinciples of systems theory:

> A system is an entity (a whole) which is composed of a set of parts (which are subsystems). These parts interact. Out of the parts interaction emerge unique properties that characterize the new entity or system as a whole. These emergent properties represent more than the simple, independent sum of the properties of the parts studied in isolation. It is hypothesized that the emergent properties appear only when the parts are allowed to interact. (p. 39)

Thus, independent theories that appear to be in competition can be integrated into a comprehensive perspective that appears to be both logical and substantiated by scientific evidence. It is proposed that this may provide the necessary body of knowledge from which the education of health professionals (i.e., athletic trainers) may be enhanced. The use of psychophysiological techniques such as imagery may increase once the educational barriers are weakened. It is hoped that this will lead to the use of psychological techniques that go beyond the traditional skills of communication and motivation.

What follows is an example of how the mind-body perspective might be applied in the development of a rehabilitation program for injured athletes. This example is offered with the understanding that it is not all-encompassing. However, it should provide a starting point from which sport medicine teams can develop programs of rehabilitation from a mind-body perspective.

The Chronology of an Injury

The following is a chronology of athletic injuries adapted from Nideffer's scheme (1987). Although his scheme included factors related to the onset of the injury as well as the athlete's coping and recovery, this chronology addresses three periods of time associated with injuries: preinjury, immediately following the injury, and during the rehabilitation program leading to the recovery and re-integration of the athlete into the competitive situation (see Table 1). Each will be described with the intended purpose of demonstrating the application of imagery techniques within the context of an integrated mind-body approach to rehabilitation.

Table I. The Uses of Imagery During Rehabilitation

The Chronology of an Injury	The Potential Use of Imagery
Preinjury	Preventive Medicine
	* enhances relaxation
	* facilitates self-regulation
	* enhances perspective toward stressors
Immediately Subsequent to Injury	Developing Awareness
	* knowledge base of the injury
	* what is to be expected during rehabilitation (instant pre-play of rehab program)
	* maintenance of positive attitudes
	* reinforce efficacy of treatment
	* knowledge of potential emotions associated with rehabilitation
During Rehabilitation	Creating the Mind-Set for Recovery
	* eliminating counterproductive thoughts
	* developing "possible selves"
	* facilitate goal setting
	* affirmation imagery
	* performance-related mental rehearsals
	* rehabilitative imagery
	* coping with pain
	* bringing closure to the injury

Preinjury

Any athlete is subject to periods in his or her life during which injury is more likely to occur. In keeping with Selye's (1974) classic work on stress, these periods are characterized by stressors that cause distress rather than eustress (an exhilarating and positive force) or stress (that energy necessary for daily existence and the body's search for homeostasis). These periods of distress may be categorized as either general life or athletic stressors. General life stressors may include the transition to college life for incoming freshmen; the homesickness experienced by athletes of all levels; or the feelings of sorrow and anguish that accompany the death of someone close. Athletic stressors might include trouble with a coach, teammate, or fans; loss of playing status; or the athletic event itself (Bramwell, Holmes, Masuda, & Wagner, 1975; Kerr & Minden, 1988; Lynch, 1988; Rotella & Heyman, 1986). The resultant injury may be the function of the fatigue associated with having to deal with these situations or the divisive effect on concentration the athlete may experience (Kerr & Minden, 1988). Inasmuch as an athlete may experience any of these, or other circumstances that have an adverse effect on his or her normal life pattern, injury is often the result.

As a form of preventive medicine that would serve to lessen the impact of stressors and, thus, reduce the potential for injury, imagery techniques that enhance relaxation and perspective toward specific situations of stress may be developed and implemented throughout the season as circumstances mandate. For example, an athlete may experience stress as the result of homesickness. An imagery experiential can be developed that puts the immediate needs of the athlete in a long-term perspective while enhancing a relaxed state of mind. It could be implemented by introducing a relaxed state, possibly with some form of Jacobsen's (1938) progressive relaxation. This may then be followed by guided imagery intended to gain perspective on the situation. This has also been described by Samuels and Samuels (1975) as developing the ability "to see . . . to look at an object from different mental points of view, as well as from different vantage points" (p. 115).

For example:

Imagine yourself as a freshman entering college. As soon as the Thanksgiving break arrives, you can't wait to get on the first plane home. Same for the December/January break. Same for the summer break.

Now, you are a sophomore. When Thanksgiving comes, you definitely want to go home, but now you'll miss some of your college friends. Same for the December/January break. Same for the summer break.

Now, you're a junior. You've established your "place" on campus. You have developed close relationships with both male and female friends. As

Thanksgiving break approaches, you weigh the pros and cons of going home or staying on campus. You decide to go home as usual. The same thoughts happen, but not as strongly when December rolls around. But with summer, you make plans to travel with your friends and tell your parents you'll see them when you finish your trip.

Now, you're a senior. You apartment or room seems more like home to you than your parents' home. Since Thanksgiving and the December break are family occasions, it's your parents who want you home more than you wanting to go. But, still, you go. Then it's summertime, and your parents are calling you to come home instead of you calling them. What does it feel like to be self-reliant, self- sufficient?

Immediately Subsequent to the Injury

Once the injury occurs, standard first aid procedures should be followed so that further complications are not created unnecessarily. The athlete should be accompanied to the physician by someone associated with the program (e.g., trainer, coach, sport psychologist, and parent) and should be given at least "the illusion of hope" at the outset (Nideffer, 1987).

Once the athlete has seen a physician, there should be an exchange of information concerning the injury between the attending medical personnel, the athlete, the team trainer/physician, and coaches. This should include specifics about the anatomy and physiology of the injured area. By using anatomical models and photographs, the abstraction of the injury is translated into more tangible and recognizable terms. In addition, the injury might be explained in lay terms that facilitate an image, for example, "the rubber bands (ligaments) need to grow back onto the bone." This knowledge is critical as it may be applied to the use of rehabilitative imagery that would be employed later (Surgent, 1991).

During Rehabilitation of the Injury

The structure of the rehabilitation program (e.g., an instant pre-play of the program) should be discussed by all parties directly involved as the sports medicine team, that is, trainers, coaches, athletes. This may include the expected time frame associated with recovery, as well as the general parameters of the physical and mental programs to be used during rehabilitation. Expectations of the athlete, such as appointments with trainers, coaches and sport psychologists; attendance at practice and games; and the criteria to be used to determine when the athlete is ready to return to practice and competition, should also be identified. In addition, *who* will make the final decision (e.g., the athlete, the coach, the physician) as to the athlete's readiness may also be discussed as part of the criteria used for return (Thomas, 1990). Of considerable importance are the factors relating to the athlete's adherence to the rehabilitation. These should be identified and discussed with the athlete. It should be pointed out that successful rehabilitation is characterized by specific behaviors associated with adherence to the rehabilitation process. Wiese et al. (1991) have identified the following: (a) the willingness on the part of the athlete to listen to the trainer, (b) the athlete's maintaining a positive attitude, and (c) intrinsic motivation on the part of the athlete. In addition, characteristics described by Duda, Smart, and Tappe (1989) include the athlete's belief in the efficacy of the treatment, the presence of a social support system, and the athlete's orientation toward task-related goals in his or her sport. Imagery experientials in which the athlete envisions the overt behaviors associated with these factors may become an integral part of daily treatments in the training room.

An example of such an application of imagery may be created by adapting the work of Lazarus (1984), who has developed procedures that depict an individual taking psychological risks. Once the behaviors associated with carrying out specific instructions from the trainer, personifying positive attitudes, demonstrating intrinsic motivation, and task-related goal setting are imagined, the athlete is then encouraged to go out and perform them.

Finally, Rotella and Heyman (1986) and Lynch (1988) have discussed the application of Kübler-Ross's (1969) work concerning the emotional recovery from the death of a loved one to the athletic setting and the recovering athlete. It is suggested that athletes may experience similar patterns of emotional reaction during their rehabilitation. These might include denial, anger, bargaining, depression, and acceptance. Were an athlete given insight into the process of recovery with imagery depicting each stage, he or she might be able to facilitate the transition from one stage to the next.

For example, an experiential entitled "Time Projection or Time Tripping" (Lazarus, 1984, pp. 131–137) may facilitate the development of an athlete's awareness concerning potential emotional reactions throughout rehabilitation. By projecting him- or herself back or forward in time and describing the emotions associated with different stages of rehabilitation from retrospective or futuristic perspectives, the athlete is encouraged to recognize various stages of recovery. For example, the athlete may recognize that he or she may become depressed during the rehabilitation, but the athlete may also recognize that depression may be part of the process that eventually leads to recovery.

In summary, the following four examples have been described to demonstrate how imagery might be applied to the first two phases of the chronology of an injury: for the pre-injury phase, (a) relaxation and perspective imagery as preventative medicine; and for the time immediately following the injury, (b) an instant pre-play of the rehabilitation program, (c) attitude and belief imagery, and (d) imagery depicting emotional stages of transition during recovery.

The Mind-Body Rehabilitation Process

The rehabilitation program for athletes should be devised by a sports medicine team composed of the attending physician, the athlete, trainers, coach, and sport psychologist. The resulting program should reflect a mind-body approach to the process of recovery (Gordon, Jaffe, & Bresler, 1984; Peper, Ancoli, & Quinn, 1979). It should address the creation of the appropriate mind-set for the recovering athlete as well as the physical dimensions of rehabilitation.

Creating the Mind-Set for Recovery

A character named Socrates from Millman's (1984) book *The Way of the Peaceful Warrior* describes the part one's mind plays in creating one's way of being. He suggests that

> "Mind" is one of those slippery terms like "love". The proper definition depends on your state of consciousness. . . . We refer to the brain's abstract processes as "the intellect.". . . The brain and the mind are not the same. The brain is real; the mind isn't. The brain can be a tool. It can recall phone numbers, solve math puzzles, or create poetry. In this way, it works for the rest of the body, like a tractor. But when you can't stop thinking of that math problem or phone number, or when troubling thoughts and memories arise without your intent, it's not your brain working, but your mind wandering. Then the mind controls you; then the tractor has run wild. (p. 62)

In essence, an athlete in rehabilitation must accomplish the same task of getting rid of a mind full of negative and counterproductive wanderings. Only then might the brain be able to do its work. These counterproductive wanderings might include certain fears associated with being injured: the fear of reinjury; the fear of the pain associated with the original injury and/or of that experienced during rehabilitation; the fear of not returning to previous level of ability; the fear of the loss of status. In addition, Ievleva and Orlick (1991) reported that recovery time for injured athletes was faster for those who did not engage in injury-replay imagery. Thus, athletes must use their intellect to guide the neuropsychological processes of the brain in such a manner as to facilitate recovery.

Developing "Possible Selves"

Upon injury, athletes are faced with what Cantor and Kihlstrom (1987) refer to as a life task. They are immediately confronted with a problem that must be resolved before normal existence can continue. In truth, the athletes must make a conscious effort to redirect their attention from playing the game to playing a new game called rehab. The game in which they must now perform becomes that associated with recovery. They must adopt a mind-set that focuses all of their energies toward that end. The immediate life task then becomes one of rehabilitation. It's a brand-new game that requires a conscious shift of attention that has as its ultimate goal their return to competition.

In addressing the task of goal setting associated with the rehabilitation process, sport psychologists might consider applying the theoretical framework of Markus and Ruvolo (1989). This framework depicts the development of possible selves. Their notion of developing possible selves addresses the potential for "personalized representations of goals" (p. 211). They discuss goal setting in terms of "constructing a possible self in which one is different from the now self and in which one realizes the goal" (p. 211). Thus, a progression of possible selves "becomes a part of the working self-concept" (Markus & Kunda, 1986; Markus & Nurius, 1986).

What is critical is the ability of the athletes to formulate and maintain the possible selves that lead toward the desired goal. They must be able to repress possible selves that are inconsistent with the task of recovery, for instance, a possible self depicting injury-replay or negative attitudes. The desired possible selves might depict the athlete as an individual having a positive outlook, descriptive self-talk, or performance-related goals. As a number of authors have suggested, the athlete should engage in affirmation imagery that portrays him or her fulfilling short-term goals (Ievleva and Orlick, 1991; Korn & Johnson, 1983). To the extent that athletes are able to accomplish these tasks their behavior will be "focused, energized, and organized by this possible self" (Markus & Ruvolo, 1989, p. 214).

For example, imagery scenarios could be patterned after the work of Maxwell Maltz concerning the self-image. Ishii (1986) describes a number of provocative experientials that focus on developing positive, assertive, and successful self-images as well as attitudes pertaining to happiness and willpower. One, in particular, places the client in an empty theater. From this setting, the client is asked to imagine a movie unfolding in which he or she handles a problem successfully. Another technique requires that the client visualize an uncrasable chalkboard on which he or she lists past successes.

The task of the sport psychologist then becomes the creation of a series of "programmed visualizations" that reflect the rehabilitative tasks and outcomes established by the sports medicine team (Samuels & Samuels, 1975, p. 229). That possible selves may depict performance goals as well as outcome goals presents the sport psychologist with the task of identifying specific scenarios depicting each. In fact, Bandura (1986, 1988) maintains that performance and outcome selves should be separated.

Korn (1983) agrees that there should be a progression from product to process goals. That is, as an initial step, athletes should imagine themselves as completely recovered and able to do all the things they were capable of doing prior to the injury. Once they have become reasonably proficient at this form of product-oriented image, they may then progress to more specific, process-oriented images.

These process-oriented possible selves should reflect instrumental selves. That is, they should represent a sequence of possible selves that depicts the athlete in the process of performing specific motor skills, each leading to a self that is one step closer to total recovery. In essence, the instrumental possible selves are intended to result in a summation effect, with the eventual result matching or surpassing the initial product-oriented image.

For example, a female basketball player undergoing rehabilitation for a knee injury consisting of a torn interior cruciate ligament with cartilage strains used the following series of possible selves over 9 months of rehabilitation:

Possible Self #1 — "Knee at 90 degrees"
"I Want to be a Success Story," e.g., following surgery, getting out of bed and out of the hospital, establishing image of desired outcome.

Possible Self #2 — "Strut Your Stuff," e.g., getting off crutches, watching other people walk, establishing own gait.

Possible Self #3 — "Hurt to get Better," e.g., progression of physical therapy, which included, in part, weight training, electric stimulation, stationary bike, stair climber.

Possible Self #4 — "Spring Forward," e.g., running @ 75 %, jumping exercises, increasing work load.

Possible Self #5 — "Let's Play," e.g., pick-up games.

Possible Self #6 — "Dribble, Drive, and Dive!" e.g., playing with no fear of failure.

Possible Self #7 — "No brace," e.g., the final stage due to school policy of mandatory use of brace following such an injury.

Other Uses of Imagery

The processes of guided and nondirected imagery can also be utilized by the athlete in the form of relaxation techniques, motor skill rehearsals, and rehabilitative experientials (Surgent, 1991). Rehabilitative imagery has been shown to have significant effects on recovery time (Ievleva & Orlick, 1991). As described earlier during the chronology of an injury, information gathered from the physician concerning the anatomy and physiology of the injury facilitates the use of rehabilitative imagery. In addition, Day (1991) has developed an educational discourse on the immune system through the use of cartoon imagery that uses immune cell caricatures to explain the function of each cell involved in the rehabilitation process. Korn (1983) described a technique of rehabilitation imagery that consists of envisioning the wounds as filling from the inside out rather than just being covered over at the surface. The filling material was cement, and the repair process was analogous to the method of repair of a hole in a concrete walkway.

Specific mind-sets that might be addressed through the use of imagery may include the following: maintenance of a positive outlook, stress control, use of positive and descriptive self-talk, and sustaining belief in the rehabilitation process. Performance-related imagery may take the form of mental rehearsal while attending practices and competitions in which the athletes imagine themselves as if they were playing. In addition, imagery has been shown to be effective in coping with pain (Achterberg, Kenner, & Lawlis, 1988; Korn, 1983; Samuels & Samuels, 1975; Simonton, Mathews-Simonton, & Creighton, 1978; Spanos & O'Hara, 1990).

Rotella and Heyman (1986) recommended the use of videotapes of past performances. This technique may serve to reinforce the symbolic learning and psychoneuromuscular processes. Imagery may also be used to facilitate closure of the rehabilitation process once the athlete has returned to competition.

Physical Rehabilitation

The use of targeted performance criteria facilitates the athlete's return to preinjury performance levels on specific tasks associated with his or her sport. They may also serve as the impetus for creating specific instrumental and performance-related possible selves. The groundwork for this, however, must be laid at the onset of training prior to the season and, most certainly, prior to injury.

At the beginning of the season's training, baseline data should be gathered for the athletes on specific tasks associated with their training, for example, maximum weight, sets, and repetitions for a variety of weightlifting routines; range-of-motion measurements for flexibility; physiologic parameters, such as heart rate, time of recovery, max VO2 for endurance; and recorded times on specific distances for indication of speed. These data provide the target criteria to which an athlete can compare his or her progress during rehabilitation.

In addition, a functional progression of specific sport skills should be identified that represent *being back* to the athlete. For example, baseball pitchers who have been out with elbow injuries may wish to use a particular pitch (e.g., breaking off a hard slider) to gauge effectiveness upon return. Tennis players may engage in the side shuffle used on the base line as an indicator that they have recovered from the pain associated with shin splints.

Each of these tasks, in addition to other methods of progressive resistance exercises and cross-training, forms the foundation for physical rehabilitation with tangible indicators of recovery. Of course, these are undertaken in proper sequence relative to the initial training-room duties prescribed by the trainers and physician (e.g., whirlpool, electrical stimulation, iced therapy).

Conclusion

Weise et al. (1991) have reported that many athletic trainers agree with the need for further education in the area of psychology and, in particular, for methods that can be applied in the athletic setting. The purpose of this chapter has been to provide an educational text that supports a mind-body paradigm for rehabilitation from psychophysiological and psychomotor perspectives, demonstrates the application of imagery within the chronology of an injury, and describes performance-related criteria used in physical rehabilitation. The chronology includes that period of time preceding the injury, the attention given to the athlete immediately following the injury, and the subsequent rehabilitation program leading to the return of the athlete to practice and competition. It is suggested that imagery techniques may be applied during the preinjury stage as a tool for preventive maintenance. During the actual rehabilitation program, the purpose of imagery is (a) to facilitate the healing process, (b) to promote the development of a positive and relaxed outlook toward recovery, (c) to create the mind-set required for optimum performance, and (d) to bring closure to the injury experience.

References

Achterberg, J., (1991, May). *Enhancing the immune function through imagery.* Paper presented to the Fourth World Conference on Imagery, Minneapolis, MN.

Achterberg, J., Kenner, C., & Lawlis, G. F. (1988). Severe burn injury: A comparison of relaxation, imagery and biofeedback for pain management. *Journal of Mental Imagery, 12*(1), 71–88.

Achterberg, J., Matthews-Simonton, S., & Simonton, O. C. (1977). Psychology of the exceptional cancer patient: A description of patients who outlive predicted life expectancies. *Psychotherapy: Theory, Research, and Practice, 14,* 416–422.

AuBuchon, B. (1991, May). *The effects of positive mental imagery on hope, coping, anxiety, dypsnea, and pulmonary function in persons with chronic obstructive pulmonary disease: Tests of a nursing intervention and a theoretical model.* Paper presented to the Fourth World Conference on Imagery, Minneapolis, MN.

Bandura, A. (1986). *Social foundations of thought and action: A social cognitive theory.* Englewood Cliffs, NJ: Prentice-Hall.

Bandura, A. (1988). Self-regulation of motivation and action through goal systems. In V. Hamilton, G. H. Bower, & N. H. Frijda (Eds.), *Cognitive perspectives on emotion and motivation* (pp. 37–61). Dordrecht, Netherlands: Kluwer Academic Publishers.

Barber, T. X. (1978). Hypnosis, suggestions and psychosomatic phenomena, a new look from the standpoint of recent experimental studies. *The American Journal of Clinical Hypnosis, 21,* 13–27.

Barber, T. X., Chauncey, H. M., & Winer, R. A. (1964). The effect of hypnotic and nonhypnotic suggestions on parotid gland response to gustatory stimuli. *Psychosomatic Medicine, 26,* 374–380.

Bramwell, S. T., Holmes, T. H., Masuda, M., & Wagner, N. N. (1975). Psychosocial factors in athletic injuries: Development and application of the social and athletic readjustment rating scale (SARRS). *Journal of Human Stress, 1*(2), 6–20.

Cannon, W. B. (1932). *The wisdom of the body.* New York: Norton.

Cantor, N., & Kihlstrom, J. (1987). *Personality and social intelligence.* Englewood Cliffs, NJ: Prentice-Hall.

Corbin, C. (1972). Mental practice. In W. Morgan (Ed.), *Ergogenic aids and muscular performance* (pp. 93–118). New York: Academic Press.

Day, C. H. (1991). *The immune system handbook.* North York, Ontario: Potentials Within.

Duda, J. L., Smart, A. E., & Tappe, M. K. (1989). Predictors of adherence in the rehabilitation of athletic injuries: An application of personal investment theory. *Journal of Sport and Exercise Psychology, 11,* 367–381.

Feltz, D. L., & Landers, D. M. (1983). The effects of mental practice on motor skill learning and performance: A meta-analysis. *Journal of Sport Psychology, 5,* 25–27.

Fiore, N. A. (1988). The inner healer: Imagery for coping with cancer and its therapy. *Journal of Mental Imagery, 12*(2), 79–82.

Gardner, H. (1985). *Frames of mind: The theory of multiple intelligences.* New York: Basic Books, Inc.

Gaston, L., Crombez, J. & Dupuis, G. (1989). An imagery and meditation technique in the treatment of psoriasis: A case study using an A-B-A design. *Journal of Mental Imagery, 13*(1), 31–38.

Gordon, J. S., Jaffe, D. T., & Bresler, D. E. (1984). *Mind, body, and health: Toward an integral medicine.* New York: Human Sciences Press.

Green, E. E., Green, A. M., & Walters, E. D. (1979). Biofeedback for mind/body self-regulation: Healing and creativity. In E. Peper, S. Ancoli, & M. Quinn (Eds.), *Mind/body integration: Essential readings in biofeedback.* New York: Plenum Press.

Greene, P. H. (1972). Problems of organization of motor systems. In R. Rosen & F.M. Snell (Eds.), *Progress in theoretical biology* (Vol.2, pp. 304–333). New York: Academic Press.

Hall, H. R. (1983) Hypnosis and the immune system: A review with implications for cancer and the psychology of healing. *American Journal of Clinical Hypnosis, 25*(3), 92–103.

Hanley, G. L., & Chinn, D. (1989). Stress management: An integration of multidimensional arousal and imagery theories with case study. *Journal of Mental Imagery, 13*(2), 107–118.

Hecker, J. E., & Kaczor, L. M. (1988). Application of imagery theory to sport psychology: Some preliminary findings. *Journal of Sport and Exercise Psychology, 10,* 363–373.

Ievleva, L., & Orlick, T. (1991). Mental links to enhanced healing: An exploratory study. *The Sport Psychologist, 5,* 25–40.

Ishii, M. M. (1986). Imagery techniques in the works of Maxwell Maltz. In A. A. Sheikh (Ed.), *Anthology of imagery techniques* (pp. 313–323). Milwaukee, WI: American Imagery Institute.

Jacobsen, E. (1938). *Progressive relaxation.* Chicago: University of Chicago Press.

Kerr, G., & Minden, H. (1988). Psychological factors related to the occurrence of athletic injuries. *Journal of Sport and Exercise Psychology, 10,* 167–173.

Korn, E. R. (1983). The use of altered states of consciousness and imagery in physical and pain rehabilitation. *Journal of Mental Imagery, 7*(1), 25–34.

Korn, E. R., & Johnson, K. (1983). *Visualization: The uses of imagery in the health professions.* Homewood, IL: Dow Jones-Irwin.

Kübler-Ross, E. (1969). *On death and dying.* New York: Macmillan.

Lang, P. J. (1979). A bio-informational theory of emotional imagery. *Psychophysiology, 16,* 495–512.

Lazarus, A. (1984). *In the mind's eye: The power of imagery for personal enrichment.* New York: The Guilford Press.

Leuba, C. (1940). Images as conditioned sensation. *Journal of Experimental Psychology, 26,* 345–351.

Lynch, G. P. (1988). Athletic injuries and the practicing sport psychologist: Practical guidelines for assisting athletes. *The Sport Psychologist, 2,* 161–167.

Markus, H., & Kunda, Z. (1986). Stability and malleability of the self-concept. *Journal of Personality and Social Psychology, 51,* 858–866.

Markus, H., & Nurius, P. (1986). Possible selves. *American Psychologist, 41,* 954–969.

Markus, H., & Ruvolo, A. (1989). Possible selves: Personalized representations of goals. In L. A. Pervin (Ed.), *Goal concepts in personality and social psychology* (pp. 211–241). Hillsdale, NJ: Erlbaum.

May, J., & Johnson, H. (1973). Psychological activity to internally elicited arousal and inhibitory thoughts. *Journal of Abnormal Psychology, 82,* 239–245.

McMahon, C. E., & Sheikh, A. (1986). Imagination in disease and healing processes: A historical perspective. In A. A. Sheikh (Ed.), *Anthology of imagery techniques* (pp. 1–36). Milwaukee, WI: American Imagery Institute.

Millman, D. (1984). *The way of the peaceful warrior.* Tiburon, CA: H. J. Kramer, Inc.

Nideffer, R. (1987, October). *Psychological aspects of injury.* Paper presented at the National Conference on Sport Psychology, Arlington, VA.

Peper, E., Ancoli, S., & Quinn, M. (1979). *Mind/body integration: Essential readings in biofeedback.* New York: Plenum Press.

Perky, C. W. (1910). An experimental study of imagination. *American Journal of Psychology, 21,* 422–452.

Porkert, M. (1979). Chinese medicine: A tradition healing science. In D. S. Sobel (Ed.), *Ways of health: Holistic approaches to ancient and contemporary medicine* (pp. 117–146). New York: Harcourt Brace Jovanovich.

Post-White, J. (1991, May). *The effects of mental imagery on emotions, immune function and cancer outcome.* Paper presented to the Fourth World Conference on Imagery, Minneapolis, MN.

Pribram, K. (1971). *Languages of the brain.* Englewood Cliffs, NJ: Prentice-Hall.

Richardson, A. (1969). *Mental imagery.* London: Routledge and Kegan Paul, Ltd.

Rotella, R. J., & Heyman, S. R. (1986). Stress, injury, and the psychological rehabilitation of athletes. In J.M. Williams (Ed.), *Applied sport psychology: Personal growth to peak performance* (pp. 343–364). Palo Alto, CA: Mayfield.

Sackett, R. S. (1935). The relationship between the amount of symbolic rehearsal and retention of a maze habit. *Journal of General Psychology, 13,* 113–128.

Samuels, S., & Samuels, N. (1975). *Seeing with the mind's eye.* New York: Random House.

Sandner, D. F. (1979). Navaho Indian medicine and medicine men. In D. S. Sobel (Ed.), *Ways of health: Holistic approaches to ancient and contemporary medicine* (pp. 117–146). New York: Harcourt Brace Jovanovich.

Schwartz, G. E. (1984). Psychophysiology of imagery and healing: A systems perspective. In A. A. Sheikh (Ed.), *Imagination and healing* (pp. 38–50). Farmingdale, NY: Baywood Publishing Company, Inc.

Selye, H. (1974). *Stress without distress*. Philadelphia: J.B. Lipincott.

Sheikh, A. A., & Jordan, C. S. (1983). Clinical uses of mental imagery. In A. A. Sheikh (Ed.), *Imagery: Current theory, research, and applications* (pp. 391–435). New York: Wiley.

Simonton, O. C., Matthews-Simonton, S., & Creighton, J. (1978). *Getting well again*. New York: St. Martin's Press.

Simpson, H. M., & Pavio, A. (1966). Changes in pupil size during an imagery task without motor involvement. *Psychonomic Science, 5,* 405–406.

Spanos, N. P., & O'Hara, P. A. (1990). Imaginal dispositions and situation-specific expectations in strategy-induced pain reductions. *Imagination, Cognition and Personality, 9*(2), 147–156.

Surgent, F. S. (1991, January). Using your mind to beat injuries. *Running and Fit News, 9*(1), 4–5.

Thomas, C. (1990, October). *Locus of authority, coercion, and critical distance in the decision to play an injured player*. Paper presented to the Philosophic Society for the Study of Sport, Ft. Wayne, IN.

Vealey, R. S. (1987, June). *Imagery training for performance enhancement*. Paper presented at the Sports Psychology Institute, Portland, ME.

Wiese, D. M., Weiss, M. R., & Yukelson, D. P. (1991). Sport psychology in the training room: A survey of athletic trainers. *The Sport Psychologist, 5,* 15–24.

SECTION 4

COUNSELING ATHLETES
WITH PERMANENT DISABILITIES

In the lead chapter of this section, **Keith P. Henschen** and **Gregory A. Shelley** employ vignettes of real-life athletic injuries that resulted in permanent physical disability. They describe counseling efforts employed in successful rehabilitative programs used with these athletes.

The second chapter, written by **Edward F. Etzel, A. P. Ferrante, Frank Perna**, and **R. Renee Newcomer**, emphasizes the need to go beyond the exclusive employment of the "medical model" in assisting disabled injured college athletes. Detailed descriptions of the roles of athletic trainers and psychological counselors are provided by way of two case studies. A number of difficulties encountered in working with this population are discussed.

In this section's last chapter, **Jane Henderson** addresses a serious problem that she asserts appears today with increased frequency, namely, suicide among athletes. She appears to be the first to write about this horrific form of self-inflicted trauma.

▲

15

Counseling Athletes With Permanent Disabilities

Keith P. Henschen
University of Utah

Gregory A. Shelley
Ithaca College

Two actual vignettes of athletes experiencing permanent disabilities are presented, and information concerning the transitional period as well as the general reaction pattern to injuries is discussed. Next, a number of general guidelines to which the sport psychologist should adhere during the various stages of the psychological rehabilitation are presented. Finally, psychological interventions that would be beneficial in each scenario are discussed. A team approach to handling athletes with permanent disabilities is advocated.

Vignette I

On a snow-covered football field in mid-December an all-pro wide receiver streaks down the sideline, with an intense concentration on the long, arching pass headed in his direction. As the ball gently nestles into the receiver's soft hands, a defensive player's helmet is planted in the middle of the receiver's back with unbelievable force. The force of the two players colliding is analogous to two cars crashing head-on at about 30 miles per hour with neither applying the brakes. At the instant of impact, the receiver suffers a severing of the spinal cord and is immediately transformed into a paraplegic.

Vignette II

On a stormy and rainy summer night an Olympic, world-class pistol shooter is involved in a tragic automobile accident. She is severely injured, with numerous broken bones and a deep concussion that leaves her in a coma for about 2 weeks. After awakening from the coma, she continues to experience migraine headaches and blurred vision. It is determined that the neurological damage is permanent and that her vision impairment is uncorrectable. She will remain, throughout her lifetime, legally blind in one eye.

These vignettes are true-life experiences and create a variety of special circumstances that must be handled by the medical science specialists. Of particular interest are the problems or challenges that these situations create for the sport psychologist. What are the similarities the sport psychology consultant must be cognizant of in both scenarios? What are the obvious and subtle differences? How, when, and where should counseling and intervention techniques be applied in each situation? Also, what are the major concerns that need to be addressed before total reintegration back into society can be achieved? The remainder of this chapter will attempt to provide salient information on how to proceed in each of these cases, as well as discuss the setbacks or problems that could possibly arise for the sport psychologist.

To begin our discussion, it should be understood, unequivocally, that sport termination trauma is real and that it often initiates a life crisis for which very few athletes are prepared. An elite athlete initially receives a great deal of publicity and support when injured. Soon the injury becomes "yesterday's news." The athlete eventually is left to deal with the trauma with the help of his or her family or intimate support group. The long-term consequences of such injuries can be devastating.

Not only is high-level athletic participation no longer probable, but the athlete's entire quality of life also is in jeopardy. Permanent physical damage may significantly hamper the person's ability to lead a productive, fulfilling life and severely limit possible career options (Ogilvie & Howe, 1986). When adjustment to new circumstances must be made, it is likely that counseling interventions will be required to assure functional transitions and recovery of what can be labeled "a new normalcy in life."

The Transition Period

Irrespective of the specific cause of the athletic termination, as illustrated by the two previous vignettes, each injured athlete must address a crucial period of adjustment with only the tools or techniques acquired in past experiences or personal growth. The demands of this transition are specific to the individual and handled differently by all those forced to experience it. Any injury is mentally, emotionally, and behaviorally challenging. The athlete's state of mental health prior to the injury will have a great influence on how the athlete reacts to the injury (Samples, 1987). It is a time when vital issues, such as permanent retirement, identity crises, and the transition from athlete to ex-athlete status, emerge. It is difficult to actually terminate any important relationship on an objective basis because the motives to do so are absent or very weak. This is exactly the difficulty in a career-ending sports injury. In general, how athletes handle this period of adjustment is most dependent upon the strength of their identification with sport, their perceptions about self-worth, and the importance they place on the expectations held for them by others. For many, the identity of being an athlete is an important part of their feelings of self-worth and interpersonal needs.

A heavy investment in the "sport identity" may be troublesome for the person making the transition from athlete to nonathlete. Such an individual has thrived on the recognition and accolades derived from competitive endeavors. When deprived of these reinforcements, the injured athlete suffers a serious loss because he or she may no longer have opportunities to develop in other areas and cultivate other talents (Ogilvie & Howe, 1986). Sports management tends to emphasize single-mindedness relative to the athletic commitment. Athletes, particularly those who compete on elite levels, are encouraged to invest heavily in training and to maintain an almost exclusive focus on sports.

In making a smooth and healthy transition from athlete to nonathlete status, the injured athlete's perceptions of self are crucial. Many athletes, even world-class competitors, do not have high levels of self-worth and, therefore, require much positive reinforcement from significant others (Henschen, 1992; Poole, Henschen, Shultz, Gordin, & Hill, 1986). Cessation of such reinforcement, heretofore provided by successful competitive experiences, may result in further decreases in self-worth and difficulty in coping with the demands of transition. Injured athletes who believe they are worthwhile and important persons exclusive of their involvement in sport are likely to adjust more easily to their status change than are those with low self-worth. It should be noted that perceptions of helplessness regarding the physical self may undermine the entire concept of self.

Loss of recognition and status, as well as the unavailability of an exciting lifestyle, may complicate the injured athlete's transition to nonathlete status. Injured athletes are no longer acknowledged in the same manner by other athletes, peers, significant others, and a previously adoring mass media. Often, so-called "close friendships" fade, and the injured athlete must rely on primary bases of support, frequently, family members. Unfortunately, members of the immediate family also are obliged to confront serious interpersonal, financial, and time-management challenges related to injury of one of its members. Consequently, the preparedness to help the athlete may be compromised. The period of adjustment to the injury (the transitional period) may be difficult for athletes due to the need to relinquish center stage, the "roar of the crowd and the smell of the grease paint," and the loss of opportunity to showcase their talent. They still must deal with unfair expectations that they have been exposed to for years: the expectation that they must "be tough," "play with pain," "never quit," etc. For example, debilitating injury to a professional athlete may result in serious loss of family income in the face of increased medical expenses.

General Reaction Pattern to Sport Injury

The period of adjustment to injury involves a number of predictable directions taken by the athlete. Although each athlete is unique in many physical and psychological ways, and so personal reactions to disabling injury will be different, even so, certain common experiences that may be referred to as stages seem to be shared by many. In the athletes' quest to accept the inevitable consequences of termination from sports, variations in defense mechanisms and coping strategies are employed. No serious physical injury occurs without psychological consequences, and these are contingent upon the personal attributes of the athletes themselves (Wiese & Weiss, 1987). According to Kübler-Ross (1969), Ogilvie and Howe (1986), and Rotella and Heyman (1986), these stages, in sequence, are depicted in Figure 1.

```
┌─────────────────┐
│     DENIAL      │
│     ANGER       │
│     GRIEF       │
│   DEPRESSION    │
│  REINTEGRATION  │
└─────────────────┘
```

Figure 1. General Psychological Reaction Pattern to Catastrophic Injury

The *denial* and/or disbelief phase is normally experienced first. Initially, the athlete is shocked, numb, and has difficulty in accepting the physical trauma. Often injured athletes will seek second, third, or as many medical opinions as they can afford, in order to disprove the inevitable diagnosis. This approach is compatible with their well-developed "athletic attitudes" that emphasizes "never giving up" and "striving to beat insurmountable odds." Sport heroes and heroines are recognized for their staunch implementation of these philosophies. However, other, less helpful attitudes also prevail that may be inhibitory, such as "Something like this cannot happen to me—only to other people." The ability to relinquish this denial and to accept the reality of the injury depends upon how well the athlete is prepared for the eventual outcome. If he or she subscribes to the myth of athletic invulnerability or invincibility, then the denial phase can be long and traumatic (Ogilvie, 1987).

When denial is no longer an effective coping strategy the athlete enters the *anger* phase. Here, emotions such as anger, rage, envy, resentment, hostility, and aggression are frequently displayed. Friends, loved ones, and family members are commonly targeted as subjects. The "why me?" and "why not you (or someone else)?" thinking is prevalent here. Often the athletes will also direct anger against themselves. Self-abuse, as well as unpredictable mood swings and resentment towards others, is evident during this phase.

Although the first two stages, denial and anger, are usually temporary, they may be experienced by the athlete with intensity and cause pain to others in the environment. Well-adjusted individuals pass through these phases relatively quickly, but individuals with more problematic adjustments may remain in the denial phase for an extended period of time or harbor extreme rage (Ogilvie & Howe, 1986).

The next phase is usually that of *grief* and bargaining. Grieving and depression are frequently extensions of each other. A grief response involves a series of feelings related to the sense of separation or loss. It is not static, but rather a dynamic state of fairly unpredictable behaviors. Again, the "why me?" attitude is prevalent with a slightly different twist. Here, acceptance of permanent change due to injury is present; however, also involved is the attempt to determine "why?" The injured party longs for "what he or she used to be" and spends a great deal of time in past memories and fantasies about the future. Factors influencing the grief reaction include the unique nature of the loss; the social system of the person who is grieving; the injured party's coping behaviors, personality, and mental health; the athlete's level of maturity and intelligence; and the athlete's social, cultural, ethnic and religious/philosophical background (Rando, 1984). Actually, the grief phase is the initial step to recovery. Almost as a last gasp effort, the individual, in the waning stages of the grief phase, resorts to bargaining. Here is where the athlete talks to a personal supreme deity and attempts to "make a deal." If he or she is completely healed, the athlete will promise to always be good, faithfully attend church, never run again, be pillars of the community, etc. This desperate effort is probably the final attempt or coping strategy used to avoid the reality that must be faced. When the injured party finally realizes that no miracles are forthcoming, then and only then is the person ready for the final phase—*acceptance* and reintegration.

The fourth phase of the general reaction pattern is *depression*. Depression in this context is usually defined as a sense of great loss. During this phase, it is common for the athlete to withdraw from teammates, friends, and family members. In other words, the depressed individual distances him- or herself from the very people who could provide the most meaningful support. Other characteristics of this phase are verbalized helplessness and perceived loneliness. Enthusiasm and vibrancy are replaced by loneliness. Confusion prevails, and a sense of purpose seems to be lost. This phase can be of short duration or can last for a long time. Its length depends on many factors, such as the injured athlete's personality and persistence of significant others in providing support.

Factors that significantly determine how quickly the injured athlete reaches the final phase (reintegration) relate to each athlete's overall physical, emotional, and psychological foundation. Once an athlete is able to accept the consequences of disability, then he or she can effectively face the challenge of reintegration into society. It would be nice to be able to describe, or present, an outline of the behaviors that would indicate that the reintegration phase is underway; however, a general description is virtually impossible because of the multitude of individual factors involved. It can be safely stated, though, that acceptance should not be mistaken for a happy stage; rather, it is almost void of feelings. Suffice it to say, that an athlete's progression through the general reaction response is dependent upon (a) prior psychological level of functioning; (b) the meaning of the disability to the athlete; (c) the nature, location, severity, and duration of the injury; and (d) the resulting changes in the individual's lifestyle (May & Sieb, 1987). The one thing that the sport psychologist should provide throughout all these stages is *hope*.

Now that we have discussed the general reaction pattern and the transitional period associated with catastrophic injury, let us examine each of the vignettes that were used to introduce this chapter, according to counseling techniques that can be used in each circumstance. It should be remembered that the following are recommended counseling methods based upon the authors' experiences and are not presented as exclusive or definitive approaches.

Vignette I (At the beginning of this chapter)

The tragedy of this scenario is only exceeded by the fact that it is condoned totally by society. What type of civilized people would sanction a contest where the outcome is disabling to an opponent? Putting that aside, the issue now becomes how to work most effectively with the injured athlete in order to facilitate his transitional period. This football player must overcome two major issues: (a) retirement from athletics and (b) adjustment to permanent disability. This first issue is relatively meaningless in this scenario. It is inevitable, and the athlete will come to this realization almost immediately upon awakening from surgery. The crucial issue for this person is not one of realizing how to become a productive ex-athlete, but rather how to deal with being a permanently disabled individual for the remainder of his life. It is not even a question of the severity of injury, because this injury is so severe that any semblance of a normal quality of life is thought (by the athlete) to be threatened.

In this case rehabilitation should involve a medical team approach with special emphasis placed in three stages: preoperative, postoperative, and long-term recovery. Prior to discussing the three stages of rehabilitation for this scenario, it should be made abundantly clear that the most effective procedures will be accomplished by a team approach. No one individual can provide all of the services necessary for this individual as he or she struggles through the stages of rehabilitation. The team should consist of family, friends, teammates, athletic trainers, medical personnel, and the sport psychologist. Each of these individuals has significant contributions to make to the injured athlete and his or her reintegration to society. Let us examine these contributions in reverse order from how they were presented previously.

In reality, the most crucial portion of the medical rehabilitation team is the sport psychologist. This professional will be the *only* individual remaining in close, personal contact throughout all the stages of rehabilitation. The sport psychologist, because of the professional relationship, will also be the sole member of the sportsmedicine team who can provide compassionate but objective evaluations and reinforcement to the injured party in an unbiased fashion. Specific procedures and techniques used by the sport psychologist will be presented as the stages of rehabilitation are discussed.

The second category of the team approach includes all the medical personnel. The operating surgeons, the personal medical doctor, and the physical therapists are part of this category. These people are all professionals and are experts at what they do—providing medical services. Sadly, these individuals are typically not trained in counseling techniques, which are essential in this scenario. That is why the sport psychologist must have the confidence and cooperation of the medical staff in order to be effective.

The athletic training staff is normally a crucial element in most injury rehabilitation situations, but this vignette is slightly different. After the initial on-the-field treatment for the injury, the athletic trainers will really have little contact with the athlete, but they can be invaluable to the sport psychologist. They can be a source of much-needed information concerning the personal aspects of the athlete which will be needed in the counseling. Nideffer (1983) identified several personality characteristics in athletes that interact with the personalities of the sports medicine team: information seeking, self-confidence, self-esteem, and extroversion or introversion tendencies. Athletic trainers can provide the sport psychologists with this personal information on the athlete, thus saving the time and energy of the sport psychologist.

Friends and teammates can also provide the injured athlete with an enormous amount of support and love, or they can be a source of potential problems. Many times friends and teammates demonstrate enormous interest in the injured athlete, but often only *initially*. As the severity of the disability becomes apparent, these same individuals may become conspicuously absent. Their visits will be frequent in the beginning, but diminish and ultimately become nonexistent over time. Many persons feel uncomfortable in the presence of disabled individuals, and the easiest solution is "out of sight, out of mind." Although sometimes difficult for the injured athlete to accept, friends and teammates have full agendas and committed lives of their own. It is often difficult for active people to spend time with inactive individuals, especially ones with disabilities. In addition, friends, relatives, and former teammates may be burdened with psychological fears and limitations that inhibit their interaction with permanently disabled persons. The sport psychologist should, therefore, prepare the injured athlete for this *abandonment* as the rehabilitation process proceeds.

Perhaps the most important members of the team approach are the family. This group can be as directly affected by the disability as the injured person. The family goes through the initial trauma of the accident, the slow transition period, and the long-term rehabilitation. Family members' lives may be as influenced by the disabling injury as the life of the athlete. The sport psychologist must be prepared to counsel family members through their transitional periods. This may prove to be very difficult. Emotions such as anger, depression, and resentment will be prevalent. In fact, the sport psychologist should recommend general family counseling in all cases involving permanent disability. A number of general guidelines should be adhered to during psychological rehabilitation:

1. athlete entry into counseling as soon as possible;
2. establishment of a positive relationship by the counselor with all family members;

3. as much positive support as possible;
4. continuity of care by the same counselors.

Constantly changing counselors, for whatever reasons, often sends an inappropriate message, so this should be avoided.

Preoperative Stage

It is very important that counseling begin immediately after the injury and prior to surgery. A great deal of psychological preparation for surgery and other invasive procedures is almost always necessary. Fear of surgery is very common, and dealing with pain is difficult. The sport psychologist can prepare an injured athlete for surgery by providing accurate information about what is to happen and what to expect. Fear is often associated with the unknown and by virtue of providing explanations of the forthcoming surgical experience, the counselor may alleviate this emotion. Training in anxiety reduction and relaxation skills is also frequently appropriate at this time. It would seem appropriate for medical personnel to provide such services to patients, but for various reasons this normally fails to occur. It is wise for the sport psychologist to anticipate providing counseling services to athletes with disabilities that the medical staff is not providing.

Postoperative Stage

In this vignette, surgery resulted in return of all bodily functions with the exception of motor activity. In other words, the football player was ultimately able to do almost everything except walk. The mandate facing the sport psychologist is to deal with the general reaction of this athlete to his tragic locomotive inability and to guide him through the period in which he accepts his serious liability. This is a difficult and time-consuming challenge. One positive psychological aspect is that in the postoperative context, problems are more accessible, closer to the surface, and more likely to be revealed. Again, postoperatively, the sport psychologist needs to first handle the transition of the athlete and then lay the foundation for reintegration into society.

Long-Term Stage

The long-term stage of counseling has two purposes: learning to deal with the disability and reintegration into society. These two aspects are interrelated, but learning to deal with the disability is the most crucial. If coping with the disability is accomplished, then reintegration is likely. The sport psychologist must assist in the cognitive restructuring of many aspects of the injured athlete's perceptions. The athlete must be convinced that he or she is still a viable, productive, and important individual, even if he or she is no longer a sports hero. Ogilvie and Howe (1986) stated that once athletes are resigned to the facts of retirement, they will experience an interesting shift in values. Instead of valuing such things as being first, travel, money, and popularity, they will redirect their emphases to reflect higher value being placed on family and friends. The counseling should focus on what the reality of the disability actually is and what the athlete will be able to do. The counselor should always present information in a positive fashion.

It is our contention that the athlete described in Vignette I will respond positively to the challenge of rehabilitation. He has, since childhood, flourished on competition and has been exposed to conflict and conflict resolution challenges in the sports arena. Challenges and competition are an integral part of his life and can be used in his rehabilitation. This athlete must be convinced that even though physical participation in sport, as once experienced, is no longer possible, nevertheless, there is still the challenge to channel many of his abilities and skills towards successful rehabilitation. The object of competition now becomes himself, his own muscles and nervous system, instead of other football players. Counseling this individual should include some, if not all, of the following interventions: cognitive restructuring, visual imagery, thought stopping, panic mitigation, relaxation, goal setting, and positive self-talk. Exactly how to employ these with this particular disabled athlete is dependent upon a variety of factors, such as personality, previous psychological training, and progress through the transition phases. Rather than describe these skills here, we indicate that previous authors have advocated and offered detailed descriptions of programs utilizing these techniques (Lynch, 1988; Rotella, 1982; Samples, 1987; Wiese & Weiss, 1987). The counseling in this scenario may continue for years.

Vignette II (At the beginning of the chapter)

This case is totally different from the last one. Here the high-level competitor is not faced with an obvious lifetime disability and, in fact, can function very effectively in society with her impairment. Counseling in this case must focus primarily on retirement from competition rather than on dealing with a restrictive permanent disability. Again, two stages of counseling are recommended: (1) the postoperative stage and (2) the long-term stage.

Postoperative Stage

The athlete in Vignette II, as is the case with almost all injured individuals, will experience the same general reaction pattern during the transition period. The emphasis during the postoperative stage will be to regain a normal level of health and to involve her husband, family, and friends in the transition period. Due to the visual demands of pistol shooting, this athlete will need to accept the termination of her competitive shooting career. She will be able to continue as a recreational shooter, but intense high-level competition is improbable. The athlete's motivation and readiness for rehabilitation and counseling in this stage will be determined by what she thinks happened, how she feels about what happened, and what she plans to do about the accident (Wiese & Weiss, 1987). Once she is physically healthy, it is quite likely she will attempt to shoot again, but understandably with poor results. The counselor must be ready for the anger and frustration that will follow. After the athlete has proven to herself that she is no longer physically capable of competitive pistol shooting, the long-term stage of counseling will commence.

Long-Term Stage

Counseling in this scenario should focus on retirement from competitive athletics. In this case the key people in the athlete's total reintegration efforts will be the counselor and the athlete's spouse. If there are "significant others" in this athlete's life, they will also be important factors. Through interaction with the athlete, the counselor must locate the influential variables that are causing her to experience frustration in the retirement process.

Previous research has identified the following factors that frequently influence the "stress" of retirement: degree of marital satisfaction, the personality of the athlete, level of self-esteem and self-concept, self-motivation and self-direction, social and emotional support, value orientation, life satisfaction, educational level, present and future financial situation, and perceived career opportunities. This list is not exhaustive but provides many of the most common factors necessary to consider when dealing with forced athletic retirement. Again, the counselor must address some of the aforementioned variables but also can aid the athlete's readjustment by teaching a number of psychological skills. These skills are taught with the intent of providing a greater quality of life. The following psychological skills could be beneficial to this athlete: relaxation, imagery, cognitive restructuring, hypnosis, positive self-talk, and concentration training. The long-term objectives for counseling this athlete involve having her accept the termination of her competitive athletic career and helping her proceed with her life in a positive manner. This injured athlete should be encouraged to remain socially integrated with her former teammates in terms of personal needs. Also, her coach should maintain his or her relationship with the athlete even though she may never compete again. The athlete should be allowed to move away from her sport (pistol shooting) at a pace commensurate with her emotional reintegration.

Conclusion

Counseling athletes with permanent disabilities is indeed a formidable challenge because each athlete's response to injury is unique. Sport trauma is real, and often initiates a life crisis for which very few athletes are prepared. Counselors should recognize the importance of the transitional period and the many psychological factors that affect readjustment. Also, the general reaction pattern phases (denial, anger, depression, grief, and reintegration) must be worked through appropriately prior to successful readjustment. Counselors also need to recognize that the way in which athletes respond to permanent disability is dependent upon their physical, emotional, and psychological foundation. An athlete's adjustment to injury is dependent upon (a) prior psychological functioning, (b) the meaning of the disability to the athlete, (c) the nature, location, severity, and duration of the injury, and (d) the resulting changes in the individual's lifestyle.

We advocate a team approach to handling athletes with permanent disabilities. Sport psychologists, medical personnel, athletic trainers, family, friends, and teammates are all important contributors to the team approach. Each of these groups has significant influences during the preoperative, postoperative and long-term stages of rehabilitation.

References

Henschen, K. (1992). Developing the self-concept in track and field athletes. *Track and Field Quarterly, 92* (1), 35–37.

Kübler-Ross, E. (1969). *On death and dying.* New York: Macmillan.

Lynch, G. P. (1988). Athletic injuries and the practicing sport psychologist: Practical guidelines for assisting athletes. *The Sport Psychologist, 2,* 161–167.

May, J. R., & Sieb, G. E. (1987). Athletic injuries: Psychosocial factors in the onset, sequelae, rehabilitation and prevention. In J. R. May & M. J. Ashen (Eds.). *Sport psychology* (pp. 157–185). Philadelphia: P.M.A. Publishing Corporation.

Nideffer, R. M. (1983). The injured athlete: Psychological factors in treatment. *Orthopedic Clinics of North America, 14,* 373–385.

Ogilvie, B. (1987). *Counseling patients with career-ending injuries.* Unpublished manuscript.

Ogilvie, B., & Howe, M. (1986). The trauma of termination from athletics. In J. M. Williams (Ed.), *Applied sport psychology* (pp. 365–382). Palo Alto, CA: Mayfield Publishing Company.

Poole, C., Henschen, K., Shultz, B., Gordin, R., & Hill, J. (1986). Psychological profiles of elite collegiate athletes according to performance level. In L. E. Unesthal (Ed.), *Contemporary sport psychology* (pp. 65–72). Orebro, Sweden: Veje Publishing, Inc.

Rando, T. A. (1984). *Grief, dying, and death.* Champaign, IL: Research Press Company.

Rotella, R. J. (1982). Psychological care of the injured athlete. In D. N. Kolund (Ed.), *The injured athlete* (pp. 138–149). Philadelphia: J. B. Lippincott.

Rotella, R., & Heyman, S. (1986). Stress, injury and the psychological rehabilitation of athletes. In J. M. Williams (Ed.), *Applied sport psychology* (pp. 343–364). Palo Alto, CA: Mayfield Publishing Company.

Samples, P. (1987). Mind over muscle: Returning the injured athlete to play. *The Physician and Sportsmedicine, 15,* (10), 172–180.

Suinn, R. M. (1967). Psychological reactions to physical disability. *Journal of the Association for Physical and Mental Rehabilitation, 21* (1), 13–15.

Wiese, D. M., & Weiss, M. R. (1987). Psychological rehabilitation and physical injury: Implications for the sportsmedicine team. *The Sport Psychologist, 1,* 318–330.

16

Providing Psychological Assistance to Injured and Disabled College Student-Athletes

Edward F. Etzel
Frank Perna
R. Renee Newcomer
West Virginia University

A. P. Ferrante
The Ohio State University

A significant number of college student-athletes regularly incur athletic injuries and disabilities. The authors discuss challenges encountered when working with this special population, the unique consequences associated with their losses in functioning, and ways of providing psychological assistance. Two cases are offered illustrating the nature and course of work with injured and disabled student-athletes.

In the summer of 1987, The National Collegiate Athletic Association's (NCAA) President's Commission hired The American Institutes for Research (AIR) to conduct a comprehensive survey of college student-athletes. The end product, The National Study of Intercollegiate Athletes (NSIA) (AIR, 1988), provided an unprecedented view of the reported experiences of both female and male NCAA Division I sport participants from 42 institutions throughout the country. Among many other things, slightly more than half of the respondents said that they had incurred an injury during their college days. As the NSIA summary results indicate, this figure would not be too shocking, given the frequency and intensity of physical activity associated with sport, if it were not also learned that 70% of football and basketball players and 50% of those who participated in other sports also said that they had experienced "intense" or "extremely intense" pressure to disregard their injuries (American Institutes for Research [AIR], 1988, p. 52). Other authors have also noted high rates of injury across intercollegiate sports (Lanese, Strauss, Leizman, & Rotondi, 1990; Zemper, 1989). Taken together, these data reveal the pervasiveness of injury experienced by college student-athletes as well as the need to help members of this special on-campus population cope with losses in functioning that they are either discouraged from addressing or denied.

Difficulties Providing Psychological Services to Student-Athletes

Assistance to injured student-athletes is typically provided by well-trained and caring athletic trainers and physical therapists, as well as by various sport medicine physicians. Their rehabilitative efforts traditionally focus on the physical trauma itself with treatments directed toward returning the student-athlete back to the field, court, track, or pool as soon as possible, unless the injury is disabling (i.e., it is a condition that is characterized by long-term or permanent losses in functioning). However, as Rotella and Heyman (1986) have pointed out, injured athletes often are not prepared to return to participation because they have had little time to adjust to loss, given the efficiency of modern rehabilitative interventions, and therefore commonly experience a wide range of concomitant psychological responses (e.g., anxiety, fear, depression). Unfortunately, these psychological responses appear to be infrequently addressed by collegiate sports medicine professionals, even in the case of distressing, disabling conditions.

Several reasons seem to underlie this rather narrow approach to rehabilitating physically impaired student-athletes. First, sports medicine professionals are usually not formally trained to consider psychological aspects of assisting the injured and disabled. They may not understand the potential usefulness of psychological consultation or intervention for the impaired student-athlete who is attempting to cope with loss of functioning. Although there occasionally are on-campus helping professionals (e.g., psychologists, counselors, or psychiatrists) who are formally or informally affiliated with the college or university sports medicine team and who could be helpful to the psychological rehabilitation of injured or disabled student-athletes, this does not seem to be the norm. What seems to be a common situation is one in which athletic department staffs are not aware of either the availability of helping professionals or the ways in which this expertise can be relevant to the rehabilitative process. If athletic department staffs are aware, they may not know how or when to refer an injured student-athlete.

Another obstacle is the prevalence and influence of the so-called "medical model" adhered to by the majority of sports medicine professionals, which does not place much emphasis on psychological approaches to the treatment of injury. Accordingly, helping professionals see fewer numbers of referrals of injured student-athletes from sports medicine professionals to on-campus psychological services than might be warranted. Limited consultations are likely to occur between sports medicine staff and mental health professionals, despite the frequency of injuries and the severity of many of them. Seeing what they believe, many sports medicine staff often may not sense the need to consult or refer an injured person.

In the end, such concern with physiology and not adjustment is seen as not helpful to injured and disabled student-athletes. Although it may be argued that sports medicine staff know the student-athletes they serve very well, adhering closely to the medical model may not provide injured people with the amount and range of care that can help in the holistic rehabilitation of those who are injured or have a disability. It has been shown that psychological support can be a very useful adjunct to medical interventions because the effects of injury are not limited to the afflicted body part(s) alone (Eldridge, 1983; Lynch, 1988).

Reluctance to involve helping professionals is somewhat understandable. Even in the 1990s, psychological treatment remains a mystery for many people. Stereotypic images of the couch and the bearded analyst persist; misconceptions about who seeks help from such people (i.e., only those who are mentally ill or crazy) contribute to the avoidance of on-campus helping professionals (even if they are affiliated with the athletic department staff) and their services. In fact, college students in general, and student-athletes in particular, tend to underutilize psychological services for many reasons (Pinkerton, Hinz, & Barrow, 1987).

Even if student-athletes know about psychological services and are referred for help, several obstacles make such assistance typically difficult to tap or completely inaccessible to them. Some of those barriers are (a) the "high visibility" of student-athletes on campus, (b) the limited amount of time available to seek outside help, (c) misconceptions about the personalities of student-athletes, (d) the restrictive nature of the athletic environment, and (e) certain attributes of student-athletes (Ferrante & Etzel, 1991).

Visibility. Student-athletes are often high-profile members of their school's community. Their names and faces regularly appear in the media. They may stand out in a crowd because of their size: A well-known personality on crutches is quite recognizable. Accordingly, student-athletes often avoid places like counseling and psychological service centers because they cannot easily seek assistance as privately as others can. There is often reluctance manifested in the forms of anxiety and shame that makes it difficult for students in general to seek help. Student-athletes' notoriety can further compound the problem.

Time demands. Whether in or out of season, student-athletes lead hectic, stressful lifestyles (AIR, 1988; Etzel, 1989). Time is a precious commodity. Although recent NCAA legislation has put a cap on the number of hours that those who participate in intercollegiate athletics may be involved in sport-related activities (i.e., 20 hours per week), historically student-athletes have spent much more than 20 hours conditioning, practicing, and competing. The National Study of Intercollegiate Athletes (AIR, 1988) revealed that in 1987–88 student-athletes reported participating in excess of 30 hours per week in their chosen sport(s). Participants in that same study reported that they spent more time participating in athletics-related activities than they did preparing for and attending classes. Clearly, there are individual differences in the amount of time devoted to participation across schools and programs of differing competitive levels. Nevertheless, when combined with the amount of time that must be devoted to academic responsibilities, daily individual responsibilities and a personal life, little time is left during a highly structured day to seek professional help from service centers that are typically open from 8 A.M. to 5 P.M. Student-athlete frustration with this situation is common. We cannot recall the number of times a student-athlete has said to us: "Doc, I just can't seem to make it in."

Misconceptions about student-athletes. Student-athletes, in particular football and men's basketball players, and members of other athletic teams on certain campuses, are often seen by the community as a spoiled, "overprivileged" group (Remer, Tongate, & Watson, 1978). Some may assume that the athletic department is taking care of all of their needs. Therefore, on-campus helping service providers who could be of assistance to those who become injured or disabled may not see a need to reach out to a group perceived as pampered or they may be reluctant to do so because they are anti-athletics. Although some student-athletes may be "spoiled," if they are young people who truly have a need for personal assistance in the wake of an injury, it should be as available to them as it is for any other student.

Restrictive environments. Over the years, many athletic departments have come to be seen by others, and often by themselves, as autonomous organizations on campus. Sperber (1990) goes so far as to say that many athletic departments are merely entertainment businesses that have essentially no real connection to the mission of their respective academic institutions. Independent-minded athletic department staff may not trust mental health professionals or other "outsiders" with the care of their student-athletes. Somehow, it is erroneously assumed that all student-athlete needs can be met by athletic department staff alone (except in times of true crisis). Indeed, the "We can take care of our own in-house" attitude appears to be held by many athletic department staff (e.g., coaches).

Student-athlete attributes and developmental tasks. Other barriers to injured college student-athletes seeking psychological assistance are various personal characteristics (e.g., behaviors and attitudes), as well as certain so-called "developmental tasks" that all college students face.

As a group, student-athletes tend to be a rather independent lot, which is understandable in view of some of the messages they may learn from influential others in the athletic world. Also, individualism is characteristic of college students in general. Indeed, one of the major developmental tasks of college students involves struggling to become an independent adult (Chickering, 1969). Over time, many student-athletes seem to acquire a sense that they can solve most (if not all) of their difficulties. They also seem to learn through sport to be strong and to minimize or deny physical and emotional pain. If one is not tough or "macho," one is somehow an inferior peer. Therefore, injured or disabled student-athletes may not ask for or seek help even though they may be experiencing considerable distress. "When rugged individualism . . . leads to, or heightens, an unwillingness to seek or accept assistance, athletes will find themselves separated from existing and potential sources of social support"(Pearson & Petitpas, 1990, p. 9). Consequently, persistent encouragement to seek outside psychological assistance on the part of referral sources (e.g., athletic trainers) is often necessary to get assistance from helping professionals for an independent-minded, injured, or disabled student-athlete.

Another developmental task that this group must work through involves learning to deal effectively with authority (Farnsworth, 1966). Those who have problems relating to powerful others often will not respond to their guidance or direction. Consequently, referral for psychological assistance may be met with resistance, even though it is in the best interest of the injured person. Therefore, if people with such difficulties who do come to obtain help are forced to do so by others (e.g., coaches or trainers), they must be handled with sensitivity so as not to alienate them.

It is not uncommon for those who do ultimately make contact with a helping professional to expect that they can obtain relief in a very brief amount of time and/or without much personal effort. Upon becoming aware of this agenda (the "quick fix"), the astute clinician must carefully educate the injured person about the nature of psychological treatment (e.g., roles of client and therapist, goal setting, responsibility for change and ways in which it may occur) so as to create realistic expectations for their work together.

Finally, for those who can have an impact on assisting injured or disabled student-athletes, it will be helpful to assume a broader view of the individuals who are both college students and participants in athletics. Student-athletes are not students or athletes first and foremost. Rather, they are developing young *people* in transition who are in the process of becoming adults. They are continuously working through the many developmental tasks that people at their stage in life are confronted with such as (a) becoming independent; (b) dealing with authority; (c) learning to deal with uncertainty and ambiguity; (d) developing personal standards, values, and a sense of purpose; (e) developing a mature sexuality; (f) developing feelings of security and competence; (g) establishing personal identity and attaining prestige and esteem; and (h) managing emotions (Chickering, 1969; Farnsworth, 1969). Further, their roles of students and entertainers frequently make the transition from childhood to adulthood more complicated (Ferrante & Etzel, 1991). Therefore, it is most useful to view their experiencing of athletic injury and disability within the context of their uniquely demanding lifestyles.

Clearly, our position underlines the importance of taking a "holistic" approach to the treatment, rehabilitation, and aftercare of injured and disabled student-athletes. We believe that the student-athlete is a *person* first, and it is from this "person-ness" that the athletic, academic, developmental, and career needs evolve. Accordingly, athletic injury can be regarded as both an obstacle and a threat to the realization of long- and short-term needs and goals. Injury and disability can leave student-athletes vulnerable to distress that can complicate and inhibit the process of physical and psychological rehabilitation. We believe that injured or disabled student-athletes can best be served by understanding their unique needs within the context of their individual histories, personalities, current experiences, and aspirations.

The Unique Consequences of Incurring an Injury for College Student-Athletes

The ways that people characteristically respond to sport-related injury and the theoretical concepts that help us to understand why they respond in these ways have been discussed in previous chapters of this book and in other resources (Astle, 1986; May & Seib, 1987; Rotella & Heyman, 1986; Silva & Hardy, in press; Tunick, Etzel, & Leard, 1991). Therefore, we will not review them here. There are, however, several points that we believe can help the reader understand how college student-athletes respond to injury and/or disability and how to better assist them as they struggle to cope with their losses.

The novelty of loss. First, when young student-athletes' physical capacities are suddenly or progressively not what they have been throughout life, it may simply be the first time this has ever been encountered. They typically have been successful, highly functioning people. The world of injury and loss is foreign territory for many student-athletes. Indeed, many young people age 18–21 often have a limited, if any, history of significant losses. They may have little appreciation of the finite nature of human capacities. When student-athletes are not capable of doing what they have taken for granted all their lives, it can be a very frustrating, unwanted revelation. For adults in a position to assist injured or disabled young athletes—adults who usually own a more extensive loss history—it may be difficult to appreciate the magnitude and complexity of the problem. Therefore, it is important that coaches, sport medicine, and helping professionals not underestimate or discount the impact of injury on student-athletes.

The effects of changed status. As is the case with noncollegiate athletes, when student-athletes become injured or disabled, their lives may change in various ways psychosocially. Over time, student-athletes often become isolated and alienated from their peers, experience changes in their social status, and may encounter new academic/developmental concerns (Ermler & Thomas, 1990; Pearson & Petitpas, 1990; Tunick et al., 1991).

Student-athletes who cannot participate in day-to-day athletic activities (e.g., conditioning, practicing, traveling, and competing) become separated from their teammates, coaches, and others with whom they normally interact. Because they can no longer function in their customary roles, injured people become gradually or suddenly estranged from their previously predictable and supportive social network. Sadly, they sometimes are intentionally ignored, set aside, or criticized by insensitive coaches or peers for being injured (which somehow implies that one is weak, less valuable, or not committed enough to "tough it out"). More commonly, the impaired student-athlete becomes gradually separated from others. The time once spent on the field or in the weight room is now spent in the care of athletic trainers in the athletic training room—if fortunate, with some time sitting on the bench watching others do the now impossible. One disabled client succinctly described the confusion and frustration of being in this unfortunate situation in the following way: "It's like I'm on the team, but I'm really not. I don't know what else to do."

Other relationships change for injured or disabled student-athletes. Although their conditions often make them the focus of public attention for a while, as time passes they fade from the spotlight, their stories become old news, and healthy others take their places. Students and media do not pay as much attention to the student-athlete as they did in the past. Social opportunities often become fewer for the former BMOC or BWOC. There are no tales to relate about the upcoming game or meet; only recollections of bygone accomplishments and the unglamorous rehabilitation process are left to tell. Special status is lost or at least diminished.

Confronted with the reality of assuming a radically different, usually unanticipated, lifestyle, injured and disabled student-athletes face different academic situations and challenges. More free time is often available to injured student-athletes whose rehabilitation activities do not consume a large part of the day (although they may witness the case of an injured yet active player who receives 4 hours of rehabilitation daily to stay in playing condition). In such situations, academic priorities can come more to the forefront and serve as a "blessing in disguise" for those who have neglected their studies. Previously flexible professors who do not appreciate the need for continued accommodation, however, may become less sympathetic to the impaired student-athlete who may still need occasional special arrangements in view of the demands and inconveniences of the rehabilitation process (Tunick et al., 1991).

For disabled student-athletes, especially those whose injury is career ending, academic priorities and career paths will probably need to be reexamined over time. When faced with this major life transition, school frequently assumes a higher priority in life. A reassessment of interests, skills, and abilities is often warranted. On-campus helping professionals who are trained in career-vocational counseling can be great assets in such cases. (See Riffee & Alexander, 1991 for a discussion of career counseling strategies for student-athletes.) In the case of disabled student-athletes, educational-vocational counseling and supportive psychotherapy can be undertaken concurrently and interactively as there is considerable overlap in the concerns seen in such cases (Pinkerton, Etzel, Rockwell, Talley, & Moorman, 1990).

Injured and disabled student-athletes may benefit from such combined psychological interventions to address questions about changing personal identity (i.e., confidence in maintaining a sense of continuity and sameness of the self) (Chickering, 1969). (The reader will recall that developing a sense of identity is one of the major developmental life tasks of college students.) When impaired student-athletes are forced to examine for themselves and for others who they are when they cannot be who they once were, they are often left with an overwhelming sense of confusion and numbness. Kir-Stimon's (1977) discussion of the mind-set of severely disabled persons at the onset of emotional rehabilitation is very similar to what we often hear injured and disabled student-athletes say to themselves:

Who am I?

I am different than I was.

I don't like me.

Nobody likes me.

I am not worthwhile.

Perhaps I never was worthwhile.

Who was I?

I have no real identity anymore.

I have changed. Nothing is the same as before.

My friends, my family, the world about me has changed.

I am lost.

(Kir-Stimon, 1977, p. 365)

Answering the question of "Who am I if I'm not an athlete?" becomes very difficult because many student-athletes have "foreclosed" on their identities early in life. That is, many have learned to identify themselves as athletes at a young age and so act in ways that are consistent with their self-perceptions (Chartrand & Lent, 1987). Therefore, it can be very disturbing to student-athletes (especially for the alarming number of male baseball, basketball, and football players who expect to become professionals) when the identity of being an athlete must be abandoned. Indeed, research indicates that many student-athletes are less mature than their nonathlete peers in terms of being able to make mature educational and career plans (Blann, 1985; Sowa & Gressard, 1983). Consequently, referring injured and disabled student-athletes to obtain professional assistance for personal-social and educational-vocational concerns is often very timely from a developmental standpoint.

Methods of Providing Psychological Assistance to Injured or Disabled Student-Athletes

Although the number seems to be growing, only a few universities today appear to have professionally trained psychologists, counselors, or psychiatrists whose duties specifically involve providing direct psychological service to student-athletes. Most of these institutions utilize professionals who are members of counseling services. Some have a staff member who serves as a liaison with the athletic department. A small number of schools have a professional who is affiliated with both the athletic department and a helping service (Ferrante & Etzel, 1991). Whatever the administrative arrangement, on-campus helping professionals who are interested in or who have been hired to provide assistance to student-athletes in general, and in particular those who are injured and disabled, face many challenges.

As mentioned above, several barriers serve to separate helping professionals from injured or disabled student-athletes who could benefit from their expertise. To begin to bridge the gaps that exist, the helping professional must have the outside support of the athletic director and the chief student affairs officer. These two influential people can assist the helping professional in the initial efforts to establish credibility within the often closed athletic community. These people have the power to create an inroad to staff and student-athletes that the helping professional may otherwise never develop alone.

Given a crack in the door, the helping professional must begin the process of educating the athletic community about the potential usefulness of psychological assistance to injured and disabled student-athletes. In general, coaches, student-athletes, sports medicine staff, and administrators do not appear to readily understand how such services can be helpful (or they may be resistant for reasons mentioned earlier). Establishing credibility is a long-term project that can be quite frustrating. Indeed, one of the authors of this chapter was reminded by an athletic department administrator: "Remember, 95% of the people here don't care about what you do."

Meeting with coaches, sports medicine staff, and each team is an effective way of introducing the professional to potential referral sources and consumers of services. With the permission of coaches and sports medicine staff, regularly attending practices and visiting athletic training rooms are also effective ways of familiarizing people with the helping professional and the services available to injured and disabled student-athletes. It may also serve to undo some of the stigma associated with psychologists (i.e., "Dr. X is an OK person who is interested in helping us and who can be trusted").

Perhaps the most important relationship to establish and nurture is the one between athletic trainers and the helping professional. Athletic trainers historically have a very special relationship with coaches and student-athletes (Compton & Ferrante, 1991). They are perhaps the most trusted people within the athletic community. Indeed, their services are clearly understood, needed, and utilized on a daily basis. This is typically not the case with mental health professionals and their services, unless such services have been used for some time. Developing close ties with the athletic training staff can be very helpful to the accessing of injured and disabled student-athletes and their coaches. Such a relationship can enhance the extent to which helping professionals are accepted and trusted by the athletic community. Also, athletic trainers can be good referral sources of student-athletes who have been injured or who have other difficulties of which the athletic trainer becomes aware (e.g., personal problems, substance use, performance decrements). Given the opportunity, presenting to student trainers on mental health issues, psychological aspects of injury and disability, communication skills, and referral methods can help develop good working relationships between helping professionals and the athletic training staff. Student athletic trainers can become effective referrers of injured and disabled student-athletes with such training.

Finally, another method of facilitating the provision of psychological assistance to injured or disabled student-athletes is to conduct needs assessments and other surveys. For example, collecting data on the psychological responses to loss of functioning can help establish the need to provide counseling or therapy. Undertaking research in collaboration with interested sports medicine staff members can provide a wealth of useful information and can further promote the cooperative efforts of athletic trainers and helping professionals.

The Effects of Injury and Disability on College Student-Athletes: Two Case Examples

The following case examples are offered to provide further insight into the psychological impact of sport injuries and the role of psychological services in the treatment and follow-up of injured and disabled student-athletes. Each case describes the general course of counseling with an NCAA Division I-A student-athlete. Due to ethical considerations relating to issues of confidentiality, these cases are presented in composite form. Although these situations may have involved both female and male clients, the following examples are referenced only in the male gender.

Case 1

A student-athlete was referred for consultation and recommendations by the director of sports medicine following extensive neurological and other medical examinations. Several months prior to the referral, the student-athlete had experienced a number of symptoms including paresthesia (i.e., numbing and tingling sensations in the hands and feet and part of the face) with accompanying motoric changes, blurred vision, and generally decreased coordination. Results of subsequent examinations revealed that the student-athlete had experienced a demyelinating episode, a phenomenon that is seen in several disorders of unknown etiology. Of these, multiple sclerosis (MS) is the most prominent. The diagnosis of MS becomes quite difficult in that it requires the occurrence of a second demyelinating episode; remission can be quite long-term (e.g., up to 25 years). Consequently, a firm diagnosis could not be made. However, the student-athlete was provided with information to help better understand his general medical situation as it existed. Then, the student-athlete was referred for psychological services, to assess his current psychological functioning and to obtain emotional support and decision-making assistance.

In the initial session, the student-athlete complained of feeling frustrated, discouraged, and intermittently angry and sad. He also reported feeling anxious in view of the "incomplete diagnosis," its potential limitations regarding the questions of his continued sport participation, and uncertainties regarding his personal functioning in the future. Further exploration of the situation revealed that his parents appeared to be denying the implications of the medical examinations. Stating that they "didn't raise a quitter," they were pressing him to continue to participate in his sport. He was also afraid of disappointing his teammates and coach and felt threatened by the possibility of not meeting their expectations. Unfortunately, the student-athlete was physically incapable of performing at the high skill level that he had previously achieved and, as a result, was experiencing considerable dissonance.

In consultation with the referring physician, it was agreed that a treatment team would be formed consisting of the physician, an athletic trainer, and a clinical/counseling sport psychologist. The treatment team plan involved (a) monitoring the student-athlete's medical progress and providing information about the condition, (b) developing and implementing a "controlled" workout/training regimen, and (c) providing supportive counseling/psychotherapy to help him cope with various stressors and assist with decision making relative to the situation.

The student-athlete's participation in regular counseling provided a confidential, professional setting in which he was continually encouraged to explore his concerns and feelings. Over the course of several months, he received help dealing with the personal-social stress surrounding the need to make important decisions (e.g., whether he should prematurely end his sports career, how to interact with his coaches and parents) without the aid of a firm diagnosis. With the assistance of the psychologist, he also was able to resolve issues surrounding his parents and their expectations, as well as the pressures of his coach and teammates.

The role of the athletic trainer and the controlled workout/training regimen held special, strategic significance to the process and outcome of the case. More specifically, the student-athlete faced a number of difficult decisions—each without the benefit of a concrete diagnosis, information that would have made decisions more clear-cut. The controlled workout setting allowed for the development of progressive training goals and the monitoring of any physiological distress, if it occurred. In that setting the student-athlete was encouraged to test progressive limits comfortably, away from the coach's watchful eye and any teammate pressures. With the support of the athletic trainer, the student-athlete was able to gain confidence and experience-based insight into his current level of functioning by seeing gradual increases in performance with or without symptoms. Having made significant progress in the controlled training program, the student-athlete ultimately rejoined his team with the permission of the physician. Although it was gratifying for him to be a part of his team again, he had experienced ongoing discouragement for some time in view of the fact that his athletic abilities were still well below their previous level. As a consequence of this dissatisfaction, following the conclusion of his season, he announced to his psychologist that he had decided to pursue a medical release and resign from the team—something he had considered and processed in counseling. His plan was to focus on academics and to continue with other campus and community involvements. The student-athlete continued his counseling relationship for some time and obtained assistance with concerns surrounding his premature retirement from sport, as well as issues concerning his personal adjustment to a different lifestyle.

Case 2

K. was an 18-year-old freshman student-athlete who was referred by an athletic trainer to the psychologist for athletics soon after the beginning of the first semester of the academic year. K. had been a very successful high school student and athlete who had no previous history of injury. He was excited about beginning college and had worked hard on a daily basis over the summer to get into shape for his first season of athletic participation. K. had only been on campus for a month when during an informal conditioning activity, he unfortunately incurred a serious orthopedic injury. The injury required immediate surgery. Although the procedure was successful, the injury left K. disabled, facing a painful rehabilitation process that would last several months.

When he came to our first session soon after the surgery, K. reported feeling depressed, angry, and very frustrated in the wake of the totally unexpected turn of events in his life. It seemed unfair to him that, despite all his hard work, he had fallen victim to this injury. K. had just begun to feel that he was becoming a part of his team when he was suddenly torn away from them. Although he had begun to receive treatment from a very competent and caring athletic trainer, he suddenly felt alone and alienated from his newfound peers. K. recognized he was still officially part of his team, but in reality he knew that he would have to wait until next season to join them as a healthy teammate. An unprecedented personal struggle against physical and psychological pain lay ahead.

Other difficulties made the effects of the injury even worse. K. had indicated that he was considering psychological assistance before his injury in view of a long-standing conflict with one of his parents with whom he had not lived with for several years. He had struggled with his parents' separation on and off over the years. This parent had been trying to reconnect with him, and he was troubled about whether to do so and, if so, how to proceed. The issue appeared to be particularly important at the time given K.'s need for emotional support from primary caregivers. As an aside, he was receiving support from a distance from the parent with whom he lived and a stepparent, support that was very helpful to his recovery.

From a developmental standpoint, K. was also confronted with the considerable task of becoming an independent person. Adjusting to school in a healthy fashion, he had begun to make the transition away from home and family. Before his injury, K. indicated that he was a happy person. After having felt homesick for a short time, the number of phone calls had dropped off and things were going well. However, his injury forced K. to have to depend on his family once again and slowed down the process of being an independent young adult. He knew that he could not solve his problems alone.

Within a few sessions we established a good working relationship. K. was encouraged to explore his thoughts and feelings about the issues mentioned earlier, and he was comfortable doing so. His mood improved progressively over time as he became engaged in school and in his rehabilitation. However, K. continually struggled with his feelings of isolation from his team. We worked on ways that he could spend time with them, if only briefly. This was quite difficult for K. to do because his rehabilitation was regularly scheduled during the team's practice sessions, and he experienced mobility difficulties. He often saw some of his teammates in the athletic training room and appreciated their contact and concern. Occasionally, K. made it out to their practice site toward the end of practices, something that was enjoyable yet frustrating and depressing, because he could do little else but watch. When the team's season started, K. could not travel with them early on; this was also a source of distress. Eventually, K. was able to travel with them as his condition improved. This was a great relief for him, which he saw as a sign of reconnecting with the peers he longed to be with.

Our work also focused on the rehabilitation process itself. K. and his athletic trainer had set challenging yet realistic goals for his recovery. Although he worked hard and made exceptional progress, he had to work through considerable daily pain. K. shared the pain he experienced, something he did not want to share with or could not do with others, with his psychologist. K. also worked together on fears he had about moving on to increasingly more challenging levels of activity. He received support and encouragement from his athletic trainer and psychologist to continue to take small steps, which he did. With each step, he gained confidence and learned to deal with uncertainty.

All the while, K.'s concern about his estranged parent became progressively less important. So much time and energy were taken up with school and rehabilitation that K. chose not to address the issue at the time. It was just too much for him. He decided to work hard in both areas until he was back to normal.

Over the course of counseling, which lasted a few months, K.'s psychologist occasionally visited him in the athletic training room as he went through his rehabilitation activities, something he appreciated. Ultimately, K. indicated that it was very helpful for him to have had someone who was available to listen to him and support him as he worked to overcome his injury and disability. He performed very well academically during his ordeal and remained a well-adjusted person upon follow-up. Interestingly, K. said he was thinking about becoming an athletic trainer.

Conclusion

The foregoing has been an attempt to present information about ways to provide psychological support to a special group of young people—college student-athletes. To assist more fully their coping with and recovery from injury and disability, it is important to understand their unique lifestyles and the developmental tasks that they must confront, as well as the barriers that exist to their seeking and/or obtaining helping services. The authors hope that our observations and suggestions will prove useful to readers who want to better understand and more effectively assist the considerable numbers of student-athletes who experience sport-related losses in functioning each year.

284

SECTION 4 • CHAPTER 16

References

Astle, S. (1986). The experience of loss in athletes. *Journal of Sports Medicine, 26,* 279–284.

American Institutes for Research (AIR). (1988). *Summary results from the 1987–88 national study of intercollegiate athletes* (Report No.1). Palo Alto, CA: Center for the Study of Athletics.

Blann, F. (1985). Intercollegiate athletic competition and students' educational and career plans. *Journal of College Student Personnel, 26,* 115–118.

Chartrand, J., & Lent, R. (1987). Sports counseling: Enhancing the development of the student athlete. *Journal of College Student Personnel, 66,* 164–167.

Chickering, A. (1969). *Education and identity.* Washington, DC: Jossey-Bass.

Compton, R., & Ferrante, A. (1991). The athletic trainer-helping professional relationship: An essential element for the enhanced support programming for student-athletes. In E. Etzel, A. Ferrante, & J. Pinkney, (Eds.), *Counseling college student-athletes: Issues and interventions* (pp. 221–230). Morgantown, WV: Fitness Information Technology.

Eldridge, W. (1983). The importance of psychotherapy for athletic related orthopedic injuries among adults. *Comprehensive Psychiatry, 24,* 271–277.

Ermler, K., & Thomas, C. (1990). Interventions for the alienating effect of injury. *Athletic Training, 25,* 269–271.

Etzel, E. (1989). *Life stress, locus of control, and sport competition anxiety patterns of college student-athletes.* Unpublished doctoral dissertation, West Virginia University, Morgantown.

Farnsworth, D. (1966). *Psychiatry, education, and the young adult.* Springfield, IL: Thomas.

Ferrante, A., & Etzel, E. (1991). Counseling college student-athletes: The problem, the need. In E. Etzel, A. Ferrante, & J. Pinkney (Eds.), *Counseling college student-athletes: Issues and interventions* (pp.1–19). Morgantown, WV: Fitness Information Technology.

Kir-Stimon, W. (1977). Counseling with the severely handicapped: Encounter and commitment. In R. Marinelli & A. Del Orto (Eds.), *Psychological and social impact of physical disability* (pp. 363–369). New York: Springer.

Lanese, R., Strauss, R., Leizman, D., & Rotondi, A. (1990). Injury and disability in matched men's and women's intercollegiate sports. *American Journal of Public Health, 80,* 1459–1462.

Lynch, G. (1988). Athletic injuries and the practicing sport psychologist: Practical guidelines for assisting athletes. *The Sport Psychologist, 2,* 161–167.

May, J., & Seib, G. (1987). Athletic injuries: Psychological factors in the onset, sequelae, and prevention. In J. May & M. Asken (Eds.), *Sport psychology: The psychological health of the athlete* (pp.157–185). Great Neck, NY: PMA.

Pearson, R., & Petitpas, A. (1990). Transitions of athletes: Developmental and preventive perspectives. *Journal of Counseling and Development, 69,* 7–10.

Pinkerton, R., Etzel, E., Talley, J., & Moorman, J. (1990). Psychotherapy and career counseling: Toward an integration for use with college students. *Journal of American College Health, 39,* 129–136.

Pinkerton, R., Hinz, L., & Barrow, J. (1987). The college student-athlete: Psychological considerations and interventions. *Journal of American College Health ,37,* 218–226.

Remer, R., Tongate, R., & Watson, J. (1978). Counseling the underprivileged minority. *The Personnel and Guidance Journal, 56,* 626–619.

Riffee, K., & Alexander, D. (1991). Career strategies for student-athletes: A developmental model. In E. Etzel, A. Ferrante, & J. Pinkney (Eds.), *Counseling college student-athletes: Issues and interventions* (pp. 101–120). Morgantown, WV: Fitness Information Technology.

Rotella, R., & Heyman, S. (1986). Stress, injury, and the psychological rehabilitation of athletes. In J. Williams (Ed.), *Applied sport psychology: Personal growth to peak performance* (pp. 343–364). Palo Alto, CA: Mayfield.

Silva, J., & Hardy, C. (in press). The sport psychologist: Psychological aspects of injury in sport. In F. Meuller & A. Ryan (Eds.), *The sports medicine team and athlete injury prevention.* Philadelphia: F. A. Davis.

Sowa, C., & Gressard, C. (1983). Athletic participation: Its relationship to student development. *Journal of College Student Personnel, 26,* 236–239.

Sperber, M. (1990). *College sports inc.: The athletic department vs the university.* New York: Henry Holt.

Tunick, R., Etzel, E., & Leard, J. (1991). Counseling injured and disabled student-athletes: A guide for understanding and intervention. In E. Etzel, A. Ferrante, & J. Pinkney (Eds.), *Counseling college student-athletes: Issues and interventions* (pp. 199–220). Morgantown, WV: Fitness Information Technology.

Zemper, E. (1989). Injury rates in a national sample of college football teams: A 2-year prospective study. *The Physician and Sportsmedicine, 17,* 100–102, 105–108, 113.

17

Suicide in Sport:
Are Athletes at Risk?

Jane Henderson
John Abbott College, Quebec, Canada

If you are reading this then I guess I did the job. It is not anyone's fault, it was my decision nobody else's. I have been thinking about suicide since grade 7 I just never had the courage to just go ahead and do it. I'm just too tired of living just to damn lazy, and I do not feel like going on. I know I will never make it to Notre Dame sure *I might be good on my team but to make it I would have to be the best in Canada, and I just don't have the talent. World Cup skiing is just something that is totally out of reach.* I have never been the best at anything to make it big in this day en age it just isn't being in the right place at the right time. I want all my friends and family to just keep going on with there normal life with out me.

(Suicide note written by a 15-year-old, captain of the football team and MVP, who killed himself by gunshot; Corbella, 1996).

Suicide is a conscious act of self-induced annihilation best understood as a multi-dimensional malaise in a needful individual who defines an issue for which suicide is perceived as the best solution. (Shneidman, 1985, p. 203)

According to the Center for Disease Control and Prevention (1995), the incidence of suicide among teenagers and young adults has nearly tripled in the United States over the last 40 years. Suicide is now the second leading cause of death among adolescents. Canada has the dubious distinction of having one of the highest teenage suicide rates in the industrialized world (Health Canada, 1994). However, completed suicides only partially reveal the extent of this phenomenon; suicide attempts are much more prevalent. It is estimated that an average of 500,000 teenage suicide attempts are made in the United States every year, or one per minute (Anthony, 1988).

Alarmingly, the suicide rate for those 15 to 19 years of age has increased by almost 30% in the last 10 years ("Suicide Among Children," 1995). After taking into consideration the suicides that are labelled accidental, such as drug overdoses or single car accidents, most experts agree that the actual number of suicides in this age-group is from 5 to 20 times higher. Suicide then, especially among teenagers, is a serious public health problem. Surprisingly, suicide experts are finding that more and more suicide victims tend to be high achievers in school and sport as well as seemingly well-balanced individuals.

Media reports of recent suicides of Olympic-level athletes in Canada, the United States, and Australia suggest that athletes as a group are being overlooked as potential suicide victims. There is a tendency among those who coach and train athletes to view them as more psychologically sound than their typical nonathlete peers, and therefore not to expect athletes to commit suicide. In fact, recent research examining college students' attributions about suicide showed that athletes who committed suicide were viewed as more competent and in less distress than were nonathletes who committed suicide (Lewis & Shepard, 1992). These young athletes were thought to be immune from typical adolescent stressors. For these reasons, suicide has not been a popular topic of research in sport. Only three articles were available on this subject at the time of this writing, with only one being empirical in nature. Presently, there are no chapters addressing this issue in any sport psychology texts. Because virtually no records are kept on the numbers of suicides in sport, either by current or past participants, little is available to sport psychologists on this topic. In contrast to the perceptions noted above, those at risk for suicidal behavior (nonathletes) have generally been thought to be suffering from severe psychopathology. However, more recent research has revealed that sociodemographic variables, such as parental loss, divorce, and disappointment, may put young people at high risk for suicide (Holinger, 1989). Other studies have emphasized the role that stressful life events may play in provoking suicide in youth (Pfeffer, 1986). Young athletes are certainly not exempt from these pressures. A case in point: Sarah Devens was captain of three sports teams at Dartmouth and probably the best woman athlete the school ever had. The stress of high expectations and her own competitive spirit may have contributed to her death by suicide (Callahan & Steptoe, 1995). Olympic world-class athletes, in particular, must face formidable stress. Paul Thomson, a member of Canada's 1988 and 1992 Olympic sailing team, died when he jumped off a bridge. It is thought that Thomson was grappling with what he felt were poor results at the 1992 Olympiad (Ireland, 1994).

Much has been written about the stress-reducing properties of exercise. Nevertheless, the relationship between exercise intensity and mood alteration remains unclear (Berger & Owen, 1992). The relationship between exercise and mood is not always a positive one. Berger and Owen (1992) conclude that although there is a need to clarify the relationship between exercise and mood, enough data exist to suggest that those wishing positive psychological benefits should avoid intense or prolonged exercise. However, athletes vying for improved performance are often subjected to gruelling and lengthy training sessions, possibly resulting in extreme fatigue and negative emotion. In combination with other stressors and interacting with certain personality traits, intense training may be detrimental to the psychological well-being of teenagers. For some athletes then, strenuous exercise along with other stressors may increase the risk of suicidal behavior.

Psychopathology may then not be the only reason teenagers and young adults, especially athletes, attempt to take their own lives. In light of the occurrence of recent suicides in sport, it appears crucial for sport psychologists to reexamine their perceptions and assumptions about the risk of suicide in athletes. One longitudinal study has determined that 69 known Major League Baseball players have committed suicide. Most of these suicides occurred during the off-season or after retirement (Coleman & Lester, 1989). Because sport represents a microcosm of society (Eitzen & Sage, 1982) and because suicide rates are increasing, especially among young adults, athletes will be at least as vulnerable to suicidal behavior as the general population will be. The rigors of an athletic lifestyle may place athletes at greater risk for suicide under some circumstances, but actually lessen the risk under others.

This chapter addresses suicide among athletes. It discusses hypothesized, causally related issues as well as preventative factors.

Why Are Athletes at Risk?

What are the conditions that might contribute to athletes' suicide attempts? It is difficult to answer this question, because no empirical data about causal factors are available. Therefore, information derived from the general population has been extrapolated to sport populations. Suicide is a very complex, multidimensional phenomenon, and probably no one factor exclusively accounts for its attempt. A multiple-risk factor approach is the most appropriate model to employ. No psychological profile of the person likely to attempt suicide has been identified; however, after-the-fact analysis of suicide victims has revealed some factors that may be involved. Similarly, there may be additional factors that would place an athlete at risk for committing suicide:

* Age-group (15–24 years)
* Biochemical fluctuations due to diet and weight loss and intense exercise
* Personal loss: relationships, injury, retirement, performance, cuts from sport teams
* Narcissistic and perfectionistic personalities
* Coaching behaviors

Age and Developmental Considerations

Most high school, college, and professional athletes are part of a high-risk age-group for suicide. Coincidentally, the prevalence of suicidal thoughts peaks among young people in the 15- to 24-year age group, which is twice the rate for other age groups (Emond et al., 1988). In the United States, suicide is the second leading cause of death for persons 15 to 24 years of age. More than 1 in every 1,000 children will attempt to commit suicide before reaching the age of 25 (Center for Disease Control, 1986). What makes this age-group especially vulnerable is the tendency for "all-or-nothing" thinking. Unlike adults, they have neither the experience nor the ability to see that all failures or defeats are not permanent.

Adolescence is a period of rapid and profound physical and cognitive emotional changes, or as Petersen and Hamburg (1986) suggest, a critical transition period. Most adolescents "successfully navigate through adolescence learning to use developing skills to solve problems" (Berman & Jobes, 1994, p.55). However, a minority of them experience great difficulty in achieving the challenging and difficult transition to adulthood. For some, suicide appears to be the only solution. Suicide experts agree that suicidal individuals tend to view suicide as impermanent and deny its reality (Allen, 1987). Rather, they view it as a continuation of pain-free life and fail to understand that suicide results in a permanent state—death. A recent study by Tousignant, Hamel, and Bastien (1988) of 2,327 secondary students in the province of Québec in Canada (average age 16.3 years) revealed that 6.7% of young people have already attempted suicide. In addition, three times as many girls as boys make the attempt; however, more boys succeed, as they tend to choose more lethal means (Garfinkle, Froese, & Hood, 1982).

Dietary Factors

Dietary practices and associated biochemical changes related to weight loss in athletes may also be factors in psychological depression, which can, in some (but not all) cases, lead to suicide. Athletes trying to lose weight might be under considerable stress, which may be associated with depressive episodes. Depression may be an antecedent of attempted suicide. It is also thought that nutritional deficiency may affect mood (Wurtman & Wurtman, 1986; Young, 1986). For instance, folate deficiency has been shown to cause a decrease in the level of the brain chemical, serotonin (Botez, Botez, & Maag, 1984), which in turn has been speculated to be linked with depression (Young, 1986).

A variety of violent impulsive behaviors have also been linked with lower than normal levels of serotonin. The National Institute of Mental Health (Waters, 1994) reports that, based upon 22 autopsies of the brain and body fluids of suicide victims, there appears to be a connection between low levels of serotonin and suicide. The precursor of serotonin is L-tryptophan, normally produced by the body but dietarily contained in many carbohydrate foods. Animal studies have confirmed that altering dietary L-tryptophan can influence serotonin levels (Wurtman & Wurtman, 1984). Sufficient levels of brain serotonin are known to be important in the regulation of eating, mood, and impulse control (Garfinkle & Kaplan, 1985). It is conceivable that athletes restricting their diets in an attempt to make weight may be placing themselves at greater risk for depression and impulsive behavior. Research examining women of normal weight who diet shows a significant relationship between dieting and depressed mood. Further study of the influence of high or low carbohydrate intake during weight loss on high-intensity physical performance in college wrestlers demonstrates that rapid weight loss is associated with low carbohydrate intake, which adversely affects the wrestlers' physiology and psychology. Their physical performance is impaired, and tension, depression, anger, fatigue, and confusion scores on the Profile of Mood States (POMS) are significantly elevated (Horswill, Hickner, Scott, & Costill, 1990).

Eating disorders have been linked with depression, but a causal relationship has not been established. Herpertz and Remschmidt (1989) have shown that adolescent patients suffering from major depression disorder have significantly lower body weight than do those without a current episode. In addition, the researchers reported a highly significant negative correlation between body weight and depressive symptoms. Highly restrained eaters of normal body weight demonstrate impaired cognitive functioning, which Green, Rogers, Elliman, and Gatensy (1994) explain in terms of anxiety resulting from the stressful effects of imposing and maintaining dietary restraint. Recent suicides and attempted suicides of successful female athletes focus attention on the problem of diet and eating disorders in sport. Gymnastics, figure skating, running, wrestling, diving, and swimming are among the sports wherein weight problems and eating disorders appear to be developing at an alarming frequency (Rosen, McKeag, Hough, & Curley, 1986).

A case in point concerns a nationally ranked distance runner who thought being thin would make her run faster. She attempted suicide by jumping into a river near her home. The runner survived, suffering paralysis, and wrote her experiences of disordered eating in a book entitled *Dark Marathon* (Wazeter & Lewis, 1989). Wazeter chronicles a life of extreme dieting and the associated irrational and obsessional thinking that followed. Although researchers are uncertain what comes first, the biochemical imbalance in the brain that causes athletes to lose weight or behavior leading to the weight loss, the argument is probably moot. There is a growing body of literature that has investigated eating disorders, especially among female athletes. Less is known about the relatively small number of males who develop eating disorders and who have been seen by doctors. However, the research of Garfinkle, Garner, and Goldbloom (1987) suggests that many of these males are competitive athletes. More research is required to clarify this issue, and the relationship between disordered eating and striving for enhanced performance deserves closer attention. A high proportion of competitive female athletes resort to dangerous weight control behavior to maintain an edge over their opponents and to satisfy expectations of coaches and judges (Black & Burckes-Miller, 1988). Even seemingly casual comments by coaches overly concerned with their athletes' weight may prompt young athletes to resort to dangerous weight control behaviors to deal with the perceived criticism (Rosen & Hough, 1988). Although many coaches express concern about this issue, very few seem to be aware of the extent of the problem and how their behavior could precipitate it (Jaffee, 1988).

A list of hypothesized risk factors for the development of eating disorders includes cultural, familial, and individual categories. These factors are believed to interact and thereby result in dieting that enhances an individual's sense of self-control and consequent self-worth (Garfinkle & Garner, 1982). Among those who may be at high risk for developing eating disorders are "women who, by career choice, must be thin to achieve." This category includes athletes (Garfinkle et al., 1987, p. 625). Coaches should approach the matter of weight control in relation to sport performance with care and insight. A negative, critical approach by the coach can have a devastating effect on the athlete's self-esteem, general behavior, and sport performance, which may lead to a cycle of disordered eating, depressed mood, and impulsive behavior.

Personal Loss

Most people show only a temporary lowering of mood after a loss or disappointment. Familial interactions and other life stressors involving loss have been identified as important sources of risk for suicide in youths.

There are many difficulties involved in collecting empirical data relative to suicide. "The people who are most important to understand are by definition unavailable to the suicide researcher" (Berman & Jobes, 1994, p. 68). Therefore, researchers rely upon retrospective study of suicide attempters or ideators. These derived data may not be generalizable to suicide completers. However, stressful events have been found to be involved in suicidal behavior in young people, including divorce or separation in the family; disciplinary problems at home or at school (Shaffer, 1974); unsupportive and disinterested fathers; stress in early years resulting in parent-child difficulties (Tousignant, 1993); physical illness or injury (Tousignant, Hanigan, & Bergeron, 1984); and various psychological disorders. Events that have been shown to trigger suicide attempts in youth include the loss of something or someone that is important to the victim and resultant humiliation (Pfeffer, 1993). Particularly relevant is the loss of a supportive person, that is, the loss of a person with whom the subject has a meaningful relationship. The importance of loss of social support as a contributor to suicidal risk is, therefore, underscored. Depression is difficult to assess and thus diagnose in adolescents who express it in a great variety of ways (Davidson & Choquet, 1981). Thus, the perceived loss these young people experience is even more important.

Checklist of Risk Factors

Many suicide theories exist that emphasize different underpinning factors, but no single understanding of the nature of suicide prevails. Therefore, a checklist of risk factors has not emerged from the literature that will describe any one suicidal adolescent. One may "read between the lines" in order to identify common themes with many of them operating synergistically. Nonetheless, the following are frequently cited as being causally related to suicide attempts in youth (Berman & Jobes, 1994):

1. Negative personal history including early life events, narcissistic injury, inadequate or negative models for coping, and biochemical vulnerabilities.
2. Psychopathology: Severe psychopathology such as schizophrenia and paranoia would generally contraindicate participation in sport. Narcissism, compulsivity, aggression, and low frustration and disruption tolerance are personality characteristics that could be related to suicide in sport.
3. Humiliation: anticipated or real, loss of self-esteem or punishment.
4. Rigidity.
5. Social isolation.
6. Hopelessness.

None of the above risk factors is likely to be the exclusive cause of suicide. However, their interaction and individual strength will determine who will and who will not commit suicide. These stressors, in and of themselves, do not pose a risk for most adolescents; however, those with weak stress management skills are vulnerable to suicide. Those who are coping with a social loss or a blow to their self-esteem seem to be especially vulnerable (Shaffer, 1974).

Athletes who have committed suicide have tended to be good students and well-known individuals. There may be, of course, the problem of recording bias and publicizing only the most sensational stories. Nevertheless, many talented athletes attempt to take their lives. Shaffer, Garland, Gould, Fisher, and Trautman (1988) note a subgroup of suicide completers who show evidence of anxiety, perfectionism, and distress at times of change and dislocation. Berman and Jobes (1994) describe these teens as the "high achieving star" (p. 93).

Accounts from coaches, teammates, and parents depict most of the young athlete suicide victims as "normal teenagers," although perfectionistic and typically the "last one expected to commit suicide." The victims tended to live with one parent or stepparent and had a confrontational or aloof relationship with the other parent. Many indications point toward a perfectionist attitude: "He (the suicide victim) was the big hockey star in lower grades, but at the regional school there were a lot of other hockey players. He was used to being the best and then he went to the middle; he wasn't used to that and he didn't think people liked him anymore" (Fine, 1990).

Injury

Another important stressor in the lives of athletes is injury. Studies investigating athletes' emotional response to injury show that more seriously injured athletes experience the most depressed mood (Smith, Scott, & Wiese, 1990), and depressed mood associated with long-lasting injury was found to be positively related to attempted suicides in athletes (Smith & Millener, 1994). Smith and Millener (1994) identified factors common to suicidal athletes in their study: (a) surgery, (b) a 6-week to 1-year rehabilitation process, (c) depleted athletic skill, (d) lack of perceived athletic competence, and (e) being replaced by another athlete in their sport positions.

Injury results in many life changes for an athlete. The psychological stress brought about by injury is well documented in sport psychology literature. It is thought that the primary stressor is loss of affiliation, or the social support system, which is an important part of much athletic life.

> After stressful events people turn to those closest to them as a source of strength. It is those closest to us who carry our burdens when we are incapable, who offer a shoulder on which to cry, shelter from adversity,

and solace from grief. Significant others share their resources to help those for whom they care through these most difficult periods of life. (Hobfall & Stephens, 1990, p. 459)

Injury brings to an abrupt end feelings of belonging and allegiance to a group that team membership fosters. For many athletes, the social status, affiliation, and high self-esteem associated with their participation in sport are not to be found in any other social institution. They are unprepared to deal with the dramatic and sudden changes in their personal sphere conveyed by injury. As Shaffer, Garland, Gould, Fisher, and Trautman (1988) have said, coping strategies for dealing with loss of affiliation and the associated changes brought about by injury should be taught to athletes.

Retirement is also a time of increased stress for athletes. A study of suicides in Major League Baseball reveals that the 69 players who committed suicide did so mostly after career termination (Coleman & Lester, 1989). Retirement, like injury, is often viewed as a loss of athletic identity and associated with diminished self-esteem. Social support mechanisms may break down, and the athlete may be insecure about his or her purpose in life. Hopelessness or powerlessness is well documented as an important precursor and indication of increased suicide risk (Berman & Jobes, 1994).

In furthering the discussion of loss or disappointment as a potential precipitator of athletic suicide, reactions associated with being cut or dropped from a team also deserve attention. Such responses may be similar to those for injury, with regard to humiliation and diminished self-esteem. As the majority of suicide victims arc male, it is interesting to note that they are much more likely than females to have experienced a specific trauma or loss of status directly before suicide. Relationship break-ups are also likely to be an issue (Thompson, 1987). Teams are similar to families in structure and social function. Loss of this "family" or "relationship" could be a heartbreaking occurrence for some, especially those youngsters whose home life is lacking in nurturing qualities. "Sometimes emotionally disturbed and alienated youngsters seek a sense of belonging in new families" (Berman & Jobes, 1994, p. 94). Injury, retirement, and being cut from the team result in loss of attachment to a number of support structures: the team, teammates, social prestige, and social relationships. Berman and Jobes (1994) and Ramsay, Tanney, Tierney, and Lang (1994) have suggested that attachment loss is an important precipitator of suicide.

Narcissism

As previously indicated, affiliation and attachment to a team provide many athletes with strengths and security that may enhance their invulnerability to suicidal behavior. Garmezy (1985) and Rubenstein, Heeran, Housman, Rubin,

and Stechler (1989) have identified stress-resistant children as those who perceive their families to be cohesive and adaptable and who belong, as valued
members, to a peer group. These children are seen as having less suicidal tendencies. Affiliation, then, serves as a protector, but what happens when the attachments to the peer group break down, as in the case of injury, retirement,
cuts, or performance decrement? What occurs depends on the psychological
resources of the athlete. High-achieving athletes may be narcissistic and ego-
centric and thereby motivated to spend many hours and years of grueling
training. Narcissism is defined as an unconscious lack of self-esteem, where
the locus of self-control is external and the need for attention is never satiated.
A certain amount of narcissism is healthy and necessary. Unhealthy narcissism develops in a child, for instance, when a parent is unable to separate himself or herself from the child and thus lives vicariously through the child's
achievements. Through the child's performance (sport), he or she strives to
satisfy the needs of the parent and is thus unable to develop a healthy sense of
self. Miller (1990), a psychotherapist writing about narcissism and the gifted
child, speaks of these children who have been praised and admired for their
talents and achievements, and who have been a source of parental pride. She
notes that instead of having a strong and stable self-assurance, the opposite is
the case:

> In everything they undertake, they do well and often excellently, they are
> admired and envied; they are successful whenever they care to be—but
> all to no avail. Behind all this lurks depression, the feeling of emptiness
> and self-alienation and a sense that their life has no meaning. Addition-
> ally, as soon as "the drug of grandiosity" fails, as soon as they are not on
> top, not definitely the superstar or whenever they suddenly get the feel-
> ing they failed to live up to some ideal image and measure, they feel they
> must adhere to, they are plagued by deep feelings of guilt and shame.
> (Miller, 1991, p. 6)

There is much dispute as to the cause of these narcissistic disturbances in
highly gifted people (Kohut, 1971; Mahler, 1968). However, it appears that as
young children, these people were unable to develop a sense of their own self,
apart from their parents and their own needs beyond the need for achievement
and admiration.

Young people with low self-esteem may be attracted to sport because it
provides an opportunity for attention and satisfies their narcissistic needs. According to Dielens (1984), participation in physical activity is linked to narcissistic tendencies because of the overemphasis on self. Sport provides a

forum for displaying the great self, to be seen and to be admired. As athletic ability improves, for some, the nagging of deep self-doubt is not alleviated. These athletes increase their training in an effort to cope with the feelings of "not being good enough." Sometimes this training becomes overtraining and is counterproductive to performance. Injury may be the result. In addition, eating disorders may be prompted by feelings of low self-esteem. A cycle of food deprivation, dieting, and ensuing performance decrease due to overtraining and lack of proper nutrition results in a depressed mood. If the child suffers an injury to self-esteem, perhaps through an ostensibly innocent remark about performance given by the coach and negatively perceived by the athlete, it might trigger the sense of "being no good." Tragically some self-destructive act could be the result.

Role of the Coach

Few would question that coaches exert a strong influence on the behavior of their athletes. Coaches should, therefore, reflect upon their own behavior, tactics, and modes of communication. Anthony (1988) suggests that some suicides occur as a direct result of a devastating experience within the competitive realm. A tragic example is the case of a high school football coach who discovered that one of his prospective players who was cut from the team had hanged himself (Anthony, 1988). Anthony (1988) suggests that coaches must be willing to undergo self-assessment with regard to their department and methods. They must be sensitive to their athletes' feelings when experiencing rejection.

The majority of teenagers who kill themselves provide an array of clues about their imminent suicidal behavior to those in a position to notice. According to Brent, Pepper, and Allman (1987), 85% of adolescent completers in their study had made noticeable suicidal threats in the week prior to their deaths. Tragically, these threats are not usually taken seriously or are totally missed by those in a position to respond. Prevention of an adolescent suicide often fundamentally depends on the awareness and sensitivity of key people in the young person's life who seriously respond to obvious or veiled suicidal cues and make referrals to those who can help (Berman & Jobes, 1994). The coach is such a person. Often, the attitude that feelings are not to be discussed prevails among athletes on a team. Thus, athletes who exhibit signs of weakness may not be taken seriously, and their signals are often dismissed by teammates and coaches. Only after their death by suicide are those who have been close to the athlete able to perceive the cries for help that had been given. Even then, these signs are too often dismissed as having been irrelevant.

Prevention of Suicide in Athletes: Understanding Vital Signs

An understanding of why talented athletes may take their own lives ultimately leads to a discussion of what one can do to prevent these untimely deaths. Sport can be a positive influence in the lives of young people, teaching them life skills that are difficult to learn in other environments. However, for some, sport may provide seriously negative consequences. Children whose role identity is contingent upon sport performance may be at risk. The lessons these children learn about themselves through participation may be self-destructive and reinforce low self-esteem.

Coaches, parents, and team officials must be aware of the indicators of suicidal ideation or impending suicide. These include verbal, behavioral, and situational factors. Recognition of an impending suicide may not surface on the competitive field, but may be hinted at in locker room talk or behavior.

Verbal behaviors may include, but are not be limited to

1. blatant statements or jokes about suicide or death;
2. a preoccupation with dying or death.

The behavioral indicators of suicidal thought are diverse and include any noticeable change in typical behavior for that person. Of note might be

1. changes in eating, sleeping, and grooming habits;
2. changes in energy level;
3. changes in school and/or sport practice habits;
4. sudden personality changes;
5. self-destructive behavior;
6. difficulty in concentration.

Situational factors in the lives of athletes that might be related to suicidal behavior have been discussed earlier in this text. To reiterate, they include

1. broken home;
2. perfectionist attitude;
3. recent significant loss; in performance, of a family member, break-up of a significant relationship, injury, termination from sport;
4. alcoholism in family, and other problems at home;
5. suicide history in family or previous suicide attempt;
6. striving for weight loss to enhance performance;
7. psychological or emotional problems.

Suicide may be prevented by parents, teammates, sport psychologists, athletic trainers, and physical therapists when they are aware of the danger signals and prepared to respond to them. Rosenberg, Eddy, Wolpert, and Broumas (1989) estimate that training of gatekeepers in the signs and symptoms of suicidal ideation could potentially reduce youth suicide by approximately 13%. Such professionals may be able to refer vulnerable athletes to well-trained experts. Many opportunities to divert suicide are missed because those in a position to notice cries for help have missed important cues. Experts believe that those who commit suicide have not decided to take their own lives until they actually do it. Suicidal individuals seek those whom they trust and feel connected to in some way, such as friends, family members, or coaches (Ramsayet al., 1994). One of the most important factors in preventing a suicide is the presence of a supportive resource. Many suicidal episodes are short-lived, and a supportive person's talking and listening may draw the suicidal individual away from self-destructive thoughts and at the same time provide the necessary hiatus to mobilize professional assistance, if required. School counselors or other community resources could be asked to provide this training to all sport personnel, including athletes. Often coaches do not want to discuss suicide, or human failings in general, because they are apprehensive about directing their athletes' thoughts improperly. However, experts agree that talking about suicide does not create or increase the risk (Ramsey et al., 1994). Open discussion and genuine concern about suicidal thoughts are a source of relief and are often effective in suicide prevention. In fact, not offering these opportunities may contribute to feelings of increased isolation, helplessness, and hopelessness (Ramsey et al., 1994). The sporting environment should be a safe place where children feel at ease to discuss and cope with emotional needs. Sadly, it is often not the case. A questionnaire attached to the athlete's medical information could be used to explore an athlete's coping resources. Some sample questions might include the following:

1. If I were cut from the team, I would _____
2. If the coach berates me, I would _____
3. Five people I could talk to if I needed to: _____
4. After a loss I generally feel _____
5. After my playing career is over, I am going to _____
6. If I should be seriously injured, I would _____

The coaching staff should be alert to athletes who are not able to name people to whom they could talk in an emergency. Additionally, by prompting athletes to think about how they might cope in various situations, the groundwork is being laid for athletes to be more prepared should these scenarios actually arise. Stress-coping resources are learned responses that must be taught to athletes.

The key to success in preventing suicide is early intervention. Every suicide threat must be taken seriously. Adults often tend to minimize the importance and intensity of adolescent feelings and respond to a young person's crisis without appreciating the feeling from the perspective of the young person (Ramsey et al., 1994). The threat of suicidal behavior is usually an act of desperation, a cry for help rather than a manipulation. Any statement or action about suicide must be taken as a serious invitation to respond. It is a normal response to feel anger or frustration in dealing with such a situation; however, the underlying reason for these feelings is often one of inadequacy. Teammates, coaches, and trainers feel they do not have the training to effectively deal with a suicidal person. The feeling may be justifiable, but should not deter one from providing empathy or referring the person to an available, competent expert who is able to offer help.

Conclusion

There are a number of practical things that the coach, trainer, or sport psychologist can do when help is needed. Ramsey et al. (1994) liken the initial intervention of nonspecialist suicidal help to a "lifeguard," that is, an intermediary between a suicidal person and professional care. Every situation is different, but it is important for the helper to know that providing any demonstration of support for the suicidal person could potentially decrease the suicidal feelings.

Involving oneself with young people in sport demands a great responsibility because these individuals have not yet fully fashioned their feelings, their ability to express themselves, and, in sum, their lives. The vulnerability of their youth makes it incumbent upon responsible adults to be trained to listen to the "music behind the words." By doing so, they will not just assist their young athletes in attaining prowess, but greatly enhance the total of their lives and preclude one of the great tragedies in the human experience, the loss of human potential, the death of a child.

References

Allen, B.P. (1987). Youth suicide. *Adolescence, 22*, 271–290.

Anthony, M. (1988a). Teenage suicide: Coaches can play important role as counselors for athletes. *Interscholastic Athletic Administration, 14*(3), 20–23.

Anthony, M. (1988b). Teenage suicide: Spreading a network of caring over field of athletic competition. *Interscholastic Athletic Administration, 14*(2), 4–6.

Berger, B., & Owen D. (1992). Preliminary analysis of a causal relationship between swimming and stress reduction: Intense exercise may negate the effects. *International Journal of Sport Psychology, 23*, 70–85.

Berman, A. K., & Jobes D. A. (1994). *Adolescent suicide assessment and intervention*. Washington, DC; American Psychological Association.

Black, D., & Burckes-Miller, M. (1988). Males and female college athletes: Use of anorexia nervosa and bulimia nervosa weight loss methods. *Research Quarterly, 59*(3), 252–256.

Blotez, M., Botez, T., & Maag, U. (1984). The Wechsler subtests in mild organic brain damage associated with folate deficiency. *Psychological Medicine, 14,* 431–437.

Brent, D. A., Perper, J. A., & Allman, C. J. (1987). Alcohol, firearms and suicide among youth. *Journal of the American Medical Association, 257,* 3369-3372.

Callahan, G., & Steptoe, S. (1995, July 24). An end too soon. *Sports Illustrated, 83*(4), 32–36.

Center for Disease Control. (1986). *Youth suicide in the United States, 1970–1980.* Atlanta: Author.

Center for Disease Control and Prevention. (1995). *Youth suicide in the United States, 1980–1990.* Atlanta.

Coleman, L., & Lester, D. (1989, April). *Boys of summer, suicides of winter.* Paper presented at the Annual Meeting of the American Association of Suicidology, San Diego.

Corbella, L. (March 16, 1996). Recalling a life too short. *The Calgary Sun.*

Davidson, F., & Choquet M. (1981). *Le suicide de l'adolescent: étude épidémiologique.* Paris, Les Éditions ESF.

Dielens, S. (1984). Narcissime et activités physiquess à la mode: profil psychologique des pratiquants d'aérobie, de jogging et de bodybuilding. *Revue de l'Éducation Physique, 241,* 21–24.

Eitzen, D. S., & Sage, G. H. (1982). *Sociology of American sport.* Dubuque, IA: William C. Brown.

Emond, A., Guyon, L., Camirand, T., Shenard, L., Pineault, R., & Robitaille, Y. (1988). *Et la santé ça va? Rapport de l'enquête Santé Québec,.* Québec: Les Publications du Québec.

Fine, S. (1990, April 2). Student gave few hints of plan to end his life, acquaintances say. *Globe and Mail.*

Garfinkel, B., Froese, A., & Hood, J. (1982). Suicide attempts in children and adolescents. *American Journal of Psychiatry, 138,* 35–40.

Garfinkel, P., & Garner, D. (1982). *Anorexia nervosa: A multidimensional perspective.* New York: Brunner/Mazel.

Garfinkel, P., Garner, D., & Goldbloom, D. (1987, October). Eating disorders: implications for the 1990's. *Canadian Journal of Psychiatry, 32,* 624–630.

Garfinkel, P., & Kaplan, A. (1985). Starvation based perpetuating mechanisms in anorexia nervosa and bulimia. *International Journal of Eating Disorders, 4,* 651–655.

Garmezy, N. (1985). Stress-resistant children: The search for protective factors. In J. E. Stevenson (Ed.), Recent research in developmental psychopathology, *Journal of Child Psychology and Psychiatry Book, Supplement No. 4* (pp. 213–233). Oxford: Permagon Press.

Green, M., Rogers, P., Elliman, N., & Gatenby, S. (1994). Impairment of cognitive performance associated with dieting and high levels of dietary restraint. *Physiological Behavior, 55,* 447–452.

Health Canada. (1994). Suicide in Canada: *Update of the report of the task force on suicide in Canada.* Ottawa, Ontario.

Herpertz-Dahlmann, B., & Remschidmt, H. (1989, August). Anorexia nervosa and depression. On the relation of body weight and depressive symptoms. *Nervenartz, 60*(8), 490–495.

Hobfall, S. E., & Stephens, M. A. P. (1990). Social support during extreme stress: Consequences and intervention. In B. R. Sarason, I. G. Sarason, & G. R. Pierce (Eds.), *Social support: An interactional view* (pp. 454–481). New York: John Wiley and Sons.

Holinger, P. (1989). Epidemiologic issues in youth suicide. In C. Pfeffer (Ed.), *Suicide among youth,* Washington, DC: American Psychiatric Press.

Horswill, C., Hickner, R., Scott, J., & Costill, D. (1990). Weight loss, dietary carbohydrate modifications and high intensity, physical performance. *Medicine and Science in Sports and Exercise, 22*(4), 470–476.

Ireland, J. (1994, May 30). When the spotlight fades, Olympic athletes fall victim to depression. *Calgary Herald,* pp.A1–A2.

Jaffee, L. (1988). Eating disorders and coach athletes relationships. *Melpomene Report, 7*(1), 12–13.

Kohut, H. (1971). *The analysis of self.* New York: International Universities Press.

Lewis, R., & Sheppard, G. (1992, Summer). Inferred characteristics of successful suicides as a function of gender and context. *Suicide and life-threatening behavior, 22*(2), 187–196.

Mahler, M. (1968). *On human symbiosis and the vicissitudes of individuation.* New York: International Universities Press.

Miller, A. (1990). *The drama of the gifted child.* New York: Basic Books.

Parker, K., & Price, F. (1996, October). *In the trenches, applied sport psychology issues at the NCAA division 1 level.* Paper presented at the Annual Meeting of the Conference of the Association for the Advancement of Applied Sport Psychology. Williamsburg, VA.

Peterson, A. C., & Hamburg, B. A. (1986). Adolescence: A developmental approach to problems and pathology. *Behavior Therapy, 17,* 480–499.

Pfeffer, C. (1986). *The suicidal child.* New York: Guilford.

Ramsey, R., Tanney, B., Tierney, R., & Lang, W. (1994). *Suicide intervention handbook.* Calgary, AB. Living Works Education.

Rosen, L., & Hough, D. (1988). Pathogenic weight control behaviors of female college gymnasts. *The Physician and Sportsmedicine, 16*(9), 140–143.

Rosen, L., McKeag, D., Hough, D., & Curley, V. (1986). Pathogenic weight control behavior in female athletes. *The Physician and Sportsmedicine, 14*(1), 79–86.

Rosenberg, M., Eddy, D., Wolpert, R., & Broumas, E. Developing strategies to prevent youth suicide. In C. Pfeffer (Ed.), *Suicide among youth* (pp. 203–225). Washington, DC: American Psychiatric Press.

Rubenstein, J. L., Heeren, T., Housman, D., Rubin, C., & Stechler, G. (1989). Suicidal behavior in "normal" adolescents: Risks and protective factors. *American Journal of Orthopsychiatry, 59,* 59–71.

Shaffer, D. (1974). Suicide in childhood and early adolescence. *Journal of Psychology Psychiatry, 15,* 275–291.

Shaffer, D., Garland, A., Gould, M., Fisher, P., & Trautman, P. (1988). Preventing teenage suicide: A critical review. *Journal of the American Academy of Child and Adolescent Psychiatry, 27,* 675–687.

Shneidman, E. S. (1985). *Definition of suicide.* New York: John Wiley & Sons.

Smith, A., Scott, S., & Wiese, D. (1990). The psychological effects of sports injuries: Coping. *Journal of Sportsmedicine, 9,* 352–369.

Smith, A., & Millener, E. (1994). Injured athletes and the risk of suicide. *Journal of Athletic Training, 29*(4), 337–341.

Suicide among children, adolescents, and young adults—United States. (1995). *Journal of School Health, 65*(7), 272–274.

Thompson, T. (1987). Childhood and adolescent suicide in Manitoba: Demographic study. *Canadian Journal, 32,* 264–269.

Tousignant, M. (1993, May). La santé mentale dans l'enquête de la Défense Nationale. *Rapport Final de Recherche.* Montréal, 1990.

Tousignant, M., Hamel, S., & Bastien, M. F. (1988). Structure familiale, relations parents-enfants et conduites suicidaires à l'école secondaire. *Santé Mentale Québec, 13,* 79–93.

Tousignant, M., Hanigan, D., & Bergeron, L. (1984). Le mal de vivre: Comportements et idéations suicidaires chez les cégepiens de Montréal. *Santé Mentale Québec, 9,* 122–123.

Waters, H. (1994, April 18). Teenage suicide: One act not to follow. *Newsweek, 123*(16), 49.

Wazeter, M., & Lewis, G. (1989). *Dark marathon.* Grand Rapids, MI: Zondervan Publishing.

Wurtman, R., & Wurtman, J. (1984). Nutrients: Neurotransmitter synthesis and the control of food intake. In J. Stunkard & E. Stellar (Eds.), *Eating and its disorders* (pp. 77–86). New York: Raven Press.

Young, S. (1986). The clinical psychopharmacology of Tryptophan. In R. Wurtman & J. Wurtman (Eds.), *Nutrition and the brain* (Vol. 7, pp. 49–88). New York: Raven Press, 49–88.

SECTION 5

APPLICATIONS: CASE STUDIES

Chapter 18
Using Qualitative Case Analysis in the Study of Athletic
Injury: A Model for Implementation
Gregory A. Shelley

Chapter 19
I Cried Because I Had No Shoes . . . :
A Case Study of Motivation Applied to Rehabilitation
Bruce W. Tuckman

Chapter 20
Conversion Blindness: A Case Report
David Pargman

This section consists of three chapters that depict case studies of injured athletes. Understandably, the format in which they are presented differs somewhat from those in the book's other sections.

In the section's first chapter, **Gregory A. Shelley** employs a qualitative research design to clarify his client's experiences associated with injury onset and rehabilitation, as well as factors that influence the athlete's perceptions about the injury experiences.

In the second chapter, **Bruce W. Tuckman** provides an account of his own battle with a debilitating athletic injury. He shares personal insights and describes a step-by-step account of his self-counseling strategies.

In the book's final chapter, its editor, **David Pargman**, describes a strategy employed to resolve conversion blindness in a high school football player. Its contents also relate to two other chapters in the book— "Ethical and Legal Issues for Sport Professionals Counseling Injured Athletes" (chapter 3), by Lou M. Makarowski, and "The Malingering Athlete: Psychological Considerations" (chapter 8), by Robert J. Rotella, Bruce C. Ogilvie, and David H. Perrin.

18

Using Qualitative Case Analysis in the Study of Athletic Injury: A Model for Implementation

Gregory A. Shelley
Ithaca College

Although athletic injury continues to be an important and growing area within the field of sport psychology, the perspectives of injured athletes have remained generally unknown. In addition, there has been little use of qualitative methodologies to assess individual injury experiences. Still, each year millions of athletes experience at least one, and sometimes multiple injuries while competing in athletic practices and competitions. From the youngest youth participants, to the masses of recreational sports enthusiasts, to elite and professional athletes, the number of sport-related injuries is staggering. In fact, as many as 17 million injuries occur each year among American athletes. (Heil, 1993)

Whether minor or serious, athletic injury can present one of the most emotionally traumatic and challenging experiences an athlete encounters (Heil, 1993; Weinberg & Gould, 1995). With so much personal identity invested in a sport, the time and commitment to training and competing, and a continued emphasis on displaying physical prowess, many athletes suffer a great sense of loss when faced with injury (Evans & Hardy, 1995; Shelley, 1995). Still, the psychological dimensions of athletic injury, including the behavioral, cognitive, and emotional components, are often overlooked or minimized by the athlete, as well as the entire sports medicine team (Pargman, 1993). Although continued attempts have been made to study the psychological impact following athletic injury, many studies have centered on assessing the potential stages or phases that injured athletes can expect to proceed through (Hardy & Crace, 1990; McDonald & Hardy, 1990) while often ignoring the unique emotional aspects of the injury experience as described by each athlete. Furthermore, there has been little attempt to qualitatively assess the psychosocial processes surrounding athletic injury and rehabilitation. The few qualitative attempts to study athletic injury that have been conducted have been retrospective in nature (Gould, Udry, Bridges, & Beck, 1997a, 1997b; Rose & Jevne, 1993). As a result, there is still a lack of research that depicts the in-depth descriptions of the injury experience as described by the injured athlete as that athlete works through injury, rehabilitation, and return to play. The unique perceptions and perspectives of injured athletes have yet to be adequately or simultaneously assessed throughout the injury, rehabilitation, and return phases.

The purpose of this chapter is to provide an in-depth description of the injury experience as perceived by a select group of injured athletes. In addition, a second purpose is to examine the factors that impacted or influenced each of these athlete's perceived injury experiences. The athletes were examined as they endured their injury (no participation), rehabilitation (limited-participation), and return to competition (return to play) within the same sport season in which their injury originated. In accordance with the outlined purpose, the following research questions were examined:

1. What are the experiences associated with the onset of and the rehabilitation from athletic injury?
2. What are the factors that impact, contribute to, or influence the perceived injury experience?

Methodology

Design

A qualitative phenomenological research design was utilized to assess the experiences and perceptions of four ($n = 4$) injured athletes. From a philosophical view, phenomenology entails describing one's experiences by attending to that individual's perceptions flowing from his or her own conscious awareness of a particular event (Husserl, 1962). Therefore, in order to study the injury experience, one must study the person in context (i.e., throughout the injury), for it is there that the person's values and true experiences become known.

An important concept in phenomenology is the concept of life-world, or the world of lived experience (Cohen, 1987). Phenomenology is meant to be the study of how people describe things and experience them through their senses (Patton, 1990). Accordingly, the focus of the present qualitative inquiry was to describe patterns of "lived experiences" as depicted by each athlete's responses to questions pertaining to his or her injury, rehabilitation, and return to play.

Instrumentation

Rose and Jevne (1993) suggested a study design that assesses the perspectives and perceptions of injured athletes as they progress through the process of rehabilitation. In response to this suggestion, in-depth, semistructured interviews were conducted with one male and three female intercollegiate, Division I athletes following their injury (no participation phase), rehabilitation (limited-participation phase), and return to practices and competitions (return to play phase). Similarly, each athlete's primary athletic trainer and position coach were respectively interviewed following the athlete's limited and return to play phases. Interviews of each athlete, his or her trainer, and coach were conducted according to the following outlined schedules (see below) and included open-ended questions as contained in respective interview guides. Questions were derived from a combination of the researcher's personal experience in working with injured athletes, athletic trainer consultations, sport psychologists' consultations, and a review of the existing injury literature.

Athlete. Each athlete was asked a series of questions specifically designed to assess his or her own unique injury experiences. Each athlete was interviewed on three separate occasions: (a) at the end of the no-participation period, (b) at the end of the limited-participation period, and (c) following the complete return to practices and competitions.

Trainers. In an attempt to triangulate and strengthen the data through multiple informants, each athlete's athletic trainer was asked a series of questions that focused on the trainer's perceptions of the athlete's injury experiences. The trainer was interviewed at the end of the athlete's limited-participation period, just prior to the athlete's attempting a return to play.

Coaches. To further triangulate the data, each athlete's coach was asked a series of questions that focused on his or her perceptions of the athlete's injury experiences (e.g., any changes noticed in the athlete's behavior or play;

concerns, worries) as they related to the athlete's return to practice and competitions. The coach was interviewed 2 weeks following the athlete's first complete return to practice.

Observations. In a final attempt to triangulate the data, field notes were kept that included nonparticipant (i.e., researcher) observations as perceived during training room visits, attendance at practice and competitions, and daily conversations with the athlete, teammates, trainers, and friends.

Athlete Case Descriptions

Athlete 1. He was a 21-year-old male starting offensive lineman (tight end) for a top 10 ranked, Division I football program. As a second-year starter, he was completing his senior season. With four games left, he suffered a sprained left knee (medial collateral ligament) with a prognosis of 2 weeks off from practice/games. He was given a probable return date that would allow him to participate in the final two football games of his collegiate career. However, there were no guarantees of his return. Because he had never suffered/experienced a serious injury in his entire football career, he was very unsure as to what his injury, rehabilitation, or return entailed. Although his football career was likely coming to a close at the conclusion of his current season, he still had one year of school to complete his bachelor's degree. He was an average student, maintaining a 2.5 GPA. He missed 20 days of practice and two games before he was given clearance for full participation and return to play.

Athlete 2. She was an 18-year-old freshman female Division I cross-country and track athlete. She was considered an average runner for her cross-country team while an above average middle distance runner for her track team. Despite her freshman status, she was looked to for her potential impact on team leadership. Coaches had high future expectations for her as she had much "untapped" potential. With 2 weeks left in her cross-country season, she suffered a plantar-fasciitis injury to her left foot and was given a prognosis of 3 to 4 weeks totally off from running. Although this was a new diagnosis, she had been diagnosed with plantar-fasciitis in the same foot 4 months prior to her current injury. Although she pushed herself very hard in everything she did, she especially struggled with not being able to run and work out. She was a 4.0 student throughout high school and her first graded term in college. She missed a total of 53 days of cross-country and indoor track before being cleared for a complete return to her outdoor track season.

Athlete 3. She was a 19-year-old sophomore female Division I cross-country and track athlete and was extremely talented (top 5 ranked Junior National Champion) in the 10,000 meters. Having performed very well in her prior meets and competitions, she suffered a 3rd metatarsal stress fracture on her right foot during the height of her indoor track season. She was given a prognosis of 4 to 6 weeks with no running followed by a slow rehab progression, starting with non-weight-bearing exercises. As a pre-med (3.75 GPA) student, she was very much a perfectionist, always striving to be better and better, in and outside of sport. She was very active prior to her injury and found herself extremely bored and frustrated with her time off from working out, practice, and competing. Although very quiet, she was a leader and captain on her track team. Due to various complications, she missed a total of 74 days before she was cleared for full participation in her summer training program and competitions. She missed the remainder of her indoor and all of her outdoor season before her return to running.

Athlete 4. She was a 21-year-old senior female Division I gymnast for a top 3 ranked gymnastics program. As a senior, she very much anticipated ending her collegiate career on a "good note" at the national tournament. About 4 weeks before the regional and national tournaments, she suffered a second-degree sprain of her left ankle. Although having been injury-prone throughout her past two seasons, she had never injured an ankle until her current injury. Her ankle injury added increased burden to an already unhappy and frustrating senior year. Although she was a good student (3.4 GPA), she was tired of school, competing, teammates, and college in general. She was very much ready to be done with her collegiate career and move on to her next phase in life. She was told that her injury would require at least 10 days away from practice before her limited return. She missed a total of 12 days before her limited return and 21 days until she was cleared for her complete return.

Data Management and Analysis

Following the transcription of each interview, data were analyzed according to the following eight procedural steps:

1. Each athlete's oral descriptions of his or her injury experiences were read in order to obtain a feel for them. The researcher attempted to get a general sense for what had been discussed.
2. From each transcript, significant statements and phrases that directly pertained to athletic injury were extracted.
3. Meanings were formulated from these significant statements and phrases as they related to the injury experience. Similar to what Glasser and Strauss (1967) defined as the "constant comparative method," significant statements and phrases were categorized into meaning units.
4. The formulated meanings were then synthesized into clusters of lower order themes. By using the constant comparative method, meaning units were systematically synthesized into lower order themes. These lower

order themes comprised the basis for the final analytical steps.

5. The clustered, lower order themes were then integrated into higher order themes by which the initial injury experience for each athlete was described.

6. To achieve final validation, the researcher asked each athlete to review the injury description.

7. The higher order themes from the trainer and coach, as well as the higher order themes from the researcher's observations, were then compared to and integrated with each athlete's higher order themes from the no-participation, limited-participation, or return-to-play phase. Although the trainer's higher order themes were compared to the athlete's limited-participation phase and the coach's higher order themes were compared to the athlete's return-to-play phase, the researcher's observational higher order themes were compared to and integrated with each of the three phases. These *exhaustive,* higher order themes comprised the final description of the injury experience for each athlete at each phase.

8. Finally, the exhaustive, higher order themes from each athlete were compared across subjects (i.e., athletes) in order to examine the *common* themes in each of the no-participation, limited-participation, and return-to-play phases. Through multiple informants (athletes, trainers, and coaches) and multiple methods of data collection (interviews and observations), final analyses were provided.

Results

A total of 20 interviews (i.e., 5 per athlete), as well as the researcher's observations, were content analyzed and integrated into common themes (i.e., Step 8 above). An analysis of the exhaustive, higher order comparisons revealed 17 common themes among the subjects. These common themes were categorized by way of the three aforementioned injury (6 themes), rehabilitation (6 themes), and return-to-play phases (5 themes).

Research Question 1: What are the experiences associated with the onset of and the rehabilitation from athletic injury?

Participants were unique in their thoughts, emotions, and feelings relative to their injury and situation; however, the following common themes and similarities emerged for each outlined phase.

No-Participation Phase

1. There existed *bitterness* concerning their current injury situations and *jealousy* toward their healthy teammates.

2. At times, there were *frustration, anger,* and *guilt* surrounding their inability to practice, work out, and help out their team and teammates.

3. Despite some support from their families, there existed *feelings of being isolated* from and *misunderstood, ignored,* and *abandoned* by coaches and teammates.

4. There was a *concern* as to what their coaches perceived in terms of their injury, their lack of playing time, and their overall injury situation.

5. Despite the newness of their injury, there existed a *sense of hope* and confidence concerning their future, overcoming their physical injuries, and once again returning to their sport.

6. There existed a *fear* of injury, reinjury, and a fear of not returning to their previous playing form.

Limited-Participation Phase

1. Athletes generally developed an *increased confidence* in and a more positive attitude toward successfully completing their rehabilitation and once again returning before season's end.

2. There continued to be an *ongoing fear* of reinjury.

3. There were *feelings of being unsupported, misunderstood,* and negatively *judged* by teammates and coaches.

4. There was *uncertainty* as to what others might be thinking as athletes questioned how their coaches were perceiving them and their injury status.

5. The athletes looked to and developed a *supportive and trusting relationship* with their trainers.

6. Despite having developed a *sense of accomplishment* in completing their rehabilitation, there remained *caution and doubt* concerning whether or not they would completely overcome their injury and once again contribute to their team.

Return-to-Play Phase

1. There was a growing *sense of confidence* in their abilities, as well as a *feeling of satisfaction* in regard to having worked hard and accomplished a return to their sport.

2. Returning to practices and competitions resulted in a definite and positive impact on the athletes as they once again started to regain their *enthusiasm and excitement* for playing.

3. There were *apprehension and doubt* concerning their return as the athletes were *cautious* about their return, *confused* about what they were

able to do, *timid* concerning their effort and intensity, and even *superstitious* about their future health and injury.

4. There was an ongoing *desire to be understood, encouraged,* and *supported* by their coaches and teammates.
5. There remained a *fear* of reinjury and a *concern* for future injury.

Research Question 2: What are the factors that impact, contribute to, or influence the perceived injury experience?

Concerning the second research question, several factors emerged that impacted or influenced the athletes' perceived injury experiences. By way of reviewing the emergent, common themes for the no-participation, limited-participation, and return-to-play phases, the following factors emerged as impacting or influencing the overall injury experience.

No-Participation Phase

The following concerns were considered: whether or not the athletes (a) compared themselves to their healthy teammates; (b) focused on their inability to work out, practice, or play; (c) remained included in the normal functioning and interaction of their teams; (d) were concerned about their coaches' perception of their injury and situation; (e) were able to positively focus on the future and overcoming their injury; and (f) focused on reinjury.

Limited-Participation Phase

The following concerns were considered: whether or not the athletes (a) focused on their confidence and developing a more positive attitude toward their return; (b) focused on reinjury; (c) were concerned about being understood and supported by teammates and coaches; (d) were concerned about their coaches' perception of their injury and status; (e) desired a positive relationship with their trainers; and (f) focused on their return and contribution to their team.

Return-to-Play Phase

The following concerns were considered: whether or not the athletes (a) focused on their hard work in relation to their rehabilitation process and return; (b) focused on their return to daily practices and competitions; (c) perceived they had control of, a role in, or an impact on their return; (d) perceived a need to be understood, encouraged, and supported by teammates and coaches; and (e) focused on reinjury.

Conclusion

The principal findings relating to the aforementioned three injury phases included the following.

1. Throughout all phases, athletes were fearful of reinjury or experiencing another future (i.e., new) injury.

It is common for athletes of all ages and ability levels to express a fear of reinjury following an initial injury. In his discussion of athletic injury, Heil (1993) speculated that fear of reinjury is always present for the injured athlete. Results from the current study support this statement in that every athlete expressed a fear of reinjury or a fear of experiencing another new injury in the future.

Although Feigley (1988) suggested that athletes may try to hide their fears because coaches might perceive such fears as a weakness, this was not apparent with any of the four subjects. Despite the athletes' limited interaction with their coaches until their return to play, none of the athletes seemed to want or try to hide their fears. In fact, two of the four subjects made it very clear to their coaches that they were dealing with such fears.

Petitpas and Danish (1995) outlined injured athletes' anxieties and fears as stemming from the loss of a daily practice routine and a normal schedule outside of sport, the ongoing pain and discomfort associated with the injury, and the uncertainties about making a complete return. All seem to be important factors impacting and influencing the perceived injury experiences of the subjects in this study.

2. Throughout all phases, athletes gained a growing sense of confidence in their abilities and once again returning before season's end.

Confidence starts with a thought about one's ability to perform a task successfully. When athletes are confident, they believe that they not only can, but will, complete a desired behavior. Confident athletes believe in themselves, and they believe in their ability to acquire the necessary skills and competencies, both physical and mental, to reach their potential (Weinberg & Gould, 1995). For injured athletes, this entails believing that they have the abilities to overcome their injury and make a successful return to their sport. All four subjects showed a sense of hope and confidence throughout their injury, rehabilitation, and return to play.

Although confidence may be difficult to witness directly, through observations, the participants did appear to gain confidence in their abilities as time progressed and they became more healthy. This was especially evident in how these athletes approached their rehabilitation exercises and limited-participation training. As the athletes became more familiar with their routines, the equipment, and their trainers, they became more confident in their abilities to perform the tasks demanded. As a result, they became more excited about completing their rehab and were more willing to take risks while performing exercises.

This is no surprise. As injured athletes get closer to their "normal" physical health, they likely develop greater confidence in their physical prowess. What is especially interesting, however, is that these athletes developed a sense of hope and confidence immediately following their injury, during the no-participation phase. It may be that because all the athletes were starters and leaders on their respective teams, they believed in themselves and their abilities to complete a successful return to practices and competitions. They may have already developed a high degree of confidence prior to their injury that simply carried over into their injury, rehabilitation, and return. Although some athletes might lose confidence after an injury because of deteriorated physical status and an inability to practice and compete (Petitpas & Danish, 1995; Rotella & Heyman, 1993; Weinberg & Gould, 1995), this was not the case with the subjects in this study.

3. **During both the no-participation and limited-participation phases, athletes felt isolated from, ignored, abandoned, misunderstood, and/or unsupported by teammates and coaches.**

At one time or another, all of the subjects felt as though they were isolated, abandoned, ignored, misunderstood, or unsupported by their coaches, teammates, or both. It is not uncommon for some coaches to pay much less attention to an injured athlete (Wiese-Bjornstal & Smith, 1993). In some case, coaches may be unsure what to do or say. Coaches may also feel as though they do not have the time to spend with the injured athlete. Still other coaches may feel that the injured athlete is primarily the trainer's responsibility. Finally, in the worst cases, the coach may pay less attention to the injured athlete because he or she is no longer useful to the team.

The very nature of athletic injury and the removal of the athlete from the immediate sporting environment often force the athlete to deal with feelings of isolation, misunderstanding, and loneliness (Heil, 1993; Shelley, 1995). Feeling isolated from and unsupported and unrecognized by their teammates and coaches may be the reason many athletes turn to their family for the support and encouragement they desire.

Although the athletes continued to struggle with their feelings of isolation and abandonment, their coaches did not generally recognize these feelings. In fact, in many cases the coaches felt as though they were adequately "caring" for the injured athlete, when in fact they were ignoring the athlete. This was evident in the researcher's observations concerning contact between coaches and injured athletes. Rarely did any coach visit an athlete in the training room or make any effort to comfort the athlete concerning these feelings. If coaches did recognize these feelings of the athlete, they made no attempt to communicate their understanding. Yet these athletes greatly desired to be understood and supported by their coaches.

Finally, Crossman and Jamieson (1985) described injured athletes as likely to overestimate the seriousness of their injury and misperceive or misinterpret the information that is available to them. If this is true and athletes misinterpret information from their teammates or trainers, it also seems very likely that they too would misinterpret information from their coaches. Taking this one step further, it may be that athletes miss some information altogether. Could coaches be providing information, even support and encouragement to athletes, yet because of some heightened fear, anxiety, worry, or concern, the injured athletes miss such information? Although this question is beyond the scope of this study, such a question demands further investigation.

4. **During both the no-participation and limited-participation phases, athletes were concerned about how their coaches were perceiving them and their injury status.**

In addition to athletes' thoughts about their injury and recovery, it has been shown that their attitudes and beliefs can greatly influence their affective experiences (Williams & Roepke, 1993). For injured athletes, attitudes or beliefs are often dictated by the feedback that they receive by way of their teammates, coaches, or trainers. In other words, injured athletes' self-image, or how they think others see them, is often dictated by their teammates', coaches', or trainers' perceptions of them. For the injured athletes who may worry about their position on a team, their loss of attention and status, and making a return to playing at less than 100% (Shelley, 1995), it is of primary importance that they understand their coaches' perceptions concerning such issues. Clearly, all of the athletes were at least somewhat concerned as to how they were perceived by their coaches.

Specifically, during the no-participation and the limited-participation phases, the participants questioned what their coaches might be perceiving in terms of how they viewed the athletes' overall injury status, their lack of or limited playing time, or their current training.

Results indicated that it was important for these athletes to know what their coaches were thinking and feeling. It could be that these injured athletes simply needed some form of reassurance that they were still a part of their team. It may also be that these athletes wanted to know that their coaches still believed in them, that they were still valued as athletes, or that things were going to work out.

Results indicated the athletes experiencing vacillating emotions. On the one hand, the athletes wanted desperately to be back to and a part of their teams. Yet, on the other hand, at least while they were limited in their participation, they were quite reluctant to be an active member of daily practices. It seems very possible that because many athletes have much of their self-esteem so closely tied to their physical prowess (Evans & Hardy, 1995), the athletes would rather not have their coaches and teammates see them practice and perform at any level other than 100%. It could be that the athletes were concerned that their peers and coaches might perceive them to be "less effective" or unable to contribute. Still, they wanted to remain a part of and united with their team.

5. **During the limited-participation and return-to-play phases, athletes developed doubts about completely overcoming their injury as they remained cautious in their preparations.**

It is common for injured athletes to feel concerned about whether they will ever completely overcome and return to their previous form (Rotella & Heyman, 1993). During the limited-participation and return-to-play phases, participants developed doubts about completely overcoming their injury as they also displayed caution in their daily preparations. Although they experienced a sense of confidence in their abilities to successfully overcome their injury and believed that they possessed the abilities to make a return to their sport (i.e., conclusion 2), there still existed at least some doubt as to whether or not they would ever completely overcome their injury. In a general sense, they were confident that they had the abilities to overcome their injury but were doubtful that they could remain healthy or even regain the health they needed to make a complete return to their sport.

Fear of reinjury may also show itself as a sense of caution and doubt concerning the future (Heil, 1993; Petitpas & Danish, 1995). It may be that as athletes work through their injuries, they begin to anticipate the worst. That is, they focus on the possibility of another injury and begin to doubt their return. As they continue to doubt their return, they likely adopt a cautious approach to their practices and competitions. Although the athletes' caution was observable on limited occasions, it was made clear by the athletes themselves, their trainers, and coaches.

It could be that once athletes have suffered an injury, they begin to question their invulnerability (Petitpas & Danish, 1995). It seems very likely that before injured athletes accept their injury, they question or even doubt their eventual return. This may be especially true for those athletes who are attempting a return in the same sport season in which their injury occurred. A same-season return often does not leave much time to overcome an injury psychologically. In fact, all of the subjects were extremely focused on, yet very hesitant about, returning before season's end.

Athletes who do question their invulnerability and possibly begin to doubt their return might become much more tentative in their play, protective of their injury, or cautious in their approach. In fact, their cautious play may even translate into performance decrements, which can lead to further frustration for the athlete (Petitpas & Danish, 1995). On several instances, coaches made comments concerning the athletes' "subpar" play or a particular athlete's frustration with not being 100% recovered.

One important point remains: At times throughout their limited rehabilitation and return to play, the athletes experienced varying degrees of doubt about whether or not they would actually make a complete return to their sport. As a result of these doubts, athletes typically exercised caution in how they prepared for and participated in practices and competitions.

Recommendations for Future Qualitative Inquiry

It would seem logical to start with a follow-up to the present phenomenological study and design. Replication, which addresses the injury experiences for athletes throughout their injury, rehabilitation, and return to play, is critical. Such future work should include more subjects, a greater mix of genders, and more interviews throughout the injury, rehabilitation, and return-to-play phases. With a greater mix of genders and number of subjects, it would then be possible to examine the applicability and generalizability of the present findings. As currently reported, results are not generalizable outside of the subject pool of participants. Also, with additional interviews throughout the no-participation and limited-participation phases, a more detailed account of athletes' perceptions, thoughts, and feelings is possible.

It is also recommended that injured athletes be studied who are coping with and working through season-ending injuries. Again with similar qualitative methodologies and study designs, the perceptions of athletes over the course of an entire year could be examined in relation to those athletes trying to make a "comeback" in the same sport season in which their injury originally occurred. It would be interesting to assess the potential changes in and intensities of the various cognitions, emotions, and behaviors of athletes dealing with injuries of varying severity and length. It may be that there is a very unique set of characteristics, perceptions, and emotions that differentiate short-term, intermediate, and long-term (i.e., season-ending) injury experiences. Along these same lines of qualitative inquiry, it is also important to further study the potential stage-like process that many athletes may experience following injury (Hardy & Crace, 1990; Rose & Jevne, 1993; Rotella & Heyman, 1993). It may be that qualitative methodologies would further explain the psychological stages or phases by which some injured athletes proceed.

With a fear of reinjury so common, it is also suggested that such fears be further delineated. Petitpas and Danish (1995) outlined specific anxieties and fears as a result of changes in daily practice routines, a new or abnormal schedule, ongoing pain, or the uncertainty surrounding the future. Although the present study begins to detail such fears, further research is warranted. Future studies should examine fears in relation to the timing and intensity of these emotions, the severity and duration of injury, and the investment on the part of the athlete (i.e., age, starting status, level of play).

The concept of confidence must also be further studied. Although the present study showed athletes to be confident in their own abilities to overcome their injuries, they still doubted their complete return to practices and competitions. Future studies should focus on the relationship between self-confidence and the athlete's perceptions concerning the probability of completely overcoming the injury and making a complete return.

Although the present study indicated that injured athletes do desire to be understood and supported by their coaches, trainers, teammates, and peers, it is yet unclear what constitutes this understanding and support. It is important that future research defines what it means for athletes to be understood and supported. It is important that professionals working with injured athletes know which behaviors and expressions are interpreted by the injured athlete as understanding and supportive. As previously stated, if athletes misperceive or misinterpret information provided to them, they may also miss some information altogether. It could be that coaches are in fact providing more support, encouragement, and understanding than what is being reported by the athlete. Future research should specifically address what injured athletes are expecting and desiring in terms of support and encouragement.

Summary

Although much more research is needed to enhance the application of the present findings, the results provide greater insight into the experiences associated with athletic injury and rehabilitation. At the same time, there is much more to be gained by continuing in this line of research. It is recommended that qualitative inquiry be continued in the future study of athletic injury. A model has been provided, and several recommendations have been made for further research. It is hoped that similar research designs add to the results and conclusions already discussed in the present case studies and further serve the athlete working through and coping with athletic injury.

References

Cohen, M. Z. (1987). A historical overview of the phenomenological movement. *Journal of Nursing Scholarship, 19* (1), 31–34.

Crossman, J., & Jamieson, J. (1985). Differences in perceptions of seriousness and disrupting effects of athletic injury as viewed by athletes and their trainer. *Perceptual and Motor Skills, 61,* 1131–1134.

Evans, L., & Hardy, L. (1995). Sport injury and grief responses: A review. *Journal of Sport and Exercise Psychology, 17,* 227–245.

Feigley, D. A. (1988, October). *Coping with fear in high level gymnastics.* Paper presented at the annual meeting of the Association for the Advancement of Applied Sport Psychology, Nashua, NH.

Glasser, B. G., & Strauss, A. L. (1967). *The discovery of grounded theory.* New York: Aldine.

Gould, D., Udry, E., Bridges, D., & Beck, L. (1997a). Coping with season-ending injuries. *The Sport Psychologist, 11,* 379–399.

Gould, D., Udry, E., Bridges, D., & Beck, L. (1997b). Stress sources encountered when rehabilitating from season-ending ski injuries. *The Sport Psychologist, 11,* 361–378.

Hardy, C. J., & Crace, R. K. (1990). Dealing with injury. *Sport Psychology Training Bulletin, 1,* 1–8.

Heil, J. (1993). *Psychology of sport injury.* Champaign, IL: Human Kinetics.

Husserl, E. (1962). *Ideas: General introduction to pure phenomenology.* New York: Macmillan.

McDonald, S. A., & Hardy, C. J. (1990). Affective response patterns of the injured athlete: An exploratory analysis. *The Sport Psychologist, 4,* 261–274.

Pargman, D. (1993). Sport injuries: An overview of psychological perspectives. In D. Pargman (Ed.), *Psychological bases of sport injuries* (pp. 5–13). Morgantown, WV: Fitness Information Technology.

Patton, M. Q. (1990). *Qualitative evaluation and research methods* (2nd ed., pp. 68–73). Newbury Park, CA: Sage.

Petitpas, A., & Danish, S. J. (1995). Caring for injured athletes. In S. M. Murphy (Ed.), *Sport psychology interventions* (pp. 255–281). Champaign, IL: Human Kinetics.

Rose J., & Jevne, R. (1993). Psychosocial processes associated with athletic injuries. *The Sport Psychologist, 7,* 309–328.

Rotella, R. J., & Heyman, S. R. (1993). Stress, injury, and the psychological rehabilitation of athletes. In J. M. Williams (Ed.), *Applied sport psychology: Personal growth to peak performance* (2nd ed., pp. 338–355). Mountain View, CA: Mayfield.

Shelley, G. A. (1995). The psychological ramifications of sport injuries. In K. P. Henschen & W. F. Straub (Eds.), *Sport psychology: An analysis of athlete behavior* (3rd ed., pp. 315–330). Longmeadow, MA: Mouvement.

Weinberg R. S., & Gould, D. (1995). *Foundations of sport and exercise psychology.* Champaign, IL: Human Kinetics.

Wiese-Bjornstal, D. M., & Smith, A. M. (1993). Counseling strategies for enhanced recovery of injured athletes within a team approach. In D. Pargman (Ed.), *Psychological bases of sport injuries* (pp. 149–182). Morgantown, WV: Fitness Information Technology.

Williams, J. M., & Roepke, N. (1993). Psychology of injury and injury rehabilitation. In R. N. Singer, M. Murphey, & L. K. Tennant (Eds.), *Handbook of research on sport psychology* (pp. 815–839). New York: Macmillan.

19

I Cried Because I Had No Shoes . . . : A Case Study of Motivation Applied to Rehabilitation

Bruce W. Tuckman
Florida State University

This is a case study of a 58-year-old marathon runner, intensely ego in-volved in his athletic activity, who developed a potentially debilitating chronic condition of the lower back that made further competitive, long-distance running impossible. The paper describes the initial manifestation of the condition and the ensuing physical rehabilitation process under-taken. It then illustrates how motivation was used to facilitate the rehabili-tation process by focusing on attitude (the belief that recovery was possi-ble), metacognition (the strategies of goal setting and planning), and drive (increasing the incentive value of the outcome). The initial strategy, estab-lishing racewalking as a substitute goal activity, was not sufficient to avoid surgery and ultimately gave way to noncompetitive jogging.

Introduction

. . . and then I met a man who had no feet. What does this little adage tell us? That no matter how badly off we are, there will always be someone else who is worse off. Remembering this may help us put our personal calamities in perspective.

This is a chapter about sports injury rehabilitation. However, there is a facet of it that must be noted. It is about injuries that are so severe that even after rehabilitation, the athlete cannot continue performing the sport at the same competitive level. The purpose of the rehabilitation, therefore, is to enable the athlete to function as a normal human being, not a supernormal one. However, the repair of the physical disability in such a case may be easy compared to the repair of the psychological disability associated with separation from the sport. Thus, considerable attention must be addressed to dealing with and overcoming the psychological impact of this separation. When we talk about meeting both the physical and psychological demands of recovery, we are talking about motivation.

The data for this chapter come from an intensive (and exhaustive) case study of a single athlete, one with whom the author is intimately familiar and extraordinarily empathetic, himself. I, myself, am the single subject of this in-depth examination of the psychological impact of physically necessitated separation from successful competition in one's sport. I will begin my journey through the topic at hand by describing my case in some detail, after which I will apply motivational principles in an effort to draw conclusions, generalizations, and recommendations that can be applied by counselors to others in similar circumstances. If I am successful, you will clearly recognize that "having no shoes," although a painful and unfortunate predicament to be in, is far better than "having no feet."

The Case: Injury

I am a 53-year-old man who makes his living by being a college professor. How then can I have the temerity to suggest that this is the case of an "athlete"? In the sense that one can be an athlete only if one derives one's livelihood from athletic performance, then this is not the case of an athlete, and the case of a "real" athlete would pose considerably more severe repercussions than this one. However, I would like to contend that an athlete is someone who bases his or her sense of self on the competitive performance of an athletic endeavor, and in that sense I am (or was) an athlete. I was a competitive long-distance runner who had been running for 21 continuous years, had competed in 32 marathons, three ultramarathons, and over 200 shorter races (ranging from 5Ks to 20 milers). On average, my training consisted of running 9 or 10 miles a day, every day, with frequent long runs and periodic sessions of interval training on the track.

Yes, I was (and still am) a college professor, but I was also as much a runner as I was a professor although nobody ever paid me so much as a dime for running. In identity terms, however, "runner" and "Bruce Tuckman" were fused and inseparable; remove the one, and you might lose the other. This inseparability of self and sport was based not only on the daily training regimen but also on the sense of success derived from competition. I never viewed myself as a "jogger," clearly a recreational term, but as a "runner," and a competitive one at that.

In early December of 1989, I ran a marathon to qualify for the 1990 Boston Marathon. Over the previous 7 years, I had been experiencing a steady decrement of my racing performance, especially at the longer distances, which I attributed primarily to a combination of the aging process and a move to a much warmer climate than that in which I had grown up. During my peak marathon years of 1981–82, at the ages of 42 and 43, my best marathon times were in the highly competitive 3:08 to 3:10 range. Since then, I had "deteriorated" to the point where I was running a 3:30—the qualifying time for Boston for someone in my age range—was a real challenge. Hence, I trained very hard for this qualifying race and, despite the cold, windy, and rainy conditions, succeeded in running a 3:29:51—thereby qualifying for Boston with 9 seconds to spare!

Soon thereafter, I began to experience severe back pain, so bad that walking and bending were difficult, to say nothing of running, but I had worked so hard to qualify for Boston that I was determined to run it, and to run it I had to train for it. So I began chiropractic treatments, sports massage, and, after a brief respite, continued to train despite the pain.

In April of 1990, I ran Boston, terribly, and soon thereafter, my back pain became debilitating again. So again I followed my prescription of a brief respite from running combined with chiropractic treatments and sports massages. Also, I stretched religiously, both before and after every run, and took a cool dunk in my swimming pool after each run. Incredibly, I continued to run about 60 miles per week simply by "gritting my teeth" for the first two miles of each workout until the back pain subsided and living with the relatively constant moderate pain and limited mobility experienced during the remainder of each day.

In the middle of February, 1991, I went to San Francisco for a week and ran there every day, up and down the hills. I also walked a lot. When I arrived home, I could no longer stand erect, and the pain was constant and intense. I knew then the "jig was up," and so I went out and bought an exercise bike and stopped running. I also went back to the chiropractor for treatments three times a week. After about 6 weeks, with no visible change in my condition, I finally broke down and went to see an orthopedic surgeon who sent me for an MRI (Magnetic Resonance Image), which takes a picture of the soft tissue, in this case my spinal discs.

The result was shattering. All of my discs were in bad shape, particularly in my lower back, added to which I had a condition called spinal stenosis or a narrowing of my spinal column at about the level of my third and fourth lumbar vertebrae. My discs were not cushioning my back very well, and my narrowed spine was putting pressure on the nerves, thereby causing the pain. Twenty-one years of running with very little rest, combined with a genetic disposition to arthritis, had combined to create an intolerable situation. I was in constant pain, had trouble walking, could not bend, and could not stand in one place for more than a few moments. I had gone from being a well-conditioned athlete to being a "cripple." Were it not for my daily exercise bike rides, an activity that was essentially pain free, I would have been ready for a padded cell.

It all seems quite ironic. Over the years that I had run, I had managed to run many running partners "into the ground." Although I would show up for every workout, they would often be "down" with some injury or another. They called me the "horse that pulls the milk wagon" because of my reliability and strength. Of course, one day the horse that pulls the milk wagon drops dead as the result of accumulated overuse and is simply replaced by another nag. Was that to be my fate? I was clearly depressed, faced with the pain and immobility of my present condition and the uncertainty of my future as an athlete. Although riding a stationary bike was clearly exercise, it was not sport. I was in need of help, both physically and psychologically.

Rehabilitation

The orthopedic surgeon told me that my condition was inoperable at this time, mainly because of the limitations the surgery would impose on my mobility. He referred me for physical therapy and told me to come back in 5 or 10 years "when I couldn't stand the pain any longer," and then he would operate. Things looked mighty glum.

So, for the first time in my life, I undertook physical therapy. I did not, at the same time, undertake psychological therapy—at least in a formal sense. Because I am myself a psychologist, I decided to manage that part of the process itself. I say this up front in order to emphasize that the psychological part of the process is no less important than the physical.

Because of the pain I was experiencing, and the association between that pain and running, I was in no way tempted to run. Instead, I decided to walk. In physical therapy I learned how to stretch and strengthen my back myself, and I was given further opportunities to strengthen it on my triweekly workouts on a machine they had (called "MEDEX") that functioned specifically for that purpose. When I began physical therapy, I could barely move 45 pounds of weight with my back. Each time I went on the machine I was determined to move up to a higher level, and, by the time I had completed 20 visits, I could move 100 pounds 30 times without pain.

Every morning immediately after arising, I would do my back stretching and strengthening exercises. This took an hour. Then, either immediately thereafter or later in the day, I would spend about an hour and a quarter walking. Because, as a runner, I had always had the typical runner's obsession with going fast, it transferred over to my walking, and I began to try to walk faster and faster. I became a racewalker. I even joined up with the few other racewalkers who were to be found in my community.

When my medical insurance ran out, I left physical therapy and joined a health club, one that featured Nautilus equipment and had a machine especially designed to strengthen the lower back. It was similar to the MEDEX I had used in physical therapy. I got the physical therapist to design a workout program for me at the health club and began going regularly on a twice a week basis. I also began using a stair climber as an occasional aerobic alternative to racewalking. I began to use swimming that way as well.

I have gotten immeasurably better. I experience relatively little back pain during normal daily activities while maintaining my weight and aerobic fitness level. Compared to those for whom improvement may not be possible (those who have had serious automobile accidents, for example), I realize how well off I am. I have even racewalked a few 5K races and have performed better each time. Racewalking is a lot less "bouncy" than running and far easier on my back. However, even on this I will exhibit extreme caution!

Applying Principles of Motivation

Other than perhaps an interesting or even an inspirational story, what is my case doing in a book like this? The answer is that I would like to use it to illustrate how motivation can be used to facilitate the rehabilitation process, particularly in cases where the athlete will never be able to return to sport at the same competitive level as before the injury.

Let me propose that motivation has the following three facets or components: (a) attitude, (b) metacognition, and (c) drive.

Attitude. This is the motivational *enabler,* particularly the attitude of self-confidence or what Bandura (1977, 1986) calls self-efficacy. Believing that one can do something is what enables one to do it (combined, of course, with a suitable amount of skill). People who have this attitude can be called self-believers, and those who do not, self-doubters (Tuckman & Sexton, in press b). Self-believers have been shown not only to outperform all others, but also to outperform even their own self-expectations (Tuckman & Sexton, in press b). Furthermore, they are largely unaffected by external circumstances, although when in a competitive situation, they perform better when they do not know where they stand relative to others (Tuckman & Sexton, 1992b). In other words, if they do not know for sure how far ahead they are, they just keep "pouring it on."

Therefore, in a rehabilitative situation, an athlete will be much more motivated to try to recover if he or she *believes* that recovery is possible. In my case, I believed that I could fix my back. That belief enabled me to get better. Where did that belief come from? According to Bandura (1977), the most effective way to improve self-efficacy is to try to do something and then succeed at it (what he calls *enactive attainment*). That, however, is like a catch-22. How can self-efficacy be both a prerequisite and a result? If a person lacks self-efficacy, that person is not likely to try something and so will never experience success. To get that person to try something and have the attempt result in success, you need to create a highly structured situation in which the necessary behaviors can be carried out with assistance and without threat of failure. Bandura (1977) calls this *participant modeling*. The person models the desired behavior for him- or herself. Of course someone else is standing by to see that it is done right.

In my case, the physical therapist was the person standing by to see that I did things right. He was instrumental in helping me to carry out participant modeling leading to success experiences, each one adding to my sense of self-efficacy or belief in my ability to recover. The physical therapist never seemed to doubt that I would be able to move more weight each time I worked out on the machine. Without telling me, he would set the weight a little higher each time, and, after I had succeeded in moving it through the desired number of repetitions, inform me of what I had just accomplished. This process helped me develop the self-confidence I needed to complete my recovery.

Mere pep talks do not have the same effect. Telling someone over and over that he or she can do something does not necessarily make it happen, nor does simply showing how or pointing out someone else who is already doing it. There is no substitute for success, but success requires support and assistance. Scale down the rehabilitation task to the level that the recovering athlete can do it, and success becomes more likely. Then follow success with positive feedback. Do not tell rehabilitating athletes what they have done wrong (a typical tendency of coaches, for example). Tell them what they have done right. Positive or encouraging feedback following performance has been shown to increase both self-efficacy and subsequent performance (Tuckman & Sexton, 1991). After each workout, my therapist would always say to me something like "You sure know how to focus your energy on that weight." Hearing that always made me feel more competent.

Metacognition. This is the *guide,* particularly insofar as it includes the strategies of goal setting and planning. Metacognition as applied to motivation means having mental or thought models for accomplishing a purpose. My purpose was to recover physically and psychologically from my disability, at least to the level of normal functioning—that being less than athletic functioning. To accomplish that, I needed to set intermediate or proximal goals and to develop plans for achieving them (Tuckman, 1990, 1992). This is particularly necessary when the injured person does not have much confidence in the likelihood of recovery—a particularly prevalent attitude at the beginning of the rehabilitation process. Having the goals and plans also helps to enhance the attitude of self-confidence, so necessary for recovery.

My short-term goals were clear, to gradually reduce the pain and discomfort while, at the same time, gradually increasing the strength in my back. Each time I went for physical therapy, I set as a goal the amount of weight I wanted to be able to move on the MEDEX machine. I always tried to select a goal that seemed challenging yet attainable. This way I had a target to aim at, and each time it was a little higher than the time before. Of course there is likely to be an ultimate limit, at which time maintenance goals need to be set.

It also helps to have a plan, a mapping out in the mind of how to meet each goal. The more detailed the plan in terms of specific days, times, and activities the better because that makes it easier to follow. Also, a good plan includes acknowledgment of likely obstacles (what I call UFO's or Unavoidable Formidable Obstacles) and strategies for overcoming them. Otherwise, a miss can cause a major setback, even perhaps be an end to the whole process. Finding an alternate exercise program, namely racewalking, turned out to be an excellent strategy for me. I could set performance goals and could plan out my weekly schedule to include physical therapy workouts and racewalking workouts. I planned for shorter walks and longer walks, slower walks and faster walks. I also planned for days when I did non-weight-bearing exercise such as swimming. Moreover, I had a contingency plan for a diminution of activity should the pain return—that being the major obstacle I could imagine.

Metacognitively, I served as my own coach so to speak, because goal setting and planning are major coaching functions . The existence of an alternative activity, though, was essential to this metacognitive aspect of motivation because it gave me something for which to plan. With competition-ending conditions such as mine, just planning to be pain free is probably not enough. It is much more motivating to plan for some other kind of performance and to believe that one can achieve it.

Drive. This is the *energizer,* the source of the effort that is required to deal with the physical and psychological demands of rehabilitation. To be motivated to do something means to expend energy or effort on it. Beyond believing that a person can prevail, and having cognitive strategies to give direction, he or she must also have drive. Without it the person is not likely to succeed.

Where does drive come from? It comes from valuing or wanting something. An individual may not know how to get it, or even believe that he or she can get it, but if the person wants it badly enough, he or she will be driven. We could say that the goal or outcome has *incentive value* for the individual. For example, some of us have children who do not work hard enough at school. We know they are smart, and they probably do too, but they just do not seem to care as much as we think they should. School seems to lack incentive value for them, and so they are not driven to do well in it.

Sometimes we try, externally, to enhance the incentive value of something, and hence the drive to achieve it, by making a reward available. Some schools reward students materially for attendance, good behavior, and improved grades. The result seems to be positive. However, in the long term, people seem to persist when at least some of the incentive value comes from within.

With athletes, especially older ones, drive is often not a problem. In fact, if anything it can be a problem in the opposite way in that the older athlete has a tendency to put in more effort than is physically productive. Because of the enormous incentive value of competitive success, the older athlete is often driven to train to excess—the end result being injury. It is a clear case of the drive factor being so strong as to overshadow the cognitive factor. Then, when the athlete is injured, the drive to recover is as strong as it ever was in order to be able to return quickly to competition. In that case, the athlete throws him- or herself wholeheartedly into the rehabilitation process, but what happens, as in my case, when the likelihood of real recovery, at least to the preinjury level, is not possible?

One possibility is that there will be little incentive value for rehabilitating oneself. Why bother to put in the effort to "get better" if "better" cannot be gotten? What needs to be done is to harness the old competitive energy or drive but redirect it. Direction is a cognitive function, not a function of drive, but because attitude, cognition, and drive all interact, a change in one cannot help but produce a change in the others. Thus, the solution may be to introduce substitute goals (cognitively) and work to attach the preinjury drive to these new goals.

In my case, the substitute goal was to become a successful racewalker. Because I could not be a competitive runner, I would invest my effort in rehabilitating myself in order to become a competitive racewalker. If my sport was also my livelihood (which, of course, it was not), I would have tried to find a substitute career, the attainment of which would have become my new goal toward which I could direct my effort.

In fact, I was faced with exactly that situation not too long ago when I in voluntarily gave up administration to return to the faculty. Because the new job lacked incentive value to me, particularly in comparison to the old one, I had nothing to which to attach my drive. In such cases, the result is typically first anger and then depression, given all that drive without an attainable goal toward which it can be directed. I used all my drive to try to find another administrative job, and it was not until I accepted the reality of my situation and was able to see its incentive value that I could get past the anger and depression.

When my back injury came along, I was able to quickly settle on a new goal, racewalking, toward which I could direct my drive. Very possibly, the job experience had taught me the value of goal substitution in avoiding the anger and depression that typically follow a loss.

Conclusion

From my case, the critical importance of a *goal* can be clearly seen. A goal serves three purposes, namely, (a) as a direction in which to go (cognitively); (b) as an incentive, thereby providing something to which drive can be attached; and (c) as something to believe oneself capable of attaining (attitudinally). Because rehabilitation is a demanding process both physically and psychologically, it requires a considerable amount of motivation. That motivation, in turn, requires the necessary attitudes, thoughts, and drives. By serving as a key to each, the goal of recovery becomes very possibly the most critical element in the process.

In the case of injuries from which complete recovery is not possible (or certainly not likely), the matter of the goal becomes even more critical. In cases where an obvious goal such as complete recovery does not exist, a substitute goal must be found. The substitute goal should help the injured athlete to detach from the former competitive activity and attach to some other desired outcome. Given the new goal, the athlete can organize beliefs, thoughts, and energies around it.

In my case, this approach worked well because my substitute goal involving racewalking. In cases where an athlete cannot or will not accept a substitute goal, the motivation required for physical recovery is likely to be lacking.

The goal also serves a very important evaluative function in the rehabilitation process. In order to determine whether or not one is getting better, there must be some mental representation of what "better" is. In my case, "better" meant being able to racewalk fast enough and properly enough to be able to enter a race without either embarrassing myself or reinjuring myself. For an injured professional athlete, the goal might be getting a job as a broadcaster or coach. Landing such a job would provide a measure of having gotten "better."

In my case I was fortunate to have arrived at a substitute goal that could meet so many of the needs that had previously been met by running competitively. Whether or not I ultimately carry through on my substitute goal, it has served its purpose in facilitating my physical recovery from serious athletic injury.

Postscript

It has now been 4 years since I wrote this article, and it is revealing to examine what has transpired during this time relative to my injury. After taking up racewalking as an alternative to running, I became very serious about it—in a competitive sense. I trained hard and began to compete on a fairly regular basis. I also began to achieve some measure of success; that is, my competitive times improved dramatically.

I must also add that racewalking, unlike running, is a more structured sport. That is to say, it has rules, two, to be exact. One is that one foot must always be in contact with the ground. The second is that each leg must straighten at the knee as it passes under your body. Most of the races I entered were running races of 5 or 10 kilometers; I just racewalked instead of running. There were no judges, so I had no way of knowing that I might have been breaking a rule. However, many runners who saw me said I was running. When I finally did enter a race for racewalkers only, where there were judges, I was told that I was breaking the first rule. It was very discouraging.

A more serious problem was that although I had no back pain while "racewalking," at other times I had back pain, and it was growing considerably worse. Indeed, by the beginning of 1995, almost 4 years after my back problem had been diagnosed and I had begun physical therapy and switched from running to racewalking, the pain got so bad that my orthopedist recommended surgery. It was major surgery involving removal of small sections of bone in four locations to reduce the pressure on the sciatic nerve. I spent 3 days in the hospital and 2 weeks rehabilitating at home. At the end of that time, I was able to resume normal walking as a form of exercise.

I realized that I had substituted one competitive sport, racewalking, for the original one, marathon running. In my new sport, I had stopped training for distance, but continued training for speed. I had created a plan, but that plan had not succeeded. My original drive was so strong that it led me to rationalize away the health dangers inherent in my new plan. I had continued to engage in physical overtraining, and it had continued to take its toll on my health. It was time to change the plan.

It was also fortunate that my racewalking was not "legal," for if it had been, it would have meant again giving up something at which I was experiencing competitive success. It was easier to give up competitive racewalking knowing that I would be disqualified from every official race I entered unless I went back to ground zero and started learning it all over again.

So, after trying it out, I decided to take up a new exercise: jogging. My new plan was to limit myself to jogging five miles a day, six mornings a week, over a relatively flat course, something I discovered I could do without pain (after building up to it). My jogging pace was about 10 minutes per mile. I would do no training and make no effort to become competitive.

I have been following this plan for 2 years now. I have also continued my own physical therapy at a health club on a twice weekly basis using the same routine established for me originally by the physical therapist. I realize that my original plan was too ambitious because I had allowed my drive to dominate my thinking. In terms of the three motivational elements, there was an imbalance. I also realize that my current plan may be too ambitious as well, because I am obviously prone to let drive dominate thought. However, I take comfort in the fact that I have managed to overcome my drive for competitive success and, as a result, have not changed either my training distance or my pace.

I can only hope that this book is not put out in a third edition, at which point I will be forced to report that I am now walking or peddling a stationary bike. The hardest thing for a person to deal with, I now realize, is achieving a balance between the three motivational components. Believing and wanting are not enough to guarantee survival—although I am sure they help. There must still be some rational thinking involved.

References

Bandura, A. (1977). Self-efficacy: Toward a unifying theory of behavior change. *Psychological Review, 84,* 191–215.

Bandura, A. (1986). *Social foundations of thought and action: A social cognitive theory.* Englewood Cliffs, NJ: Prentice-Hall.

Tuckman, B. W. (1990). Group versus goal-setting effects on the self-regulated performance of students differing in self-efficacy. *Journal of Experimental Education, 58,* 291–298.

Tuckman, B. W. (1992). The effect of student planning and self-competence on self-motivated performance. *Journal of Experimental Education* (in press).

Tuckman, B. W., & Sexton, T .L. (1990). The relation between self-beliefs and self-regulated performance. *Journal of Social Behavior and Personality, 5,* 465–472.

Tuckman, B. W., & Sexton, T. L. (1991). The effect of teacher encouragement on student self-efficacy and motivation for self-regulated performance. *Journal of Social Behavior and Personality, 6,* 137–146.

Tuckman, B. W., & Sexton, T. L. (in press a). The effects of informational feedback and self-beliefs on the motivation to perform a self-regulated task. *Journal of Research in Personality.*

Tuckman, B. W., & Sexton, T. L. (in press b). Self-believers are self-motivated; self-doubters are not. *Personality and Individual Differences.*

20

Conversion Blindness: A Case Report[1]

David Pargman
Florida State University

This chapter reviews and discusses distinguishing features of two psychological conditions related to sport injury: malingering and conversion reaction. In addition, it presents a case study of a high school football athlete who experienced conversion blindness. This chapter also includes a description of the counseling approach employed to resolve the conversion blindness. Professionals who work with athletes must carefully examine their preparedness to serve clients' presenting problems related to conversion blindness and to consider making professional referrals.

Introduction

Injury may result in several undesirable psychological changes in athletes. Among these are fear of reinjury (Ievleva & Orlick, 1991); mood disturbances, such as increases in depression, tension, and anger (Grove, Stewart, & Gordon, 1990); changes in self-efficacy (Connelly, 1991); and grief responses

---

1. From "Conversion Blindness: A Case Report" by D. Pargman in *International Journal of Rehabilitation and Health*, 1996, 2(1), 57–65. Reprinted by permission.

(Gordon, Milios, & Grove, 1991). According to Danish (1986), athletic injury not only threatens physical well-being but also impinges upon athletes' self-concepts, belief systems, social and occupational functioning, values, commitments, and emotional equilibrium.

Factors underlying sport injury and injury rehabilitation are, therefore, important concerns of those who work with rehabilitating athletes. Consequently, sport injury research has been ongoing for some time, and a substantial body of literature is presently available (Anderson & Williams, 1988; Bramwell, Minoru, Wagner, & Holmes, 1975; Brown, 1971; Coddington & Troxell, 1980; Jackson et al., 1978; Pargman, 1976, 1993; Pargman & Lunt, 1989; Yukelson, 1986). More recently, inquiries have focused on assessment of psychological techniques, strategies, and programs designed to enhance recuperation from or adjustment to consequences of sport-related injury (Fisher, Domm, & Wuest, 1988; Flint, 1993; Green, 1992; Wiese & Weiss, 1987; Wiese-Bjornstal & Smith, 1993).

There have been only a few published studies, however, that address two of these psychological conditions related to sport injury, namely, malingering and conversion reaction. Unfortunately, no data are presently available that provide insight into the incidence of these conditions within the sport context. Nonetheless, it is reasonable to conclude that they indeed occur. A brief review of these conditions will likely be helpful to those who either counsel or rehabilitate athletes because health care professionals often erroneously confuse the two conditions with one another. This chapter, therefore, addresses this need and also presents a case study of a high school football player who experienced conversion blindness.

Malingering

Although difficult to ascertain, malingering has received some attention in the literature. Articles in the sport psychology literature have addressed malingering since the mid-1960s. In general, *malingering* is a term applied to persons who deceive others, relative to their having personally received some injury (Travin & Protter, 1984). In the case of the malingering athletes, the purpose of the deception is to avoid practice or competition (Kane, 1984; Ogilvie & Tutko, 1966; Rotella, Ogilvie, & Perrin, 1993). Thus, the motivation is a clearly defined behavior. Its essence is gain derived from being allegedly infirm or somehow engaged by a serious problem (Lees-Haley, 1986). Labbate and Miller (1990) recommended considering malingering as an adaptive response to adverse circumstances requiring an external incentive for having an injury.

In their conscious feigning of disability and symptoms thereof, individuals with initial malingering motives may ultimately mimic a wide array of somatic disorders. Vander Kolk (1991) made the point that malingering does not occur as often as someone might believe. Clinical reports in this area have found that outright malingering is rare (Beals & Hickman, 1972; Fordyce, 1979; Harper, 1985; Shaffer, 1981).

Conversion Reactions

Malingering is not the same as conversion hysteria. In fact, they may be "opposite ends of a range of psychologically based conditions . . . " (Stewart, 1983, p. 308). Conversion reactions (also referred to as hysterical impairments under the DSM-IV heading "Somatoform Disorders") supposedly have psychological or psychiatric bases, although dispute is still ongoing relative to their precise nature (Shalev & Munitz, 1986). In the conversion condition, functional capabilities of an organ or system become seriously compromised or completely inhibited despite the origin or system's structural integrity. Victims are thus unable to, or profess to be unable to, execute various motor or sensory functions (Overholser, 1990). Freud and Breuer (1985) first discussed such unconscious mental defense mechanisms that account for repression of unacceptable wishes followed by their "conversion" into somatic dysfunction. Unconscious factors of which they have little or no awareness or control prevent such individuals from executing certain motor or sensory functions. In the attempt to repress the unacceptable desire, underlying energy gets directed towards a somatic symptom.

It is of utmost importance that conversion reactions be diagnosed only after careful medical examination has excluded authentic pathology (Stewart, 1983). Slater and Glithero (1965), upon following up on patients diagnosed as suffering from "hysteria," found 30% of them to be seriously ill. Fishbain and Goldberg (1991) examined misdiagnosis of conversion disorder in a psychiatric emergency service. They discovered that, of three individuals diagnosed with conversion, zero actually suffered from this disorder. This misdiagnosis, followed by one patient's death, prompted litigation threats in all three cases. The diagnoses of these three cases resulted from using DSM-III criteria. It is, therefore, important to note that lack of medical evidence along with the use of DSM-IV criteria does not guarantee absence of organic damage. Thus, a premature or unfounded diagnosis of hysterical dysfunction may result in serious consequences to a diseased athlete. On the other hand, unnecessary medical interventions, such as surgery and inappropriate drug therapy, may be preventable if conversion disorder accurately and promptly gets diagnosed.

The Exaggeration/Malingering/Conversion Continuum

Vander Kolk (1991) developed a model of disabled-client coping styles. This model diagrams exaggeration on one end of a continuum and conversion at the opposite end, with malingering in the middle. The exaggeration end of this continuum represents a conscious or voluntary effort to exhibit stronger symptoms than expected, although this exaggeration is not consistent or extreme. Moving down the continuum, one would find the malingering coping style, which represents frequent and significant exaggeration of a problem. Malingerers are consciously trying to extract some reward for their behavior. At the far end of this continuum, one will find conversion, which is unique in that it is primarily a subconscious disorder. These individuals are not consciously attempting to manipulate others. They are, instead unconsciously coping with perceived personal threats. Vander Kolk (1991) noted that it is best to consider this as a fluid model because individuals do not necessarily fit into any one style of coping and self-assessment.

Case Report

Irrespective of professional interest (clinical psychologist, sport psychology consultant, physical therapist, athletic trainer, etc.), ethical practitioners have an obligation at the outset to consider the following two questions when attempting to help an athlete:

1. Do I recognize or know the problem brought to me by this athlete?
2. Am I an appropriate resource for helping this athlete resolve his or her problem?

With reference to the second question is the issue of referral. Responsible consultants examine their repertoire of professional skills and resources and determine whether it is best to refer a client elsewhere.

What follows is an account of a sport psychology consultant's response to an athlete who sought his assistance in dealing with conversion blindness resulting from a sport injury. Response to the aforementioned two questions resulted in a "Yes, I recognize and understand the problem brought to me by this athlete," and "Yes, I am an appropriate resource for helping this athlete resolve his problem."

Marvin

The subject was a 17-year-old high school football athlete who had lost all left-eye vision as a consequence of trauma sustained during football practice.

Sounding very distressed and eager that I meet with his son, his father phoned for an appointment. During the telephone conversation, my professional background and expertise became clarified.

Marvin's skeletal height was approximately 6 feet, 5 inches, and he weighed about 290 pounds. His musculature was of such an impressively developed stature that it prompted silent speculation about steroid use (abuse). Marvin's physical stature was easily comparable to that of Division I-A college football athletes that I frequently encounter professionally. He sat before me poised, relaxed, and confident and responded in an unusually grammatically correct communicative style (for a high school junior). Employing a noteworthy, rich vocabulary, he proceeded to share with me the details pertinent to his problem.

About 14 days prior, while scrimmaging in afternoon practice, Marvin, who plays both offensive and defensive tackle, collided with another athlete. Their helmets banged together forcefully, and Marvin became disoriented for a brief time period. Very soon thereafter, he realized that he could not see in one eye. While driving home from practice, he noted that his perceptual abilities seemed impaired and, as a result, his automobile veered frequently and frighteningly to one side of the road. Although his primary care physician, whom he visited late in the evening, and an ophthalmologist and neurologist, whom he consulted the next day, all assured him that his vision would return in 2 or 3 days. It had not.

Marvin described a comfortable and harmonious family environment, with his mother and father fulfilling traditional parental roles. His father owned and operated a business in a mid-sized southeastern city, and his mother helped out at the business by working in the office. Inquiry into intrafamilial dynamics revealed no apparent problems. Marvin felt that he and his dad were extremely close and the best of friends. They often hunted and fished together. Marvin helped in sundry ways at his father's business whenever time permitted and enjoyed collaborating with him on minor construction projects around the house and business location. Marvin and his father often met for lunch and, according to Marvin, they looked forward to spending time together.

Marvin considered himself to be a good athlete and good student. A review of his achievements on the playing filed and in the classroom provided support for these perceptions. He was taking a substantial number of math and science courses, which he enjoyed and in which he did well. He expressed respect and admiration for his classroom teachers and coaches and felt that he and they shared a comfortable relationship.

In addition to his professed strong and meaningful relationship with his father, Marvin also acknowledged feelings of closeness with one of his former football coaches (Steve) who, at the time, was working as an instructor/manager at the local health and fitness club where Marvin did his weight training. Steve was a real close friend, advisor, and confidant, although Marvin's father was clearly his "Number 1, real friend."

Marvin was steadfast in expressing his affinity for football. He reiterated his enjoyment of body contact and maintained that he found pleasure in hitting and hurting other people. This, he asserted, was his job, and it was his role as a football athlete to "build aggression and channel it" into activity on the playing field. As Marvin put it, "It is really important for me to play football." [I ultimately came to realize the authenticity of this remark and later realized that it was this perceived importance, although fueled by an extrinsic source (Marvin's father), that was the key factor in Marvin's conversion reaction.]

A question directed at Marvin about his sleeping patterns readily elicited a description of a dream sequence that had been frequently occurring since the accident. These dreams involved a red dragon that accompanies Marvin in many of his activities, including fishing. When asked by Marvin to reveal its identity, the dragon provided Marvin's initials (M.P.). Marvin, therefore, concluded that he and the red dragon are one and the same. Or, as Marvin described it, "He is me; he is another side of me." The dragon also often inquired if Marvin's vision had returned. We did not pursue additional inquiry into Marvin's associations with the dragon figure.

Mr. P.

Because Marvin's father accompanied him to the initial visit with me, I also interviewed Marvin's father alone briefly. Mr. P. confirmed Marvin's perceptions about their close relationship and enjoyment in working and recreating together. Moreover, Mr. P. described, in greater detail than his son, Marvin's high level of athletic ability and potential as a Division I football athlete. Mr. P. had played college football for a year and was an assistant coach on Marvin's high school team. He had coached his son in various capacities in previous years as the boy ascended different playing levels.

Mr. P. suggested that phone calls to his son's physicians would be helpful in my obtaining more detailed medical accounts of Marvin's condition than he could offer at the moment. He, therefore, provided the names and telephone numbers of these persons.

The first meeting with Marvin and his father concluded with establishment of a second appointment one week hence. During this interim, I contacted Marvin's primary care physician and ophthalmologist in order to ascertain the medical nature of his visual disability. In no uncertain terms, both physicians affirmed the visual capability of Marvin's eye. Both physicians assured me that the neurologist who had extensively examined Marvin, but whom I had been unable to reach, agreed to the absence of any medical problem and that an MRI technique applied to the apparatus in the left eye yielded negative findings. According to the ophthalmologist, "it was impossible for Marvin not to see in the bad eye."

Upon the recommendation of the neurologist and ophthalmologist, Marvin sought an additional consultation with a team of eye specialists at an out-of-town teaching hospital. Marvin obtained this "second opinion" during the time between my first and my second visit with him. The consultation replicated the findings of the original neurological and ophthalmological examinations.

On the day preceding my second meeting with Marvin, his father telephoned to confirm his son's forthcoming appointment. I had, by this time, formulated relevant hypotheses regarding causal and remediative considerations about Marvin's left-eye blindness and requested that Mr. P. visit me in my office prior to his son's appointment. At our session, I inquired into Mr. P.'s feelings about his son's inability to continue playing football. He revealed considerable disappointment. It was clear that Mr. P.'s sense of personal loss was at least comparable to that presumably felt by his son, and perhaps even more intense.

Mr. P. spoke of Marvin's athletic potential and the high probability of his winning a college scholarship. According to Mr. P., Marvin's talents were considerable and his football future was exceedingly bright. I concluded that Marvin's father had fueled a significant portion of Marvin's motivation for participating in football. It occurred to me that Marvin's alleged interest in football primarily revolved around satisfying his father, that is, not disappointing Dad. I entertained the hypothesis that Marvin wanted out of football and that the loss of left-eye vision was his escape route.

I proposed to Mr. P. that he could play a vital role in the restoration of his son's vision. I delineated for him the nature and implications of the "conversion blindness" hypothesis and proposed a problem-solving approach. Mr. P. would find a way to communicate to Marvin the "permission" for him to disengage from football. I assured him that I was aware of how difficult it would be for him to do this, Mr. P. responded agreeably and expressed his wish to do anything that would help his son, although he was insecure about his ability to express the critical message with conviction. He had, for years, entertained images and aspirations related to Marvin's potential collegiate and even professional achievements.

Having secured from Mr. P. his commitment to proceed along these lines, I suggested a role-playing session in which he would play the father and I, the son. It was necessary to disabuse Mr. P. of his inclination to use the word "quit" during the mock discourse. Throughout the role-playing session, he often said something to the effect of "It's OK, son, you can quit if you wish," or "I don't mind if you quit football, son. It's all right with me." I considered it inappropriate to permit Marvin to think of himself as a quitter. We, therefore, practiced alternate ways of expressing Mr. P.'s approval of Marvin's disengagement from football. I provided a variety of responses and rebuttals that Marvin could conceivably return. The session ended with Mr. P. affirming his determination to "let Marvin off the football hook" in a manner that reflected sincerity, caring, and support for his son's decision—whatever it might be.

Marvin had previously scheduled an appointment with me for 3 days after his father's visit. As he entered my office, he exclaimed excitedly, "Got my sight back, Doc." With the understandable enthusiasm of one who has regained possession of a function as precious as vision, Marvin elaborated upon the talk with his dad that occurred during the past 3 days. "I was able to tell Dad that I don't want to do football anymore, and he said it was all right with him." Marvin appeared relaxed and self-assured. He described, in detail, his dislike for football, how it was no fun anymore, how he would break out in a sweat when he dressed for practice, and how happy he was to feel relieved of his burden. He spoke of his abiding affinity for weightlifting, how much he loves it, and how he is likely to continue in this activity for the rest of his life. Much of this rhetoric at this time was in a stark contrast to the way he previously described his involvement in football. During this exchange, it appeared that Marvin made an effort to convince me of his honesty and basic goodness. I speculated that he was eager for me to understand that he really had lost his vision (for a while) and that he had not fabricated his affliction.

Discussion

This chapter presents a clinical case report exemplifying conversion symptoms in a high school football player. The literature indicates that conversion appears under a variety of conditions, particularly in stressful situations (Shalev & Munitz, 1986), although it seems to be a rarely described condition among athletes.

In the case reported here, the wish to disengage from football was unacceptable to the young athlete. He, therefore, used a football injury (that he would likely have been able to overcome in a few days) to subconsciously express his wish to disengage from playing football. The clinical response was to countermand this repression, permit its recognition, and lead the athlete to an understanding that disengagement from football was acceptable to his father. The athlete's father accepted the assigned responsibility of legitimizing the repressed wish. This chosen clinical response is consistent with the recommendation made by Sullivan and Buchanan (1989) to provide conversion disorder clients with a nonthreatening means of relinquishing symptoms.

Professionals who rehabilitate athletes must be familiar with mechanisms of the conversion condition in order to serve injured athletes. Conversion responses are dynamically differential to malingering behavior, and although the two may interact in some individuals, they require different clinical responses. Thus, therapeutic treatment programs designed to help injured athletes who are using inaccurate self-assessment coping styles may require use of both physical therapy and psychological interventions.

This case appears to have resolved quickly, much to the satisfaction of both athlete and author. However, complex cases warrant referral to professionals specifically trained to diagnose and respond to conversion reaction.

References

Anderson, M. B., & Williams, J. M. (1988). A model of stress and athletic injury: Prediction and prevention. *Journal of Sport and Exercise Psychology, 10,* 299–306.

Beals, R., & Hickman, N. (1972). Industrial injuries of the back and extremities. *Journal of Bone and Joint Surgery, 54*(8), 1593–1610.

Bramwell, S. T., Minoru, M., Wagner, N. N., & Holmes, T. H. (1975). Psychosocial factors in athletic injuries. *Journal of Human Stress, 1*(2), 6–20.

Brown, R. (1971). Personality characteristics related to injury in football. *Research Quarterly, 42,* 467–470.

Coddington, R., & Troxell, J. R. (1980, December). The effect of emotional factors on football injury rates—A pilot study. *Journal of Human Stress, Vol# 6,* 3–5.

Connelly, S. L. (1991). *Injury and self-esteem: A test of Soenstrom and Morgan's model.* Unpublished master's thesis, South Dakota State University, Vermillion, SD.

Danish, S. J. (1986). Psychological aspects in the care and treatment of athletic injuries. In P. F. Vinger & E. F. Hoerner (Eds.), *Sport injuries: The unthwarted epidemic* (2nd ed., pp. 345–353). Boston, MA: PSG.

Fishbain, D. A., & Goldberg, M. (1991). The misdiagnosis of conversion disorder in a psychiatric emergency service. *General Hospital Psychiatry, 13,* 177–181.

Fisher, A. C., Domm, M. A., & Wuest, D. A. (1988). Adherence to sports-injury rehabilitation programs. *The Physician and Sports Medicine, 16,* 47–52.

Fordyce, W. (1979). *Use of the MMPI in the assessment of chronic pain.* Minneapolis, MN: National Computer Systems.

Freud, S., & Breuer, J. (1985). Studies on hysteria. In *Complete psychological works of Sigmund Freud* (Vol. 2, pp. 1–323). London: Hogarth Press.

Gordon, S., Milios, D., & Grove, J. R. (1991). Psychological aspects of the recovery process from sport injury: The perspective of sport physiotherapists. *The Australian Journal of Science and Medicine in Sport, 23,* 53–60.

Green, L. B. (1992). The use of imagery in the rehabilitation of injured athletes. *The Sport Psychologist, 6,* 416–428.

Grove, J. R., Stewart, R., & Gordon, S. (1990). *Emotional reactions of athletes to knee rehabilitation.* Paper presented at the Annual Meeting of the Australian Sports Medicine Federation, Alice Springs.

Harper, R. B. (1985). The rehabilitation counselor as an expert witness in personal injury litigation. In L. J. Taylor, M. Golter, G. Golter, & T. Backer (Eds.), *Handbook of private sector rehabilitation*. New York: Springer.

Ievleva, L., & Orlick, T. (1991). Mental links to enhanced healing: An exploratory study. *The Sport Psychologist, 5*(1), 25–40.

Jackson, D. W., Jarrett, H., Bailey, D., Kausek, J., Swanson, J. J., & Powell, J. W. (1978). Injury prediction in the young athlete: A preliminary report. *American Journal of Sports Medicine, 6*(1), 6–14.

Kane, B. (1984). Trainer counseling to avoid three face-saving maneuvers. *Athletic Training, 19,* 171–174.

Labbate, L. A., & Miller, R. W. (1990). A case of malingering. *American Journal of Psychiatry, 47,* 257–258.

Lees-Haley, P. R. (1986). How to detect malingerers in the work-place. *Personnel Journal, 65,* 106–110.

Ogilvie, B., & Tutko, T. (1966). *Problem athletes and how to handle them*. London: Pelham Books.

Overholser, J. C. (1990). Differential diagnoses of malingering and fictitious disorders with physical symptoms. Special issue: Malingering and deception: An update. *Behavioral Sciences and the Law, 8,* 55–65.

Pargman, D. (1976). Visual dissembling and injury in college football players. *Perceptual and Motor Skills, 42,* 762.

Pargman, D. (1993). Sports injuries! Overview of the problem. In D. Pargman (Ed.), *Psychological bases of sport injuries* (pp. 5–13). Morgantown, WV: Fitness Information Technology.

Pargman, D., & Lunt, S. (1989). The relationship of self-concept and locus of control to the severity of injury in comparatively lower ability level collegiate football players. *Sports Medicine Training and Rehabilitation, 1,* 203–208.

Rotella, R. J., Ogilvie, B. C., & Perrin, D. H. (1993). The malingering athlete: Psychological considerations. In D. Pargman (Ed.), *Psychological bases of sport injuries* (pp. 85–97). Morgantown, WV: Fitness Information Technology.

Shaffer, J. (1981). *Using the MMPI to evaluate mental impairment in disability determination*. Nutley, NJ: Hoffman-LaRoche.

Shalev, A., & Munitz, H. (1986). Conversion without hysteria: A case report and review of the literature. *British Journal of Psychiatry, 148,* 198–203.

Slater, E., & Glithero, E. (1965). A follow up of patients diagnosed as suffering from "hysteria." *Journal of Psychosomatic Research, 9,* 9–13.

Stewart, T. D. (1983). Hysterical conversion reactions: Some patient characteristics and treatment team reactions. *Archives of Physical Medicine and Rehabilitation, 64,* 308–310.

Sullivan, M. J. L., & Buchanan, D. C. (1989). The treatment of conversion disorder in a rehabilitation setting. *Canadian Journal of Rehabilitation, 2*(3), 175–180.

Travin, S., & Protter, B. (1984). Malingering & malingering like behavior: Some denial and conceptual issues. *Psychiatric Quarterly, 56,* 189–197.

Vander Kolk, C. J. (1991). Client credibility and coping styles. *Rehabilitation and Psychology, 36*(1), 51–56.

Wiese, D. M., & Weiss, M. R. (1987). Psychological rehabilitation and physical injury: Implications for the sports medicine team. *The Sports Psychologist, 1,* 318–330.

Weise-Bjornstal, D. M., & Smith, A. M. (1993). Counseling strategies for enhanced recovery: The role of sports medicine team members. In D. Pargman (Ed.), *Psychological bases of sport injuries* (pp. 149–182). Morgantown, WV: Fitness Information Technology.

Yukelson, D. (1986). Psychology of sport and the injured athlete. In D. B. Bernhart (Ed.), *Clinics in physical therapy* (pp. 175–195). New York: Churchill Livingstone.

Index

T

V

W

Coventry University